PELVIC LOCOMOTOR DYSFUNCTION

A Clinical Approach

George G. DeFranca, DC
Director
West Boylston Chiropractic Office
West Boylston, Massachusetts

with

Linda J. Levine, DC
Director
Hadley Center for Neck and Back Pain
Hadley, Massachusetts

AN ASPEN PUBLICATION®
Aspen Publishers, Inc.
Gaithersburg, Maryland
1996

Library of Congress Cataloging-in-Publication Data

DeFranca, George G.
Pelvic locomotor dysfunction: a clinical approach/
George G. DeFranca, with Linda J. Levine.
p.   cm.
Includes bibliographical references and index.
ISBN 0-8342-0756-7
1. Pelvis—Diseases—Chiropractic treatment.
I. Levine, Linda J. II. Title.
[DNLM: 1. Joints—injuries. 2. Lumbosacral Region—injuries.
3. Movement Disorders—physiopathology.
4. Pelvic Pain—physiopathology. 5. Joints—injuries—case studies.
6. Pelvic Pain—rehabilitation—case studies.
WE 750 D316p 1996]
RZ265.J64D44 1996
617.5'5—dc20
DNLM/DLC
for Library of Congress
95-47220
CIP

The authors have made every effort to ensure the accuracy of the information herein. However, appropriate information sources should be consulted, especially for new or unfamiliar procedures. It is the responsibility of every practitioner to evaluate the appropriateness of a particular opinion in the context of actual clinical situations and with due consideration to new developments. The authors, editors, and the publisher cannot be held responsible for any typographical or other errors found in this book.

Editorial Resources: Jane Colilla

Library of Congress Catalog Card Number: 95-47220
ISBN: 0-8342-0756-7

Printed in the United States of America

1   2   3   4   5

I dedicate this book to my three beautiful daughters, Monica, Jacqueline, and Jessica, who continually inspire me to look at the world with childlike wonder and curiosity. I hope this book reminds them of the many values that I have learned, including perseverance, honesty, self-sacrifice, and humility. It is my wish that they will grow to reflect these same values in their own lives.

Table of Contents

Foreword

Pelvic Locomotor Dysfunction: A Clinical Approach is the first text solely dedicated to joint and muscle dysfunctions of the pelvic and hip regions. Dr DeFranca should be commended for compiling such a refreshing, highly readable, and easily understood book. In addition, he has written with a thoroughness that does not overwhelm the reader yet maintains the very substance of this very important topic. The anatomy, biomechanical function, clinical assessment and differential diagnosis are thoroughly discussed and fully referenced. The first part of the book discusses anatomy and function and lays the groundwork for the clinically oriented second half of the book. In addition, Dr Levine's chapter on exercise is very apropos in the discussion of treating these disorders and provides practical information in this regard.

Dr DeFranca's style of writing instills interest and excitement to any practitioner involved with treating these conditions and his book is a practical contribution to the reader's library. The many illustrations used bring the material more fully to life and enhance understanding of the various concepts presented.

This book fully discusses, among other things, the importance of sacroiliac joint movement, despite years of contrary writing and thinking. It also raises the consciousness of the reader to the key role that sacroiliac and hip joint dysfunctions play in lower back and leg pain syndromes. Anyone who has practiced joint manipulation and has witnessed the relatively quick relief afforded to patients that are incapacitated with excruciating back and leg pain knows that the sacroiliac joint is a common etiology. As this book brings to light the importance of pelvic and hip joint dysfunctions, maybe world-renowned back pain specialists will soon discuss this population of patients at their conferences.

Finally, experienced spine specialists, chiropractic and medical general practitioners, physical therapists, and students can go to this "sure to become" classic on the subject of pelvic and hip joint dysfunctions and learn how to help the millions of sufferers this book so aptly describes.

—Leonard "John" Faye, DC, FCCSS (C) Hon

Preface

Sit down before fact as a child. Be prepared to give up every pre-conceived notion. Follow humbly wherever nature leads you or you will learn nothing.

—Thomas Huxley

Approximately 17 years ago, I was abruptly introduced to pelvic joint dysfunction, thanks to a wrenching football injury that caused me to suffer considerable low back and leg pain. Little did I know then that this chance encounter would change the direction of my life. I was given several different diagnoses by practitioners of varying disciplines. Most of them placed a great deal of concern and attention on the radiographic finding of an L-5 spondylolisthesis that I had. In retrospect, my clinical workup was wanting. My treatment was symptomatic and palliative at best. All I knew was that I was unable to play sports, let alone sit for classes.

After 3 months of pain, diminished physical activity, and frustration, I went to a chiropractic doctor at the insistence of my father. What I later came to know as sacroiliac joint dysfunction was identified and corrected by Dr Herman Cohen of Elizabeth, New Jersey. I was amazed at my rapid recovery and ability to return to sports, while thankful for what seemed a fortuitous meeting with a man who understood pelvic joint dysfunction. Why was it by chance that I found the right treatment? What about the L-5 spondylolisthesis, I thought? Surely such an impressive-sounding title should cause some pain. Why did the bed rest, hot packs, medications, and exercises I was told to do fail? What about other people with similar problems experiencing similar results of failure? Why was my problem missed by numerous others from whom I sought help? These questions formed the basis for my writing this book. The book's purpose is to draw attention to a most important and often neglected area of the body and its ability to cause patients pain: functional disturbances of the pelvic joints and muscles.

It seems ironic that structures so strategically placed in the musculoskeletal system as the pelvic joints would receive such little recognition as to their importance in back pain and disturbances of the locomotor system. Being placed between the legs and trunk, they must adapt to changes in posture and locomotion. The body's most powerful muscles originate and insert near them. The extreme mechanical forces they are subjected to daily are evidenced by the powerful ligamentous support they necessitate. Surely the potential for injury and dysfunction is great.

Yet the importance of pelvic joint dysfunction and its role in the genesis of back pain are too often overlooked. Consequently, functional examination of these most important structures is ignored. To the detriment of the patient subject to clinical bias and unawareness, a diagnosis of disc disease, lumbar facet syndrome, arthritis, muscle spasm, or even stress is often bestowed. As a result, exercises, hot moist packs, drugs, injections, repeated lumbar rotary manipulations, massage, and bed rest continue to no avail and will persist in doing so until other possibilities are entertained. Other possibilities should include the examination and treatment of functional disorders of the pelvic joints and their related structures. The aim of this book is to present practical approaches to the more common disorders related to this area.

By *functional disorders*, I am referring to disorders in which the anatomical parts are structurally sound, being devoid of pathological changes, but are unable to perform painlessly the tasks for which they are designed. For whatever reason, be it use, abuse, or trauma, the parts just function poorly. Pelvic joint dysfunction pertains to loss of normal function due to a lack of mechanical play within the joint in question.

The term *pelvic joints* pertains to the two sacroiliac joints, the pubic symphysis joint, and the sacrococcygeal joint. The sacroiliac joints recently have received more attention and much controversy regarding their function and the role they play in back pain. Accordingly, they are given more attention in this book. The hip joints are included in this discussion due to their biomechanical interdependence with the pelvic joints. In addition, since no joint is an isolated entity separated from the rest of the musculoskeletal system, the related soft tissue structures and their assessment are also considered.

At the risk of seeming too restrictive in focus, I have limited this work to the discussion of the pelvic region. This is not to exclude the importance of the rest of the musculoskeletal system, nor is it to foster a reductionistic and segmented thinking. It is simply to highlight the clinical importance of the pelvic joints in back pain. The sacroiliac and hip joint, being synovial, and the sacrococcygeal and symphysis pubis joints, being amphiarthrodial, react the same way to use, abuse, dysfunction, and pathology as do similar structures found elsewhere in the musculoskeletal system. This holds true for muscular, ligamentous, and other tissues found in the pelvic region. Hence, myofascial trigger points, ligament sprains, and joint dysfunctions found in the pelvis will be similar to those found in the same tissues of, for example, the knee or shoulder.

This book emphasizes the common clinical problems that affect the pelvic region regarding functional locomotor disturbances. Accordingly, joint and muscle dysfunctions are discussed at length, with less attention given to the less commonly seen organic pathologies.

The first two chapters discuss the anatomy and function of the pelvic region, with clinical comments interspersed where necessary. Chapter 3 focuses on the clinical history, followed by a discussion on general principles of assessment and the examination process in Chapters 4 and 5 respectively.

Chapters 6 and 7 are concerned with a variety of manual techniques used to treat joint dysfunction. Two separate chapters were written to emphasize the differences between mobilization (Chapter 6) and manipulation (Chapter 7).

The soft tissue structures, as well as the clinical considerations of their treatment, are briefly presented in Chapter 8. Chapter 9 discusses the treatment of the soft tissue disorders, mostly represented by myofascial pain syndromes, friction massage, and facilitation techniques for muscle shortening.

Chapter 10 discusses various clinical observations associated with pelvic locomotor disturbances. It is followed by Dr Linda Levine's chapter on stretching and exercises.

Finally, an appendix is included to illustrate typical clinical presentations and their management.

Acknowledgments

I wish to acknowledge the following people for assisting me in the preparation of this book, knowing that they deserve more credit than is provided by the mere mention of their names. I am greatly indebted to my father, George DeFranca, Sr, because it was his influence that inspired me to pursue my chosen professional career; to Marie DeFranca, the wonderful mother of my children, for allowing me the freedom to undertake this endeavor and for the support and understanding that I needed to work on this book; and to the late John McM Mennell, MD, whose guidance and input aided greatly in the initial phases of this book.

I am especially indebted to Linda J. Levine, DC, for her friendship and long hours of honest editing and manuscript proofreading, in addition to the contributions she has made to this book. I am also indebted to Len Faye, DC, whose teachings have influenced me and my clinical reasoning on a profound level; to my sister Carol DeFranca, DC, DABCO, for her artistic touch and sisterly loving support I am forever in deep gratitude; and to my sister Diann Kelly, who was instrumental in much of the manuscript typing and conversion to computer disks.

I am most thankful to my staff, Alison Ripa, Stacey Wheeler, and Kristal Dubovick, for their much appreciated support and tolerance of my ways, which afforded me an environment in my office in which I could work effectively. I would like to thank long-time friends and colleagues Mike Glaiel, DC, for his photography and Gary Gorman, DC, for his patience in holding the various positions until we got them right. I thank Peter Viteritti, DC, for his suggestion that the topics of mobilization and manipulation be placed in their own respective chapters to elucidate the often unappreciated differences between them; and I thank Dominick Fiore, DC, for providing me with references concerning Chapter 5.

Introduction

At the turn of the century, the sacroiliac joints were considered a common source of low back pain and even sciatica.[1,2] However, Mixter and Barr's milestone report on herniated discs causing low back and leg pain touched off the era of the "disc theory" as the cause of low back pain.[3] Hence, medical interest was diverted away from the sacroiliac joint as a cause of low back pain, and attention given to it was diminished.

Unfortunately, the sacroiliac joint shared a similar reputation of clinical insignificance with the proximal tibiofibular and acromioclavicular joints. For a long time it was held that sacroiliac joint movement was negligible, if any, and that whatever movement was there was insignificant. It was also thought that no one group of muscles directly and actively moved the joint. How could a joint that did not move be of any significance, let alone one whose function was not directly affected by any set group of muscles? Yet the sacroiliac joint does move, and there are muscles that span the joint, either directly or indirectly, that can influence the joint. What about the piriformis, gluteus maximus, and psoas muscles?

Clinical interest is shifting back to the pelvic joints. Sacroiliac joint disorders are a common occurrence in clinical practice, causing much low back and leg pain. Low back and leg pain are commonly thought to be of lumbar radicular etiology; however, sacroiliac joint dysfunction is a very common cause of low back, buttock, and proximal posterior thigh pain—what is loosely called "high sciatica." It is actually a misnomer, since the sciatic nerve is not involved, and essentially pertains to the site of pain distribution. Focus needs to be shifted away from the less common, although more dramatic, causes of low back pain. From their experience of tending to many patients with low back and leg pain syndromes, Bourdillion and Day state: "The sacroiliac joint appears to be the single greatest cause of back pain. The range of motion is small and difficult to describe but, when normal joint play is lost, agonizing pain can be precipitated."[4(p229)]

Although the prevalence for sacroiliac joint dysfunction in the general population is not known, many authorities recognize its common occurrence. Of the last 100 patients seen for low back pain in my own practice, 36 were diagnosed and successfully treated for sacroiliac joint dysfunction. Bernard and Kirkaldy-Willis[5] found sacroiliac joint lesions to be the etiologic factor in 23% of over 1200 patients in a chronic low back pain clinic. Barbor[6] and Bourne[7] have conducted studies suggesting that sacroiliac problems are the cause of low back pain 50% to 70% of the time.

Sacroiliac and hip joint dysfunction is often found in school-aged children. This is due to the prolonged sitting posture encountered in school. Low back pain in children is more common than is thought and leg pains attributable to pelvic joint dysfunction are often passed off as "growing pains." Does it make sense that the body would painfully remind us that, as children, we are growing? The same pains that are called "growing pains" in children are called "I'm getting old" pains in adults. Mierau et al studied the prevalence of sacroiliac joint hypomobility in 403 school-aged children aged 6 to 17 years, and "a high degree of association was found between SI hypomobility and LBP."[8(p83)] Those demonstrating sacroiliac joint dysfunction constituted 29.9% of the elementary schoolchildren (ages 6 to 12) and 41.5% of the secondary schoolchildren (ages 12 to 17). When asked about a history of low back pain, 26.3% of the entire student body (N = 403) responded positively for prior occurrence. Interestingly, 83.1% of those children with a history of low back pain were found to have sacroiliac joint dysfunction.

Sacroiliac joint involvement in ankylosing spondylitis, Reiter's syndrome, psoriatic arthritis, and inflammatory bowel disease is well recognized. However, these processes are associated with actual tissue pathology and, although not rare, are seen less often than the joint and muscle dysfunctions discussed in this text. The reader is referred to more complete works on the subject. This does not relieve us of the obligation to be aware of and rule out such entities, as well as other pathologies; however, the aim is to shift our focus of attention to functional disturbances of the pelvic structures. Bear in mind that pathologies can masquerade as joint and muscle dysfunctions and need to be differentially diagnosed.

Pelvic joint dysfunction, particularly sacroiliac joint disturbances, can exacerbate lumbosacral congenital anomalies, especially pseudoarthrosis of an L-5 transverse process with the ilium or sacral ala. Attention is usually given to the anomaly, and patients are made to feel as if they will forever have a "bad" back because they were born with a "defect." In actuality, the body has been existing happily with the anomaly for years and considers it a normal part of the anatomy. Sacroiliac joint dysfunction can force compensatory changes at the anomaly, which, as in any other joint, may react with hypermobility and inflammation. Sacroiliac joint manipulation is usually corrective, the irritated anomaly calms down, and harmony is restored. At times the anomalous joint itself becomes dysfunctional and needs to be manipulated. It is also recognized that pregnant women experience lower back pain that is often attributed to sacroiliac joint involvement, owing to the physiologic changes that occur within the pelvic joints themselves.[9–13]

What is the basis of one's assessment of the locomotor system? This is an important question to consider because the correctness of the diagnosis rests upon its answer. A fundamental concept in the assessment of functional disturbances of the locomotor system is to appraise the cardinal function of the tissues in question. The locomotor system is a living, moving, dynamic structure that needs to be examined as such. Anatomical studies (X-ray, computerized tomography, magnetic resonance imaging) are important and useful, but they lack the ability to yield information regarding the functional integrity of the locomotor apparatus. We are not dealing with bones that simply "go out of place," requiring some treatment to "put them back in place" readily.

Unfortunately, 90% of the time and effort in dealing with the clinical investigation of lower back pain is spent looking for conditions that account for 10% of the problem. An examination of the average patient in extreme pain, even when unresponsive to prior conservative treatments, usually reveals negative neurologic and orthopedic findings. Add to this negative X-ray, computerized tomography, magnetic resonance imaging, and laboratory findings, and you have a very confusing mess. This situation does not surprise the experienced clinician who fights in the trenches daily with the never-ending battle of lower back pain presentations. The fact is, 90% of the problem when dealing with lower back pain is one of aberrant function as compared to overt structural disease or pathology. How many clinicians scratch their scalps in exasperation when confronted with a patient who suffers from severe low back pain yet exhibits negative findings on clinical investigation? Again, one needs to ask, "What is the basis of assessment?" Are we matching the basis of our assessment with the functional capabilities of the part in question? For example, joints function to move through active, passive, and joint play ranges of motion. The testing of their ability to move correctly through these parameters is therefore prerequisite to diagnosis and effective treatment. How can this functional status be surmised from X-rays or magnetic resonance imaging?

A problem confronting clinicians is the almost irresistible urge to fall prey to two incorrect assumptions. The first incorrect assumption states that if all "high-tech" testing is negative for a particular problem, then the problem does not exist. Unfortunately, most high-tech testing, being better able to detect structural pathology and advanced disease, is poorly suited to reveal the more commonly seen problems of dysfunction. Consequently, patients with functional disturbances of the locomotor system are told that their test results are negative and that nothing is wrong. As a result, they are left to fend for themselves and hope their pain will go away. It usually does not, and they find themselves turning to unorthodox methods of treatment or even psychotherapy.

The second incorrect assumption is that if a defect is visualized on high-resolution scanning procedures, such as computerized tomography or magnetic resonance imaging, then it must be the source of pain. As stated before, anatomical studies are inadequate for demonstrating problems of function. Second, false-positive results are common with these procedures. In a study conducted by Weisel et al, 35% of an asymptomatic patient population had their computerized tomography results interpreted as being positive for disc bulging. These subjects had no prior history of lower back pain or spinal injury.[14] Jensel et al[15] observed disc bulges in 52% and disc protrusions in 27% of a group of asymptomatic people. They suggest that these findings in patients with low back pain may be coincidental.

X-ray findings correlate poorly with the subjective complaints of patients. Patients who are in the most excruciating pain often demonstrate perfectly good-looking X-rays. Conversely, patients who demonstrate gross degenerative changes radiologically often have minimal, if any, subjective complaints. The point is that patients, not test results, need to be listened to, examined, touched, and functionally assessed. After all, what are we treating? Living patients or X-rays and magnetic resonance images?

In reflecting on how we live in modern society, it should not surprise us that we often suffer from joint and muscle dysfunctions, particularly as they pertain to the pelvic area. We sit far too much, assuming postures that tend to shorten certain muscle groups selectively, causing weakness and imbalance in the locomotor system. We stuff our feet, and in some cases cram them, into containers we call shoes. We walk on hard, level surfaces that yield little variation in contour, affording meager amounts of adaptive opportunities for the mobile foot to exercise itself. Many of us fail to partake in regular active exercise, forfeiting the benefits gained from moving the locomotor system and enhancing cardiovascular and pulmonary functions. Many tend to eat foods that in some cases seem hardly enough to sustain life, let alone health. Most people rarely partake in even a minimal amount of stretching exercises designed to lengthen taut, shortened tissues and to loosen stiff joints. If one observes the animal kingdom, it becomes readily apparent that after lying down, an animal will arise only to stretch its spine and limbs thoroughly—usually, by the way, in extension. If all this is not enough, we subject ourselves to much physical and psychological stress, which undoubtedly has far-reaching effects on both soma and psyche.

Throughout our lives, we expose ourselves to a variety of traumas that contribute to locomotor disturbances. Often these do not heal to full functional capacity. Consequently, yesterday's injuries, especially if improperly diagnosed and treated, become the painful legacies of today and tomorrow in the form of osteoarthritis, fibrotic joint capsules, and myofascial trigger points.

Yet despite all this abuse from daily living, the human locomotor system, equipped with an efficient cybernetic nervous system, adapts again and again to maintain order. Unfortunately, the system has a tendency either to overadapt or to underadapt. The result is excessive or inadequate neuromuscular responses, with functional abnormalities being perpetuated for months, if not years. For instance, a muscle that is shortened and tight from injury may reciprocally inhibit its antagonist, creating an imbalance of tension across the articulation they affect. This imbalance can exist for years, creating further adaptive or maladaptive responses, all mediated by the nervous system. Unfortunately, this adaptive process continues long after the pain from the initial trauma has disappeared. This is the inherent problem in just treating a patient's pain and ignoring the underlying problems of dysfunction. The pain from most musculoskeletal conditions, especially low back pain, self-remits. But although the inflammation and pain may have subsided, the insult to the system has been neurologically recorded, only to be replayed again. Soft tissue fibrosis and other inflammatory sequelae contribute to dysfunction and a greater possibility of recurrence. Therefore, in addition to treating signs of inflammation, ensuring proper joint motion and muscle length and strength will aid in functional restoration.

Being made up of moving parts linked through kinematic chains, the locomotor system exhibits interdependence in physiologic as well as dysfunctional states. This, coupled with the body's ever-present need to maintain homeostasis, demands the recognition and understanding of compensatory reactions occurring frequently in the musculoskeletal system. The pelvic ring, with its articulations and related soft tissues, lends itself readily to such reactions. Being positioned between the trunk and lower extremities, the pelvis must adapt readily to their constant dynamic changes or else manifest itself in dysfunction. As such, the pelvis can be the site of painful compensatory reactions from distant or local dysfunctions. For example, lower extremity joint problems, particularly of the hip joint, can be clinically silent in themselves, yet foster painful sacroiliac joint disturbances due to compensatory mechanisms. Just as often, primary pelvic dysfunctions can be painful or silent and cause symptomatic secondary dysfunctions to develop elsewhere. For instance, it is common to have a painful, hypermobile lumbar facet problem in response to stiff sacroiliac or hip joints. Remarkable as it may sound, it is not uncommon for the midthoracic or upper cervical regions to compensate painfully for a dysfunctional pelvis. Treatment directed solely at the painful area often misses the mark.

Local lesions do not remain isolated islands of dysfunction without causing neurophysiologic reactions elsewhere. Often the primary biomechanical fault is clinically silent, causing the clinician to be led astray when assessing the symptomatic presentation. Hence, listening to the musculoskeletal system's deceptive "cries of wolf" via painful secondary reactions commonly results in misdirected therapy. An appreciation should be gained for the body's ability to compensate and therefore to hurt somewhere other than the primary lesion's site. One must pay astute attention to the "whispered" messages of the locomotor system, for they are communicated to the aware and observant clinician in the form of subtle soft tissue changes, minute dysfunctional movements, and reflex phenomena, yet they confound those seeking "shouts" of direction. Thus, inexperienced hands that blunder through a hurried examination yielding negative findings, and worse yet, a clinical mind closed to or ignorant of these subtle messages of dysfunction can only hope to conclude that nothing is wrong, that a lesion does not exist, or worse, that the patient is in need of psychological counseling.

Some practitioners employing manual methods cling to outdated "bone-out-of-place" theories, according to which manipulation simply pops bones back into place. For example, the often-touted examination finding of a posterior innominate bone is used as an indication to manipulate the innominate back into what is thought to be a normal position. Yet in this author's experience, and, to be sure, in the experience of countless others, manipulative corrections based on abnormal bony alignment result in the annoying persistence of the bony misalignment. The posterior innominate remains posterior and probably will if that is where it needs to be for that patient. Symmetry is not the rule in human structure. Bony prominences are bent, missing anomalously, or differing in shape even from side to side. Posterior superior iliac spines differ in size and shape and are often difficult to palpate accurately. On the other hand, one cannot indiscriminately manipulate joints just because they are restricted or fixated and feel that all one has to do to achieve health in a patient is create a pop that frees up a restricted joint. Some people exist very nicely even though they harbor asymptomatic joint and muscle dysfunctions that are like an accident waiting for a place to happen.

Manual treatment is more analogous to computer programming than to mechanical engineering. There is much more involved than just "cracking" a joint or stretching a tight muscle. The nervous system is the great mediator of function. Prudent assessment and appreciation of the complexities of the neuromusculoskeletal apparatus and the confusing ways, both known and unknown, in which it manifests dysfunction are needed.

With clinical consciousness shifting toward the examination and treatment of function, and with studies[16–21] now demonstrating the value of joint manipulation in low back pain patients, acquiring the expertise necessary to assess functional disturbances will become paramount.

REFERENCES

1. Goldthwait JE, Osgood RBA. A consideration of the pelvis articulations from an anatomical, pathological and clinical standpoint. *Boston Med Surg J.* 1905;152:592–634.

2. Abel AL. Sacroiliac strain. *Br Med J.* 1939;1:683–686.

3. Mixter WJ, Barr JS. Rupture of the intervertebral disc. *N Engl J Med.* 1934;211:210–213.

4. Bourdillion JF, Day EA. *Spinal Manipulation.* 4th ed. Norwalk, Conn: Appleton & Lange; 1987.

5. Bernard T, Kirkaldy-Willis W. Recognizing specific characteristics of nonspecific low back pain. *Clin Orthop.* 1987;217:266–280.

6. Barbor R. Back pain. *Br Med J.* 1978;2:566.

7. Bourne IHJ. Back pain: what can we offer. *Br Med J.* 1979;1:1085.

8. Mierau DR, Cassidy JD, Hamin T, et al. Sacroiliac joint dysfunction and low back pain in school aged children. *J Manipulative Physiol Ther.* 1984; 7:81–84.

9. Fast A, Shapiro D, Ducommun EJ, et al. Low back pain in pregnancy. *Spine.* 1987;12:368–371.

10. Davis P, Lentle BC. Evidence for sacroiliac disease as a common cause of low backache in women. *Lancet.* 1978;2:496–497.

11. Fraser DM. Postpartum backache: a preventable condition? *Can Fam Physician.* 1976;22:76–78.

12. Sandoz RW. Structural and functional pathologies of the pelvic ring. *Ann Swiss Chiro Assoc.* 1981;7:101–160.

13. Young J. Relaxation of the pelvic joints in pregnancy: pelvic arthropathy of pregnancy. *J Obstet Gynaecol Br Empire.* 1940;47:493–524.

14. Weisel SW, Tsourmas N, Feffer HL, et al. A study of computer-assisted tomography: the incidence of positive CAT scans in an asymptomatic group of patients. *Spine.* 1984;9:549–551.

15. Jensel MC, Brant-Zawadzki MN, Obuchowski N, et al. Magnetic resonance imaging of the lumbar spine in people without back pain. *New Engl J Med.* 1994;331:69.

16. Nwuga VCB. Relative therapeutic efficacy of vertebral manipulation and conventional treatment in back pain management. *Am J Phys Med.* 1982;61:273–278.

17. Kirkaldy-Willis W, Cassidy JD. Spinal manipulation in the treatment of low back pain. *Can Fam Physician.* 1985;31:535–540.

18. Meade TW, Dyer S, Browne W, et al. Low back pain of mechanical origin: randomized comparison of chiropractic and hospital outpatient treatment. *Br Med J.* 1990;300:1431–1437.

19. Shekelle PG, Adams AH, Chassin MR, et al. *The Appropriateness of Spinal Manipulation for Low Back Pain: Indications and Ratings by an All-Chiropractic Expert Panel.* Santa Monica, Calif: Rand; 1992. R-4025/3-CCR/FCER.

20. Manga P, Angus D, et al. *The Effectiveness and Cost-Effectiveness of Chiropractic Management of Low Back Pain.* Ottawa, Canada: Pran Manga and Associates, University of Ottawa; 1993.

21. Triano JJ, McGregor M, Hondras MA, Brennan PC. Manipulative therapy versus education programs in chronic low back pain. *Spine.* 1994;20:948–955.

Chapter 1

Anatomy

Chapter Objectives

- to describe the osseous, muscular, and articular anatomy of the pelvic and hip regions
- to discuss the importance of the thoracolumbar fascia
- to discuss topographical landmarks for palpation
- to discuss common musculoskeletal congenital anomalies of the pelvic region

The anatomy of the pelvis is both interesting and complex. The word *pelvis* means "basin" in Latin, and the name is appropriate, for the pelvis resembles a hollow container bearing viscera and allowing the ingress and egress of neurovascular and muscular structures.

OSSEOUS ANATOMY

The osseous pelvis consists of three articulating structures forming a *three-joint complex*. The sacrum, a triangular-shaped bone, is wedged between the posterior aspects of the paired innominates at the sacroiliac joints (Figures 1–1 and 1–2). The innominates meet anteriorly at the pubic symphysis, an amphiarthrosis, to complete the three-joint complex. The sacrum articulates with the L-5 vertebra above and the coccyx below.[1]

Sacrum

The sacrum is usually made up of five fused segments that retain vestigial remains of vertebral elements (Figure 1–3). It is widest at its base, and its uppermost surface articulates with L-5. The anterior aspect of the sacral

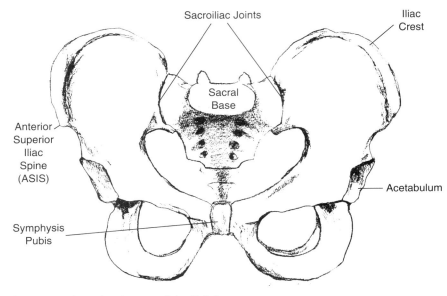

Figure 1–1 Anterior Aspect of the Pelvis

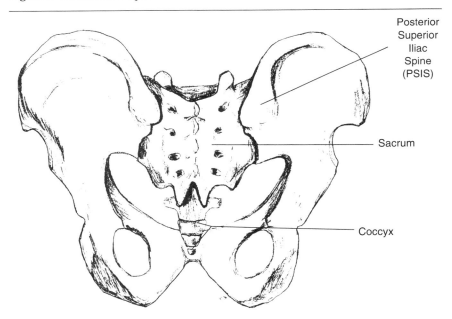

Figure 1–2 Posterior Aspect of the Pelvis

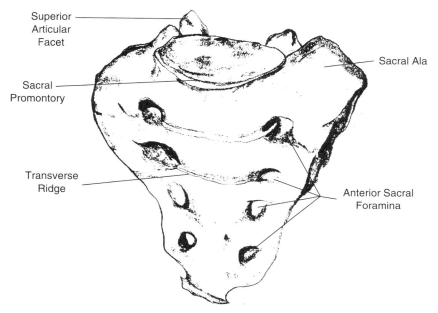

Figure 1–3 Anterior Aspect of the Sacrum

base is very pronounced and is called the *sacral promontory*. The ventral surface is marked by four transverse ridges marking the boundaries of each sacral segment. Each ridge ends laterally at the *ventral sacral foramina* on each side. The foramina transmit the ventral primary rami of the sacral nerves and the related blood vessels. The ridges of bone between the ventral sacral foramina provide origin for the piriformis muscle.

Dorsally, the spinous processes of the first four segments are retained as the *median sacral crest* (Figure 1–4). The first sacral segment is the largest and still bears functional superior articular processes that face dorsomedially to articulate with the inferior articular processes of L-5. The remainder of the articular processes form the *intermediate sacral crest* that is located just medial to the *posterior sacral foramina* in the form of four small tubercles aligned in sequence. The transverse process of the first sacral segment and its costal element fuse to form the large *sacral ala* wing. The rest of the transverse processes fuse with their costal elements to form the *sacral lateral mass*. The *lateral sacral crest*, being just lateral to the posterior sacral foramina, marks the legacy of the transverse processes as an interrupted line of tubercles. The inferior articular processes of the fifth sacral segment remain as the *sacral cornua*. The fifth segment's spinous process and lamina fail to fuse in the midline and thus form a permanent defect known as the *sacral hiatus*. The bony, nonarticular inferolateral aspect of the sacrum is termed the *inferior lateral angle*.

Viewed laterally, the sacrum exhibits a ventral concavity (Figure 1–5). The *sacroiliac articular facet* can be seen on the lateral aspect of the lateral mass, formed by the coalescence of the embryonic costal and transverse processes of the first and second sacral segments. The joint's surface is likened to the shape of a side-lying letter L, with the shorter limb being cephalad, vertically oriented, and contained within the first sacral segment. The caudal, more horizontal limb is borne by the second and half of the third sacral segments. The facet's gross appearance resembles that of an ear and hence earned the name *auricular surface*. Posterior to the joint surface proper is a roughened area serving as the attachment site for the powerful interosseous ligament.

Innominate Bone

The *innominate bone* is formed by three fused bones and conveys a shape that resembles no other known object; hence, the early anatomists chris-

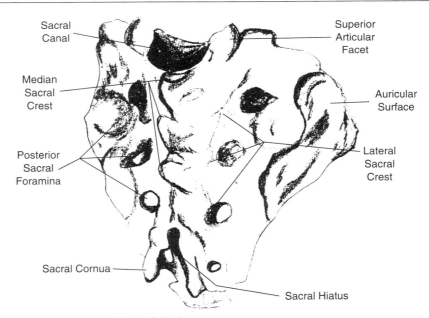

Figure 1–4 Posterior View of the Sacrum

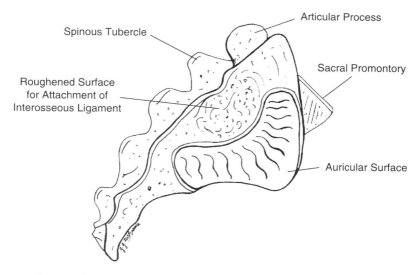

Figure 1–5 Sacrum, lateral aspect. Note articular facet and roughened attachment for interosseous ligament.

tened it *innominate*, meaning "nameless" (Figures 1–6 and 1–7). It is an oddly shaped bone formed by the fusion of the *ilium, ischium,* and *pubic bones,* which meet to form the cup-shaped *acetabulum* on its lateral aspect. The *acetabulum,* which in Latin means "a little saucer for vinegar," faces downward, outward, and forward to articulate with the femoral head.

The *ilium* is identified by its flaring crest, which begins anteriorly at the *anterior superior iliac spine,* proceeds posteriorly in an S-shaped fashion, being slightly concave medially in front and concave laterally in back, and terminates at the *posterior superior iliac spine.* Viewed laterally, the *iliac crest* presents as a convex arch forming the prominence of the hip. The lateral aspect of the ilium is broad, being convex anteriorly and concave posteriorly. The anterior superior iliac spine marks the most anterior aspect of the ilium and serves as attachment for the lateral part of the inguinal ligament. Below this is the *anterior inferior iliac spine.* A shallow groove separates the anterior inferior spine from an eminence and allows the passage of the iliopsoas tendon.

The posterior superior iliac spine is the large protuberance on the most posterior aspect of the ilium. Just inferior is the *posterior inferior iliac spine,* which is on level with the lower aspect of the sacroiliac joint. The internal surface of the ilium is smooth, large, and concave. Posteriorly lies the au-

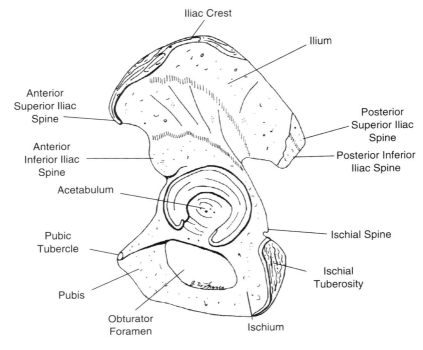

Figure 1–6 Innominate Bone, Lateral Aspect

ricular surface, which articulates with the sacrum at the sacroiliac joint. Just posterior to this is a large, roughened area where the powerful interosseous sacroiliac ligament inserts.

The *pubic bone* meets its counterpart in the midline via the *superior* and *inferior rami* to form the body of the pubic bone and gives shape to the anterior aspect of the pelvis. The paired pubic bones meet to form the *pubic symphysis joint* in the midline (Figure 1–8). Just lateral to the pubic symphysis on the superior aspect of the superior ramus is a rounded border called the *pubic crest*, whose lateral aspect gives rise to the *pubic tubercle*.

The *ischium* forms the most inferior part of the pelvis and has a thick body, large tuberosity, and thin ramus. The posterior aspect of the ischial body gives rise to the *ischial spine*, to which the sacrospinous ligament attaches. The inferior aspect of the ischium is the large *ischial tuberosity*, upon which the pelvis rests during sitting. The ramus ascends and meets with

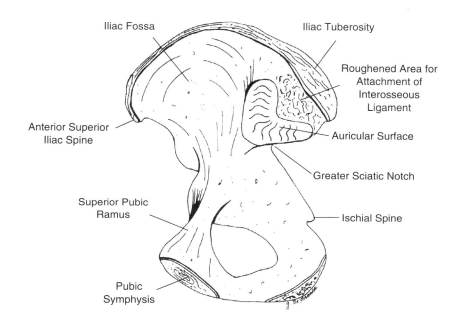

Figure 1–7 Innominate bone, medial aspect. Note articular facet.

the inferior ramus of the pubic bone to complete the ring-shaped *obturator foramen*.

Coccyx

The *coccyx* is a small bone formed by the fusion of usually four segments (Figure 1–9). The coccyx as a whole faces up and forward with its ventral surface. Usually the first coccygeal segment remains separate from the rest. The first three segments retain rudimentary bodies, transverse processes, and articular processes. The segments progressively diminish in size to where the last segment is represented by a small button of bone without any processes discernible. The coccyx is widest proximally at its base, through which it articulates with the last sacral segment via an articular facet. Rudimentary pedicles and articular processes form the *coccygeal cornua,* which extend superiorly to articulate with the sacral cornua.

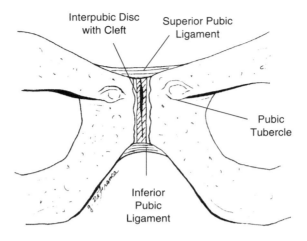

Figure 1–8 Pubic Symphysis

Vestigial transverse processes arise from the first coccygeal segment and can even fuse with the sacral inferior lateral angle.

ARTICULAR/LIGAMENTOUS ANATOMY

The pelvis proper contains three joints: the paired, posteriorly placed sacroiliac joints and the midline symphysis pubis, found anteriorly. Powerful ligamentous support lends integrity to the pelvic ring. The lumbar spine, femur, and coccyx also articulate with the pelvis. The ligaments and joints associated with the pelvis can therefore be categorized into the following six groups: (1) lumbopelvic, (2) sacroiliac, (3) sacroischial, (4) pubopubic, (5) sacrococcygeal, and (6) femoroacetabular.

Lumbopelvic

The sacrum attaches to L-5 in much the same manner as other segments in the spine are joined, except that the *supraspinous ligament* usually stops at the L4-5 level.[2] Additionally, the strong *iliolumbar ligament* attaches L-5 to the ilium. Shellshear and Macintosh[3] describe five parts to the iliolumbar ligament (Figure 1–10).

Kapandji[4] refers to a superior band of the iliolumbar ligament that connects the L-4 transverse process to the iliac crest in conjunction with an

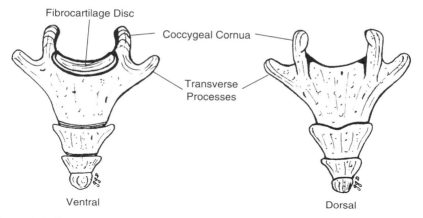

Figure 1–9 Coccyx

inferior band of ligament that attaches the L-5 transverse process with the iliac crest. Kapandji also mentions that on occasion a subdivision of the inferior band attaches to the sacrum. Luk et al[5] have shown that the iliolumbar ligament does not exist at birth but only gradually develops near the end of the first decade. The initial histological appearance of this ligament is muscular, with full ligamentous differentiation occurring in the second decade. It is thought that in response to biomechanical stresses at the lumbosacral junction imposed by the erect posture, the lower quadratus lumborum muscle fibers undergo a metaplastic transformation into the iliolumbar ligament.[5] Luk et al state that the iliolumbar ligament consists of two separate bands, both originating from the tips of the L-5 transverse process and running lateral and posterior to insert on the iliac crest.

Sacroiliac

The following information regarding the developmental anatomy was obtained mostly from work performed by Bowen and Cassidy.[6]

Literature Review

A literature review of the sacroiliac joint is full of controversy, confusion, and contradiction. Bowen and Cassidy[6] review the literature in their discussion of the age-related anatomical changes occurring in the sacroiliac joint. The first researchers to show that the sacroiliac joint was a true joint with a synovium were Albinus and Hunter[7] in the early 1700s, although Meckel was the first to write about this in an anatomy text in 1816.[8]

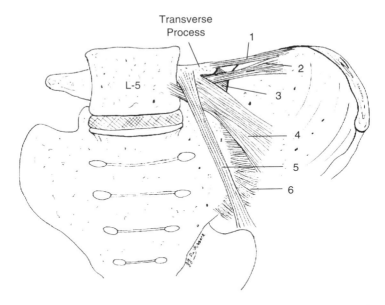

Figure 1–10 Iliolumbar ligament and its five parts: (1) superior iliolumbar ligament, (2) anterior iliolumbar ligament, (3) posterior iliolumbar ligament, (4) inferior iliolumbar ligament, and (5) vertical iliolumbar ligament. The anterior sacroiliac ligament is shown at (6).[3]

However, it was Von Luschka in 1863 who initially described the sacroiliac joint as a true diarthrodial articulation.[9] Albee[10] in 1909 regularly observed a joint space, synovial membrane, and well-formed articulation. Confirming Albee's findings in 1924, Brooke[11] moreover described fibrous and even bony ankylosis as evident, especially in male sacroiliac joints.

Sashin[12] was the first to describe age-related changes, but specimens from the first two decades were not included in his study. He described degenerative changes as present early in life, more commonly in males. Upon studying 257 specimens, he observed 85% and 50% of the male and female pelvises respectively to have osteophytic changes at the sacroiliac joints in the 40- to 49-year-old group. All male specimens aged 50 to 59 years had osteophytic changes, and 60% of them had sacroiliac joint ankylosis compared to only 14% in the female specimens.

Schunke[13] in 1938 commented on the anatomy and development of the sacroiliac joint and mentioned the histologic difference in the sacral and iliac articular cartilage. He observed that the sacroiliac joint cavity developed between the second and seventh months of fetal life. He also noted changes occurring in puberty consisting of grooves and ridges in the articular topography.

In 1951, Illi[14] described and named an intracapsular sacroiliac ligament and described sacroiliac motion based on cineradiography studies. In 1954, Weisl[15] mapped the uneven contour of the sacroiliac joint and described the sacral surface as two eminences separated by a saddle-shaped trough in the young adult.

In 1957, Solonen published a very thorough study of sacroiliac morphology.[16] He demonstrated distinctive variations in joint types that reacted differently to mechanical loading. He showed how radiography of the sacroiliac joint is inaccurate due to its complex morphology by comparing casts taken of the joint with radiographs. His dissections brought to light the differing innervation of the ventral and dorsal aspects of the joint. The ventral aspect receives innervation from L-3 to S-2, whereas the dorsal aspect receives it from S-1 to S-2.

In his anthropological study, Delmas identified two drastically different anatomical and functional types of sacroiliac joints.[17] When the vertebral column's curvatures were pronounced, the sacroiliac joint tended to lie horizontally and appeared markedly bent on itself. This *dynamic* shape, as it was called, is associated more with hyperlordotic states, seen more often in women. It tends to be more mobile and therefore predisposed to instability. The increased mobility is associated with a longer interosseous ligament allowing for motion but decreased stability. This type of sacroiliac joint occurred in 25% of the subjects studied and is an example of overadaptation to the biped posture. Its mobile characteristic resembles that of a typical synovial joint. Another 25% of the subjects demonstrated sacroiliac joints that were more vertically aligned and associated with spinal curves that were not overly pronounced. This configuration was termed the *static* type and was commonly found in men and children. The interosseous ligament was shorter and therefore afforded more stability but less mobility. Sandoz[18] commented that this type of sacroiliac joint is prone to fixation rather than instability. Its configuration is closer to that of primates and resembles an amphiarthrosis more than a diarthrosis. The remaining 50% of the subjects demonstrated a type of sacroiliac joint that was intermediate between the dynamic and the static types, representing a compromise between stability and mobility.

In 1981, Bowen and Cassidy dissected 40 autopsy specimens and commented on the gross and microscopic anatomy of sacroiliac joints from embryonic life to the eighth decade.[6] Their goals were to document age-related changes and to establish a common ground for understanding sacroiliac joint anatomy.

Gross Anatomy of the Sacroiliac Joint

The sacroiliac joint is considered a *diarthrosis* due to the following: carti-
lage-covered articular surfaces, joint capsule, joint space with fluid,
synovium, and ability to move. The joint can be divided into a ventral synovial or auricular part and a dorsal or ligamentous part that is
postauricular.[8] Sacroiliac joint morphology tends to be very variable. The
vertical and anteroposterior joint planes vary,[16] as do the sacral and iliac
articulating surfaces.[13] The sacral auricular surface is larger than its iliac
counterpart, being longer and narrower. The joint surfaces are flat and
smooth from birth until puberty, when ridges and grooves develop to impart an irregularity to the surface. The sacral side has been described by
Weisl[15] as having two elevations separated by a saddle-shaped depression. The cranial and caudal aspects of the sacral surface are elevated, with
the central depression yielding a concave appearance. The iliac surface
displays a ridge that runs longitudinally throughout its length and serves
to interdigitate with the sacral articular groove. The sacral cartilage is up
to three times thicker than that of the iliac side. Hyaline cartilage is present
on the sacral side, in contrast to the fibrocartilage present on the iliac surface.[6,13] Both the sacral and iliac surfaces are nearly parallel at the first and
second sacral segments, yet course medially at about the S-3 level.[16]

The ligaments directly supporting the sacroiliac joint can be grouped
into anterior and posterior parts. The thin *anterior sacroiliac ligament* appears to be a thickening of the anterior joint capsule (Figure 1–11).
Solonen[16] and Sashin[12] describe it as a thickening of the sacral and iliac
periosteum. The dorsal ligamentous structures consist of the powerful *interosseous ligament* and the *posterior sacroiliac ligament*. The deep, thick interosseous ligament is the main ligamentous restraint connecting the
sacrum to the ilium (Figure 1–11). It is attached just posterior to the auricular surface of both the sacrum and ilium. The ligament is so strong that on
forcible disruption of the joint in cadaveric dissections, the bony attachments give way and the ligament remains intact.[12] The joint capsule blends
in with the interosseous ligament. The posterior sacroiliac ligament is a
thin structure that is separated from the interosseous ligament by the dorsal rami of the sacral nerves and related blood vessels. It passes from the
intermediate and lateral sacral crests and passes obliquely in several fascicles to the posterior superior iliac spine and iliac crest.[1]

Through his dissections, Illi[14] observed a *superior intracapsular ligament*,
which later came to bear his name. Its existence has been controversial
ever since its discovery, since other researchers were not able to confirm
his findings. However, in 1990 Freeman et al[19] found its existence in 75% of

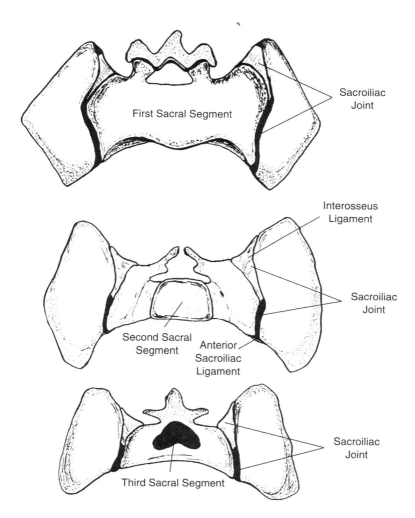

Figure 1–11 Cross section of sacroiliac joint. Note massive interosseous ligament.

their dissections of 31 human pelvises. They attribute their corroboration of Illi's findings to their dissection approach from the inferior aspect of the sacroiliac joint. Most other researchers approached the sacroiliac joint from the anterior and often inadvertently destroyed the intracapsular ligament during dissection. In their study, Freeman et al confirmed the presence of a superior intracapsular ligament running from posterosuperior on the ilium to anteroinferior on the sacrum. Its diameter ranged from 1 to

8 mm. On gross observation, it appeared to be a dense, fibrous band of connective tissue. On histological study, the band of tissue was ligamentous in nature, inserting directly into the hyaline cartilage on the sacral articulating surface. On the iliac side, the ligament blended in with the interosseous ligament. The ligament's biomechanical significance is questionable owing to its small size.

Developmental Anatomy of the Sacroiliac Joint

Embryology. Studies on the embryonic development of the sacroiliac joints are limited. Schunke[13] states that the sacroiliac joints emerge and form between the second and seventh months of fetal development. He shows how at 8 weeks the joint is represented by mesenchyme between the ilium and sacrum organized onto three layers. At 10 weeks, a cavity is formed in the middle layer. At 13 weeks, the ilium ossifies and the iliac cartilage thickens. By 8 months, a well-developed joint cavity is apparent.

In their dissections of fetal sacroiliac joints, Bowen and Cassidy observed the anterior joint capsule to be thin and pliable, with the joint stabilized mostly by the posterior interosseous ligament.[6] They further noted the sacroiliac joints to be especially mobile owing to their smooth and flat articular surfaces. Microscopically, the sacral articular cartilage was consistently three to five times thicker than that of the iliac side. The sacral chondrocytes were arranged in a pattern consistent with hyaline cartilage, whereas the iliac articular cartilage resembled a fibrocartilaginous appearance, with more collagen fibers present among the chondrocytes.

First Decade. Bowen and Cassidy[6] noted that the sacroiliac joint grew in size in accordance with somatic growth after birth. The capsule became defined, fibrous, and resilient, yet maintaining much pliability. The joint surfaces retained their planar, smooth appearance and demonstrated gliding movements easily in any direction. Microscopically, the joint capsule exhibited an outer capsular layer consisting of dense, fibrous connective tissue and an inner synovial lining only two or three cells thick. Loose areolar connective tissue was found just under the synovial layer. The iliac and sacral surfaces maintained their respective fibrocartilage and hyaline cartilage appearances.

Second and Third Decades. The teenage years see the development of corresponding grooves and ridges occurring between the sacral and iliac surfaces. The iliac surface develops a convex ridge running throughout its length, and the sacral surface displays a corresponding groove. Bowen and Cassidy[6] noticed motion to be limited to a nodding in the sagittal plane. The capsule appeared thicker and stronger, in addition to being stiffer. Microscopically, the capsule appeared more collagenous and the synovial layer thicker. Crevices were more apparent in the articular cartilage, particularly on the iliac surface. The iliac surface started to roughen and demonstrate fibrous plaques as early as 17 years, and all specimens displayed this by the middle of the third decade. The sacral surfaces yellowed near the end of the third decade, but no degenerative changes were apparent.

Fourth and Fifth Decades. The iliac ridge was consistently observed and prominent in Bowen and Cassidy's[6] dissections, and marginal bony proliferation was seen along the sacral facet. Movement was still apparent at the sacroiliac joint, and the joint capsule appeared less pliable. Plaque formation and erosions of the articular cartilage were very prevalent and consistently seen. Microscopic examination at this time demonstrated thickening of the synovium and capsule, with more of a fibrous nature apparent. Degenerative changes of the articular cartilage were visible, with advanced fibrillation and erosion seen more on the iliac side of the joint.

Sixth and Seventh Decades. Degenerative changes continued to be more pronounced. Osteophytes became larger and started to bridge the joint. The capsule became increasingly thicker and less pliant, with the joint surface becoming more irregular due to more crevices and erosions of the articular cartilage. Mobility was still present but restricted. Fibrous material was seen connecting the joint surfaces. Microscopically, advanced cartilage degeneration was seen, articular cartilage was thinner on both sides of the joint, and erosions and crevice formations were seen in increasing amounts, particularly on the iliac side of the joint. Amorphous, cellular material was seen in larger quantities in the joint space.

Seventh and Eighth Decades. Marked bony proliferation was evident, and this limited joint motion substantially. Also contributing to decreased joint motion was the large amount of intra-articular fibrous interconnections present. Articular cartilage degeneration was marked, and both sides exhibited considerable cartilage thinning. Microscopically, marginal joint capsule calcification was observed. The ground substance of both sacroiliac joint surfaces contained more collagen. Cartilage erosions were prominent, and some even extended to the subchondral bone. The iliac side of the joint demonstrated more advanced evidence of degenerative changes. Bowen and Cassidy found only one specimen with true intra-articular bony ankylosis.[6]

Sacroischial

The most powerful ligaments of the body bind the sacrum to the ischial aspect of the pelvis. The *sacrotuberous* and *sacrospinous ligaments* act as a mighty counterforce preventing the weight of the trunk from torquing the sacral base anteriorly and inferiorly by anchoring the sacral apex (Figure 1–12). The *sacrotuberous ligament* takes a wide origin from the posterior superior iliac spine, the lower sacral transverse tubercles, the lower nonarticular lateral aspect of the sacrum, and the cranial part of the coccyx. It narrows as it descends and runs laterally, only to thicken again as it inserts into the medial aspect of the ischial tuberosity.

The *sacrospinous ligament* originates from a broad base attached to the lower lateral aspect of the sacrum and proximal coccyx and runs by way of a short, triangular band slightly down and forward to insert on the ischial spine. These two ligaments divide the sacrosciatic notches into the *greater* and *lesser sciatic foramina.*

On the whole, there is a marked difference in pelvic ligaments between males and females after puberty.[16,20] Strength is sacrificed for mobility in the female pelvis, especially during pregnancy.

Pubopubic

The paired *pubic bones* meet in the midline to form the *pubic symphysis,* an amphiarthrosis (Figure 1–8). The oval ends of the pubic bones are capped by a thin layer of hyaline cartilage and are connected by a layer of fibrocartilage forming the *interpubic disc.* The longitudinal axis of the joint slants obliquely anterior, running from the inferior to the superior. A slitlike cavity is consistently found in the superoposterior aspect of the joint after the first decade of life.

The ligaments supporting this joint consist of the anterior and posterior pubic ligaments and the superior and inferior pubic ligaments. The stronger *anterior ligament* closes the anterior aspect of the joint and is interlaced with fibers from the aponeurosis of the external oblique and rectus abdominis muscles. The thinner and weaker *posterior pubic ligament* courses between the pubic bones behind the joint. The *superior pubic ligament* runs between the pubic tubercles and supports the joint superiorly. The *inferior pubic ligament,* also called the *arcuate pubic ligament,* forms a thick, strong arch at the inferior aspect of the medial ends of the pubic bones.

Sacrococcygeal

The joint between the sacrum and coccyx is amphiarthrodial and analogous to an intervertebral joint with corresponding ligamentous support

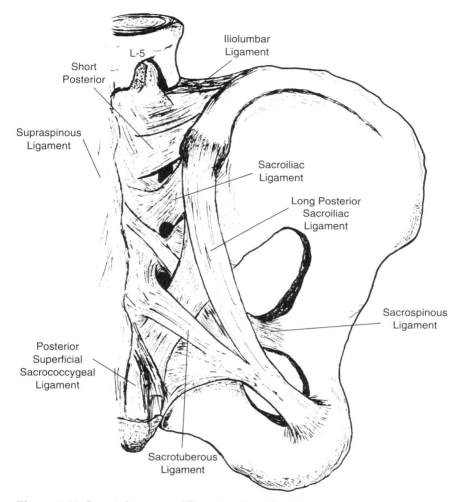

Figure 1–12 Sacrotuberous and Posterior Sacroiliac Ligaments

(Figure 1–13). Occasionally it can be synovial, with the coccyx and sacrum freely articulating.[1] The sacral articulating surface is convex, whereas that of the coccyx is concave. A thin, interposed fibrocartilaginous disc is present. Corresponding to the anterior longitudinal ligament is the *ventral sacrococcygeal ligament*, connecting the sacrum to the first coccygeal segment. The *deep dorsal sacrococcygeal ligament* corresponds to the posterior longitudinal ligament and connects the sacrum to the coccyx posteriorly. Joining the margin of the sacral hiatus to the coccyx is the *superficial dorsal*

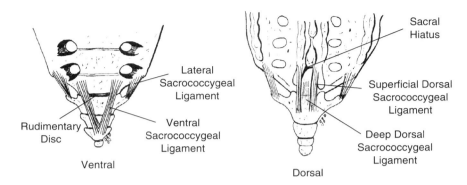

Figure 1–13 Sacrococcygeal Joint

sacrococcygeal ligament, which forms the roof of the distal sacral canal. Analogous to the intertransverse ligaments are the *lateral sacrococcygeal ligaments*, joining the transverse processes of the coccyx to the inferior lateral angle of the sacrum.

Femoroacetabular

The hip joint is anatomically and functionally linked to the pelvis and, as such, needs to be considered. The pelvic bowl rests on the femoral heads through the femoroacetabular joints. This joint is a large ball-and-socket diarthroidal articulation that is powerfully supported by very strong ligaments and a deep articular coaptation. The *acetabulum* is a cup-shaped depression on the lateral aspect of the innominate bone formed at the union of the ilium, ischium, and pubic bones (Figure 1–6). It faces laterally, inferiorly, and anteriorly and receives the rounded head of the femur.

The margin of the acetabulum is enhanced by the fibrocartilaginous *labrum*. The interior of the acetabulum is lined by a horseshoe-shaped piece of articular cartilage for articulation with the head of the femur. The deeper aspect of the acetabular fossa is nonarticular and surrounded by the horseshoe-shaped cartilage. The bony acetabulum, labrum, and articular cartilage are notched inferiorly at the acetabular notch. This notch is spanned by the transverse ligament, which affords continuity to the acetabular shape. The notch allows the transmittal of neurovascular structures into the acetabulum.

The round *femoral head* articulates with the acetabulum. It makes up two thirds of a sphere and has a pitted indentation called the *fovea* located below and behind its center. The fovea affords attachment for the ligament of the head of the femur, the biomechanical function of which seems to be insignificant. The neck of the femur supports the spherical head and forms a 125-degree angle, called the *angle of inclination*, with the shaft of the femur in the frontal plane. In the horizontal plane, the neck forms a 15-degree angle with the femoral shaft, called the *angle of anteversion* or *declination*. Therefore, the femoral head is projected medially, superiorly, and anteriorly. As a consequence, the acetabulum and femoral head both face anteriorly. Thus, during standing, the anterior aspect of the femoral head is exposed, leaving a small surface area for weight bearing posterosuperiorly. An increased or decreased angle of inclination is referred to as coxa valga or coxa vara respectively. A hip with an increased angle of anteversion is termed *anteverted*, and one with a decreased angle is called *retroverted*. Anteversion creates a toe-in gait, whereas retroversion yields a toe-out appearance. When speaking of the effects of version on the attitude of the lower extremity and foot, one needs to do so by considering the hip to be in its functional position during weight bearing.

The *greater trochanter* is a large protuberance of bone at the union of the femoral neck and shaft extending upward and laterally. It provides attachment and leverage for the powerful hip abductor muscles. The piriformis and small lateral rotators also insert on the greater trochanter, except for the quadratus femoris, which inserts below on the trochanteric crest. On the opposite side of the femoral shaft and slightly inferior is the *lesser trochanter*, a smaller bony prominence that serves as insertion for the iliopsoas muscle.

The capsuloligamentous support around the hip consists of extremely powerful structures designed to limit posterior pelvic tilting in the erect posture (Figures 1–14 and 1–15). The *capsule* originates from the rim of the acetabulum and labrum, runs parallel like a sleeve with the intracapsular femoral neck, and inserts on the intertrochanteric line in front, just proximal to the intertrochanteric crest behind.

Three extracapsular ligaments exist and are named according to their bony attachments. The *iliofemoral ligament*, also referred to as the *Y ligament of Bigelow*, originates from underneath the anterior inferior iliac spine and proceeds downward in the shape of an inverted Y to attach to the femur. Both limbs of the ligament wrap around the femoral neck, the lateral limb attaching to the greater trochanter and the medial limb attaching near the lesser trochanter. This ligament tightens in extension and internal rotation. The *ischiofemoral ligament* originates just behind and below the acetabulum and runs upward and laterally to insert on the femoral neck, where it meets the greater trochanter. It, too, tightens on extension and

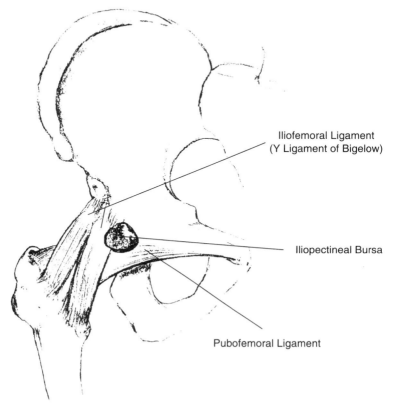

Figure 1–14 Hip Joint, Anterior Aspect

internal rotation. The *pubofemoral ligament* arises from the pubic bone near the acetabulum and attaches to the femur near the lesser trochanter. It functions mainly to limit internal rotation. Essentially, all the major ligaments around the hip joint tighten with internal rotation.

Question for Thought

- In terms of range of motion and gait, what would you expect to see clinically if capsular fibrosis and shortening were to occur in the hip joint?

The *ligament of the head of the femur*, also called the *ligamentum teres*, arises from the nonarticular acetabular fossa near the acetabular notch and runs

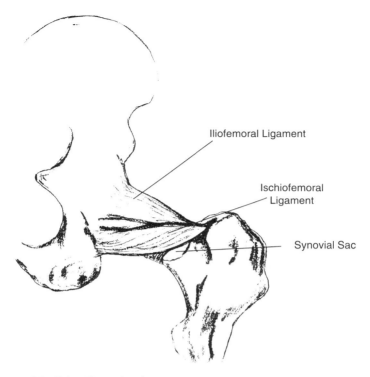

Iliofemoral Ligament

Ischiofemoral Ligament

Synovial Sac

Figure 1–15 Hip Joint, Posterior Aspect

to the fovea on the femoral head. Its function seems insignificant, other than providing a means for neurovascular structures to reach the femoral head and to spread synovial fluid over it.

MUSCULAR ANATOMY

Approximately 45 muscles attach to the pelvis. Pelvic joint and muscular dysfunctions commonly occur together. An understanding of the anatomy and function of the muscles attaching to the pelvis is essential in examining and treating pelvic locomotor disturbances.

Abdominals

Anteriorly, the abdominals consist of four muscles: the two obliques, transversus abdominis, and rectus abdominis. The *external oblique* arises from the lower eight ribs and descends in its lowest and posterior part to run vertically and insert into the lateral lip of the front half of the iliac crest (Figure 1–16). The middle and upper fibers run medially and downward to end in an aponeurosis that inserts onto the pubic bone between the pubic symphysis and pubic tubercle and ends in the midline as the linea alba. Its lower medial border is folded upon itself to form the *inguinal ligament* and extends between the anterior superior iliac spine and pubic tubercle. Acting bilaterally, it causes trunk flexion. Unilateral contraction causes lateral flexion and rotation of the trunk to the opposite side. It is innervated by the ventral rami of the lower six thoracic nerves.

The *internal oblique* arises from the lateral two thirds of the inguinal ligament, a segment of iliac crest near the anterior iliac spine, the middle third of the intermediate line on the iliac crest, and part of the thoracolumbar fascia. It arches medially and inferiorly to insert onto the pubic crest and midline linea alba. Its middle and lateral fibers run upward to insert into the lower three ribs. It functions bilaterally to flex the trunk. Contracting unilaterally, it rotates the trunk ipsilaterally, acting synergistically with the contralateral external oblique, and laterally bends the trunk to the same side.

The *transversus abdominis* originates from the lower six rib cartilages, thoracolumbar fascia, anterior three fourths of the internal lip of the iliac crest, and lateral third of the inguinal ligament. Its fibers run horizontally to insert into the linea alba medially. It functions as a girdle to support the abdominal viscera.

The *rectus abdominis* originates from the fifth, sixth, and seventh costal cartilages and xiphoid process and descends to insert on the pubic crest and symphysis. It is interrupted along its length by horizontal tendinous intersections. It strongly flexes the trunk, approximating the xiphoid and pubic symphysis. For the most part, the abdominal muscles are innervated by the lower six or seven thoracic nerves. The internal oblique abdominis and the transversus abdominis also receive innervation from the L-1 level.

Iliopsoas

The *psoas major* muscle originates from the ventral aspect of the lumbar transverse processes and the lateral aspect of the 12th thoracic and lumbar vertebral bodies and discs (Figure 1–17). It enters the pelvis and traverses over the pelvic brim behind the inguinal ligament. It proceeds in front of the hip joint capsule, becoming tendinous and receiving most of the iliacus tendon laterally. This blend of tendons inserts onto the lesser trochanter of the femur. The psoas receives its innervation from the first three lumbar nerves.

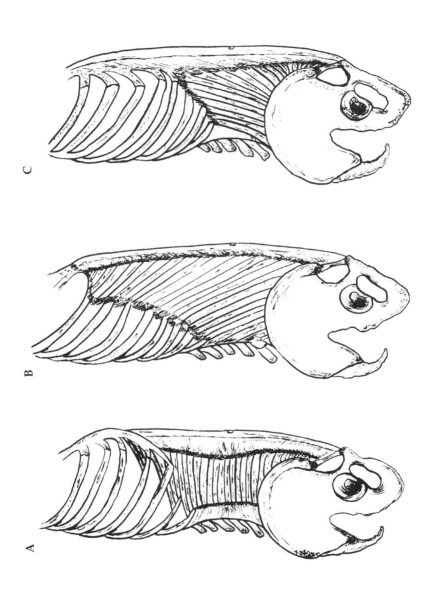

Figure 1-16 Abdominal muscles. **(A)** Transversus abdominis; **(B)** external oblique; **(C)** internal oblique.

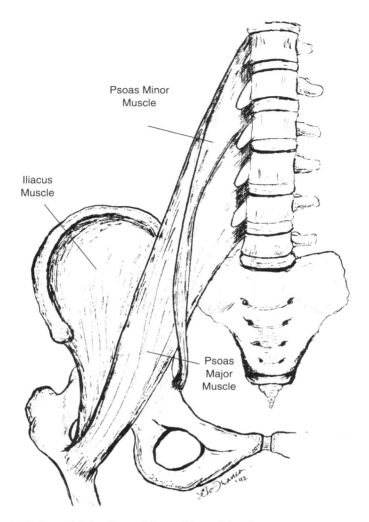

Figure 1–17 Psoas Major, Psoas Minor, Iliacus Muscles

The *iliacus* is a large triangular muscle that originates from the internal surface of the iliac bone and descends to combine mostly with the psoas major muscle. However, some fibers continue on to insert directly onto the femur just below and in front of the lesser trochanter. The iliopsoas is a strong hip flexor and assists in lateral femoral rotation. It has powerful effects on the lumbar spine due to its attachments. Unilateral contraction bends the spine ipsilaterally and rotates it contralaterally. Kapandji[4] notes that its attachment to the summit of the lumbar lordosis causes trunk flexion relative to the pelvis and accentuates the lordosis. The iliacus receives innervation from the femoral nerve.

The *psoas minor* muscle is a small muscle originating from the T-12 to L-1 disc. It inserts near the iliopubic eminence in the form of a long, slender tendon. Its presence is inconstant, and therefore its function seems insignificant.

Lower Back Region

The pelvis receives attachments from muscles originating from the posterior aspect of the trunk and spine. Even the upper extremity is linked to the pelvis via the latissimus dorsi muscle attaching to the thoracolumbar fascia.

Thoracolumbar Fascia

This tough, diamond-shaped expanse of connective tissue is strategically located to afford insertion for a variety of trunk muscles.[21] The *thoracolumbar fascia* actually consists of aponeurotic expansions from the internal oblique, transversus abdominis, serratus posterior inferior, and latissimus dorsi muscles. In the lower back, the thoracolumbar fascia splits into three layers (Figures 1–18 and 1–19). The *posterior layer* covers the erector spinae muscles, being attached medially to the lumbar and sacral spinous processes and supraspinous ligaments and laterally to the aponeurotic expanse of the deep abdominal muscles and latissimus dorsi muscle. The *middle layer* of the fascia covers the posterior surface of the quadratus lumborum muscle and attaches medially to the lumbar transverse processes and below to the iliac crest. Laterally, it joins with the posterior layer, thus investing the erector spinae muscles. The *anterior layer* of the fascia covers the anterior surface of the quadratus lumborum muscle. It is attached medially to the anterior surfaces of the lumbar transverse processes and laterally to the posterior and middle layers and the aponeuroses of the transversus abdominis and internal oblique muscles. The posterior and middle layers join laterally to form the *lateral raphe*, a dense union of fascia.[22]

Because the abdominal muscles insert into its lateral aspect, tension can be generated within the thoracolumbar fascia to help stabilize the lumbar spine during abdominal muscle contraction.[22-25] Hukins et al[26] discuss how the posterior and middle layers of the fascia restrict radial expansion or bulging of the erector spinae during active contraction. This was found to increase the axial tension within the muscle by almost 30%, which in turn increased the muscle's extensor moment proportionally.

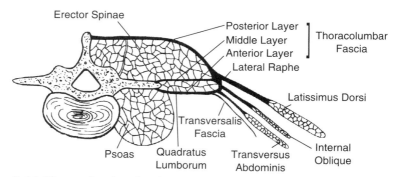

Figure 1–18 Thoracolumbar fascia, cross section. Note lateral placement of quadratus lumborum muscle.

After detailing the anatomy of the thoracolumbar fascia, Bogduk and Twomey explain how it can exert an "antiflexion" effect on the lumbar spine.[27] Approximately 57% of the force applied to the lateral raphe via abdominal muscle and latissimus muscle activity is transferred to the lumbar spinous processes through the thoracolumbar fascia.[28] Owing to its fiber arrangement, the thoracolumbar fascia transfers this force so as to approximate the spinous processes and therefore resist lumbar flexion.[29] This phenomenon has been termed the *gain* of the thoracolumbar fascia[24] and is one of three ways the thoracolumbar fascia can stabilize the lumbar spine in flexion. The second way is by attaching the L-4 and L-5 spinous process to the ilium by fibers of the deep lamina of the posterior layer. These attachments are tensed in flexion and assist the interspinous and iliolumbar ligaments. Gracovetsky et al[23] have termed the third function of the thoracolumbar fascia the *hydraulic amplifier mechanism*. As previously mentioned with regard to the research of Hukins et al, it involves the posterior layer's restriction of the radial bulging of the contracting erector spinae because of its retinacular function. This, in turn, increases the extensor moment of the erector spinae muscle group.

The importance of the above information comes to light when we consider the function of the trunk muscles and ligaments during lifting mechanics, which are covered in the next chapter.

Questions for Thought

- What is the relationship between the abdominal muscles, the latissimus dorsi, and the thoracolumbar fascia?
- How can this information be used in a low back rehabilitation exercise program?

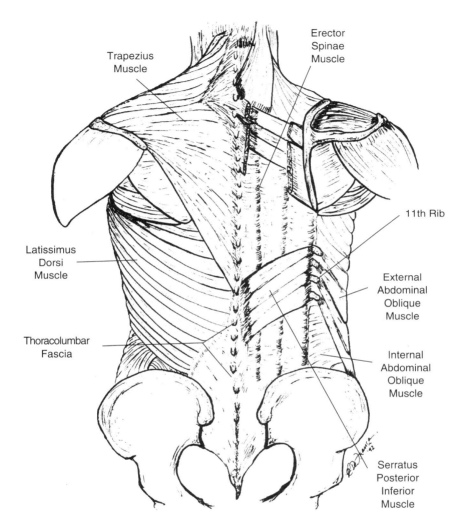

Figure 1–19 Posterior Trunk Muscles

Erector Spinae

In the past, it has been customary to think of the back muscles as one large mass arising from the sacrum and ilium from a common aponeurotic origin and traveling cephalad to various attachments on the spine and ribs. However, recent studies involving the anatomy and innervation of the lower back muscles have helped elucidate the arrangement of these muscles.[29–32] These new findings make it reasonable to view the origin and insertion of the erector spinae in a manner opposite to what conventional thinking has posited.

The lumbar erector spinae consists of the *iliocostalis lumborum* and the *longissimus thoracis* and forms the muscular, bulging prominence in the low back. Each of these muscles is subdivided into a lumbar and thoracic part, depending on their cephalad origin. The lumbar part of each muscle is made up of fascicles emanating from the lumbar vertebrae. The thoracic part arises from thoracic vertebrae or ribs.[29,32] The finding that the erector spinae muscle consists of separate lumbar and thoracic fibers[29,32] represents a major breakthrough in the anatomical and biomechanical understanding of this region. The iliocostalis lumborum is innervated by the lateral branches of the lumbar dorsal rami. The longissimus derives its innervation from the intermediate branches of the lumbar dorsal rami.

Lumbar Part of the Longissimus

The lumbar longissimus consists of five slips of muscle originating from the medial aspect of the lumbar transverse processes (Figure 1–20). These lumbar fascicles insert into the ilium near the posterior superior iliac spine. The longissimus functions mainly to impart posterior sagittal rotation during bilateral contraction. Contracting unilaterally, it serves to flex laterally the lumbar spine to the same side. Owing to its attachments, it is at a mechanical disadvantage to provide axial rotation, and its extensor action is not as strong as that of the multifidus.

Lumbar Part of the Iliocostalis

In contrast to the longissimus, which attaches at the medial aspect of the transverse, the lumbar iliocostalis originates from the tip of the lumbar transverse processes (Figure 1–21). Thus, its fascicles are arranged similarly to those of the longissimus, except that they are more laterally placed. The fascicles insert into the iliac crest just lateral to the posterior superior iliac spine. Unilateral contraction will cause lateral flexion of the lumbar spine, with the transverse processes providing a good mechanical advantage. Because of their attachment to the tips of the transverse processes, the fascicles are at an advantage to produce axial rotation, but the amount they produce is overshadowed by the indirect action of the oblique abdominal muscles rotating the trunk via the thorax. Contracting bilaterally, the lumbar iliocostalis fascicles exert a posterior sagittal rotation through the lumbar vertebrae, along with a posterior translatory force, especially at lower levels, due to the more horizontal inclination of their fibers.

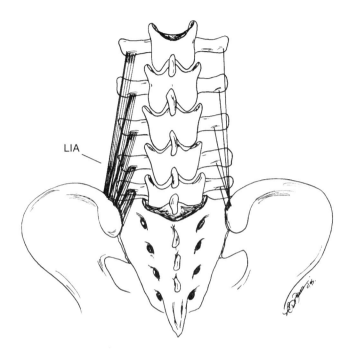

Figure 1–20 Longissimus muscle, lumbar part. On the left, the five muscular fascicles are drawn. The lumbar intermuscular aponeurosis (LIA), formed by the lumbar fascicles of the longissimus, is shown. On the right, the attachments and span of the fascicles are shown. *Source:* Adapted from *Clinical Anatomy of the Lumbar Spine* by N. Bogduk and L.T. Twomey, p. 79, with permission of Churchill Livingstone, © 1987.

Thoracic Part of the Longissimus

The thoracic part of the longissimus originates from the transverse processes and ribs from T-1 to T-12 and inserts onto the spinous processes of L-3 through S-3 and along the sacrum on a line ending just medial to the posterior superior iliac spine (Figure 1–22). The long ribbonlike tendons form the bulk of the *erector spinae aponeurosis* and cover, but are not attached to, the lumbar fibers of the longissimus and iliocostalis. Contracting bilaterally, they increase the lumbar lordosis acting through the erector spinae aponeurosis. Unilateral contraction can cause ipsilateral lateral flexion.

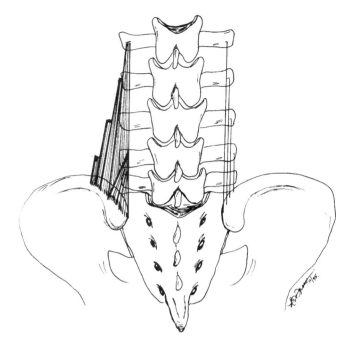

Figure 1–21 Iliocostalis muscle, lumbar part. On the left, the four fascicles of the lumbar part of the iliocostalis are shown. Their span and attachments are depicted on the right. *Source:* Adapted from *Clinical Anatomy of the Lumbar Spine* by N. Bogduk and L.T. Twomey, p. 81, with permission of Churchill Livingstone, © 1987.

Thoracic Part of the Iliocostalis

The thoracic part of the iliocostalis arises from the lower seven or eight ribs and inserts into the sacrum and ilium (Figure 1–23). Its tendons are also long and ribbonlike and add to the lateral aspect of the erector spinae aponeurosis. By spanning the lumbar spine, they create a "bowstring" effect and with bilateral contraction can increase the lordosis.[27] Unilaterally contracting, they cause lateral flexion of the lumbar spine by acting through the thorax. They also function to derotate the trunk when it is rotated contralaterally.

The *erector spinae aponeurosis* consists mostly of fibers from the thoracic part of both the longissimus and iliocostalis muscles. Contrary to earlier concepts, the lumbar part of each of these muscles remains separate from the aponeurosis[29,32] and can function independently from it.

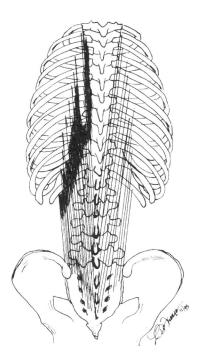

Figure 1–22 Longissimus muscle, thoracic part. On the left are shown the intact fibers of the muscle. The darkened areas represent the short muscle bellies of each fascicle. Note the short rostral and long caudal tendons, the latter of which form the erector spinae aponeurosis (ESA). On the right is shown the span of individual fascicles. *Source:* Adapted from *Clinical Anatomy of the Lumbar Spine* by N. Bogduk and L.T. Twomey, p. 83, with permission of Churchill Livingstone, © 1987.

Multifidus

The *multifidus* is a deep, large lower back muscle featuring segmentally arranged fascicles originating from each lumbar spinous process and attaching to the mammillary processes, sacrum, and iliac crest below (Figure 1–24). In the past, the muscle was viewed in the reverse, with the muscle running from below upward and inserting onto the spinous processes. Recent studies of the anatomy and innervation patterns of this muscle contend that the multifidus arises as separate bundles from each lumbar

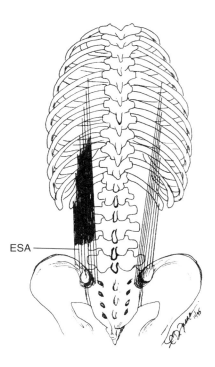

ESA

Figure 1–23 Iliocostalis muscle, thoracic part. The left depicts the intact fascicles, and the right shows their span. The caudal tendons of the fascicles collectively form the erector spinae aponeurosis (ESA). *Source:* Adapted from *Clinical Anatomy of the Lumbar Spine* by N. Bogduk and L.T. Twomey, p. 83, with permission of Churchill Livingstone, © 1987.

spinous process and radiates downward in a segmental fashion to insert on lumbar mammillary processes and the pelvis. All the fascicles arising from a given spinous process are innervated by the medial branch of the dorsal primary ramus that exits below that vertebra.[30,33]

The multifidus consists of small, short laminar fibers and larger, longer spinous fascicles. The laminar fascicles run caudally and span two lumbar levels to the mammillary process. They originate from the dorsal caudal aspect of the lamina. The L-5 fascicle inserts onto the sacrum just above the first dorsal sacral foramen. The larger fascicles arising from the spinous processes insert as five overlapping layers spanning three, four, and sometimes five segments below. The fascicles from the L-2 through L-5 spinous

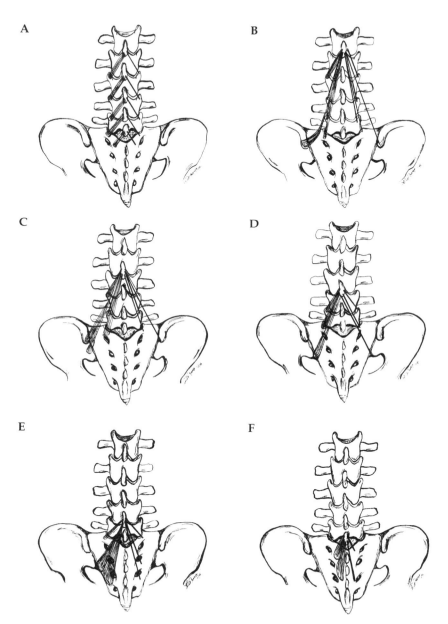

Figure 1–24 Fascicles of the multifidus muscle. **(A)** Laminar fibers. **(B)** to **(F)** Fascicles from L-1 to L-5. *Source:* Adapted from *Clinical Anatomy of the Lumbar Spine* by N. Bogduk and L.T. Twomey, p. 76, with permission of Churchill Livingstone, © 1987.

processes insert onto the sacrum, posterior superior iliac spine, and part of iliac crest.[34]

The spinous process attachment of the multifidus acts as a strong lever to impart posterior sagittal rotation, ie, extension, at each lumbar segment. The motion imparted at each segment is actually the rocking component of extension.[32] The attachments of the multifidus do not afford good mechanical advantage to impart any considerable torque in axial rotation. However, it is thought that they function to stabilize or dampen any opposing flexion caused by the abdominal muscles during trunk rotation.[35]

Quadratus Lumborum

As its name implies, the *quadratus lumborum* is a quadrangular-shaped muscle in the lumbar region. It is very important, complex, and an often-forgotten structure in the lower back, especially with regard to low back pain syndromes. In referencing Eisler, Travell and Simons[36] review the anatomy of the quadratus lumborum muscle. The quadratus lumborum consists of three layers attaching to the middle third of the iliac crest and iliolumbar ligament, the upper four lumbar transverse process tips, and the 12th rib (Figure 1–25). Thus, the fibers are oriented in three directions going from (1) the iliac crest to the 12th rib (iliocostal fibers), (2) the iliac crest to the lumbar vertebrae (iliolumbar), and (3) the lumbar vertebrae to the 12th rib (lumbocostal). The iliocostal fibers are the most posterior layer and run vertically and slightly medially as they course upward to insert on the 12th rib. The diagonally running iliolumbar fibers form the middle layer and cross with the most ventral layer, the diagonally running lumbocostal fibers. Travell and Simons[36] comment that the quadratus lumborum, owing to its layered structure and orientation of its fibers into three groups, should be thought of as three muscles when one is stretching it. The muscle appears thicker nearer its costal attachment and presents a smooth lateral border. The medial border appears serrated due to the interdigitations of the diagonal fibers attaching to the transverse processes. Being sheetlike, it lies in the frontal plane just lateral to the lumbar spine and forms part of the posterior abdominal wall. The quadratus lumborum derives its innervation from the 12th thoracic and upper three or four lumbar ventral rami.

The quadratus lumborum functions primarily as a lateral flexor of the lumbar spine by either initiating bending to the ipsilateral side or controlling it to the contralateral side by eccentric (lengthening) contraction. Acting bilaterally, the quadratus lumborum muscles extend the lumbar spine.[37,38] In discussing lower motor neuron lesions, Knapp[39] states that paralysis of both quadratus lumborum muscles makes walking impos-

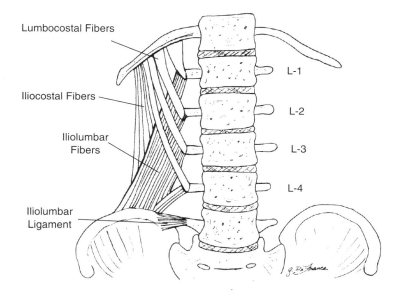

Lumbocostal Fibers

Iliocostal Fibers

Iliolumbar Fibers

Iliolumbar Ligament

L-1

L-2

L-3

L-4

Figure 1–25 Quadratus Lumborum Muscle

sible, even with braces. This indicates the important role the quadratus lumborum plays in stabilizing the lumbar spine while a person is upright. With the spine fixed in place, unilateral contraction raises the ipsilateral hip (hip hiking). The quadratus lumborum also assists respiration by stabilizing the 12th rib and its diaphragmatic attachment and is active in forced exhalation and coughing.[40,41] The quadratus lumborum is under active tension during sitting, lying, and walking positions.[42] During gait, the quadratus lumborum shows increased EMG activity just before and during ipsilateral and contralateral heel strike.[43]

Hip and Gluteal Region

The gluteal region is marked by the prominent rounded contour of the large *gluteus maximus* that characterizes the muscular development associated with mankind's upright posture (Figure 1–26). Having the largest cross-sectional area, the gluteus maximus is the strongest and most powerful muscle in the body.[44] It originates from the posterior aspect of the iliac crest near the posterior superior iliac spine, the erector spinae aponeurosis, the dorsal surface of the lower sacrum, the lateral aspect of the coccyx, and the sacrotuberous ligament. The larger upper fibers of the muscle descend obliquely and laterally to insert into the iliotibial tract with the tensor fascia lata muscle. The lower fibers insert onto the gluteal tuberosity of the proximal femur.

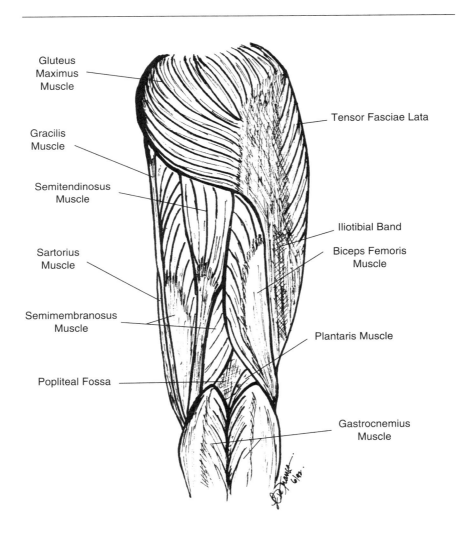

Figure 1–26 Posterior Hip and Thigh Muscles

The gluteus maximus functions to extend and laterally rotate the hip joint. Its upper fibers assist in hip abduction, and its lower fibers assist adduction.[45] The gluteus maximus is minimally active during normal walking. However, its action is essential during running, jumping, walking up a grade, and recovering from a deep squatting position. It aids in stabilizing the pelvis in the sagittal plane. The gluteus maximus plays an integral role in initiating trunk raising from the stooped position. Through its insertion into the iliotibial tract, it lends dynamic lateral knee stability. It is innervated by the inferior gluteal nerve.

The *gluteus medius* is the main abductor of the hip and is very efficient as such due to its size and highly advantageous lever arm (Figure 1–27). It originates from the lateral aspect of the iliac crest, with its anterior two thirds uncovered by the gluteus maximus. It inserts into the lateral aspect of the greater trochanter. It mainly abducts the hip joint. However, its anterior fibers assist in flexion and medial rotation of the hip joint, and its posterior fibers assist extension and lateral hip rotation.[45] This muscle is very important in stabilizing the pelvis in the coronal plane, exemplified by the maintenance of a level pelvis during a one-legged stance.

The *gluteus minimus* is the little sister of the gluteal family, having a force equivalent to one third that of the gluteus medius. It lies deep to the gluteus medius, originating from the lateral aspect of the iliac crest, and inserts onto the anterior surface of the greater trochanter (Figure 1–27). It essentially is a hip abductor but also functions to flex and medially rotate the hip joint. Both the gluteus medius and the gluteus minimus are innervated by the superior gluteal nerve.

The *tensor fascia lata* is the long-lost member of the gluteal family, having migrated anteriorly on the pelvis and taken with it its shared innervation with the gluteus medius and gluteus minimus, the superior gluteal nerve (Figures 1–26 through 1–28). It is about one half as powerful as the gluteus medius, yet its lever arm is longer, making it a strong hip abductor.[44] It originates from the anterior aspect of the iliac crest's lateral lip and the lateral aspect of the anterior superior iliac spine. It inserts into the anterior aspect of the iliotibial band at the junction of the middle and proximal thirds of the thigh. In addition to hip abduction, it acts to flex and medially rotate the hip joint. It extends the knee and laterally rotates the lower leg via the iliotibial band.

The *iliotibial band* is a thickened, tough part of the dense lateral thigh fascia, the fascia lata (Figure 1–28). The tensor fascia lata and the gluteus maximus insert into its proximal aspect to form the deltoid of the hip.[44] The iliotibial band inserts into the lateral aspect of the lateral tibial condyle on the tubercle of Gerdy. Owing to its lateral insertion below the knee

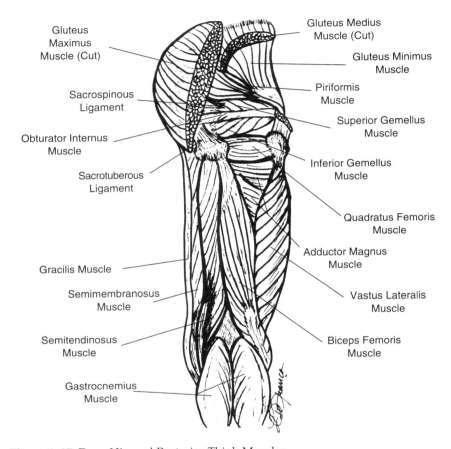

Gluteus
Maximus
Muscle (Cut)

Sacrospinous
Ligament

Obturator Internus
Muscle

Sacrotuberous
Ligament

Gracilis Muscle

Semimembranosus
Muscle

Semitendinosus
Muscle

Gastrocnemius
Muscle

Gluteus Medius
Muscle (Cut)

Gluteus Minimus
Muscle

Piriformis
Muscle

Superior Gemellus
Muscle

Inferior Gemellus
Muscle

Quadratus Femoris
Muscle

Adductor Magnus
Muscle

Vastus Lateralis
Muscle

Biceps Femoris
Muscle

Figure 1–27 Deep Hip and Posterior Thigh Muscles

joint, the iliotibial band affords dynamic lateral stability, assisting the lateral collateral ligament of the knee.

Lateral Rotators of the Hip

Muscles causing lateral rotation of the hip are numerous and powerful (Figure 1–27). The most important of these is the *piriformis* muscle. It originates from the underside of the sacrum and runs laterally through the greater sciatic foramen to insert into the upper aspect of the greater trochanter. In the normal physiologic position of stance, the piriformis produces lateral rotation, flexion, and abduction.[44] However, inversion of

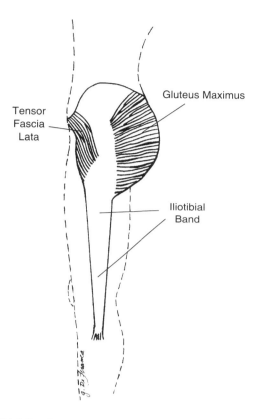

Tensor
Fascia
Lata

Gluteus Maximus

Iliotibial
Band

Figure 1–28 Iliotibial Band

function occurs when the femur is flexed past 60 degrees: the piriformis then causes medial rotation, extension, and abduction.[44] At 60 degrees, it mostly abducts. It is innervated by the ventral rami of L-5, S-1, and S-2.

The quadratus femoris, obturator internus and externus, and gemelli superior and inferior are small muscles that function to rotate the hip joint laterally. The *quadratus femoris* arises from the lateral aspect of the ischial tuberosity and inserts into the intertrochanteric area of the femur. In addition to laterally rotating the hip joint, the quadratus femoris can adduct it. It is innervated by the nerve to the quadratus femoris.

The *obturator internus* originates within the pelvis from the margin of the obturator foramen and obturator membrane. It exits the pelvis via the lesser sciatic notch, makes a sharp bend below the ischial spine, and passes posterior to the hip joint to insert into the medial surface of the greater trochanter. The obturator internus tendon is joined by the small *gemelli superior* and *inferior* muscles as they originate from near the ischial spine and proximal part of the ischial tuberosity respectively. The obturator internus and superior gemellus are innervated by the nerve to the obturator internus. The inferior gemellus is innervated by the nerve to the quadratus femoris. In addition to laterally rotating the hip, the obturator internus and gemelli abduct the flexed thigh.

The *obturator externus* arises from the external surface of the obturator membrane and the bony margin of the obturator foramen. It travels backward and upward to wind around the back of the hip joint and pass behind the femoral neck to finally insert into the trochanteric fossa. Because of its winding course, the obturator externus can still laterally rotate the hip joint while the femur is flexed, as during sitting. It is innervated by the posterior branch of the obturator nerve.

These small rotator muscles appear to be analogous to the rotator cuff muscles of the shoulder by also functioning to stabilize the hip joint posteriorly. Thus, their strength and function should be addressed during the treatment of painful hip syndromes.

Hip Adductors

The hip adductors are considerable in number and are powerful (Figures 1–29 and 1–30). They help stabilize the pelvis in the lateral direction, working in conjunction with the hip abductors. The largest and most powerful of the adductors proper is the *adductor magnus*. It originates from the inferior pubic ramus medially and the ischial ramus and inferolateral aspect of the ischial tuberosity laterally. The most medial fibers run horizontally a short distance to insert on the upper femur medial to the gluteus maximus attachment at the gluteal tuberosity. The ischial ramus fibers run inferolaterally to insert along the linea aspera and medial supracondylar line of the femur. Most of the fibers from the ischial tuberosity run straight inferior, forming a separate muscle belly that inserts on the adductor tubercle. This part of the muscle is sometimes called the "third adductor." The adductor magnus acts to adduct the hip and powerfully extend it as well.[46] In a personal communication, Travell commented on how the adductor magnus acts as a hamstring muscle due to its peculiar attachments. The adductor magnus is innervated by the obturator nerve and the tibial division of the sciatic nerve.

The *adductor longus* originates from the front of the pubic bone and descends to insert on the linea aspera in the middle third of the femur. The *adductor brevis* arises from the outer surface of the inferior ramus of the

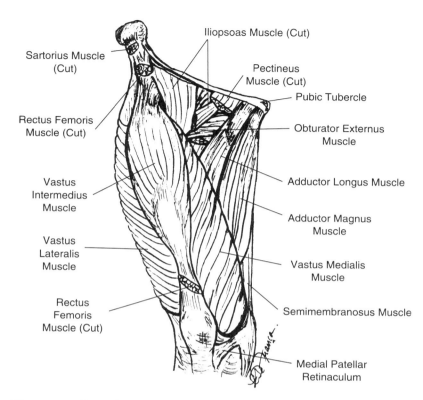

Sartorius Muscle (Cut)

Iliopsoas Muscle (Cut)

Pectineus Muscle (Cut)

Pubic Tubercle

Rectus Femoris Muscle (Cut)

Obturator Externus Muscle

Vastus Intermedius Muscle

Adductor Longus Muscle

Adductor Magnus Muscle

Vastus Lateralis Muscle

Vastus Medialis Muscle

Rectus Femoris Muscle (Cut)

Semimembranosus Muscle

Medial Patellar Retinaculum

Figure 1–29 Deep Anterior Thigh Muscles

pubis and passes downward and backward to insert on the proximal femur between the lesser trochanter and linea aspera. The above two muscles adduct and flex the hip joint and are innervated by the obturator nerve.

The *pectineus* is an often-overlooked adductor muscle. It arises from the superior ramus of the pubis and the bone near the pubic tubercle and courses downward, backward, and laterally to insert on the proximal femur, covering the adductor brevis. It functions to adduct and flex the thigh and is innervated by the femoral nerve and accessory obturator nerve.

The *gracilis* muscle is a long, superficial adductor of the hip originating from the inferior ramus of the pubis and inferior half of the symphysis pubis. It runs inferiorly to insert on the proximal aspect of the medial tibia

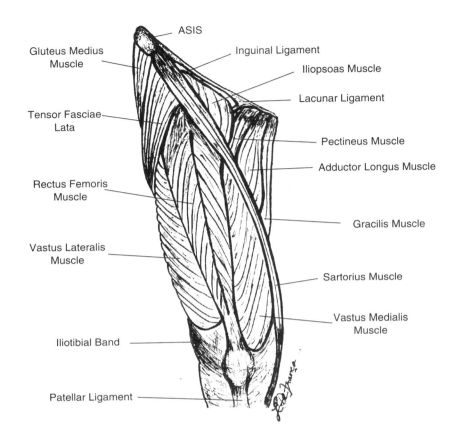

Figure 1–30 Anterior Thigh Muscles

just below the condyle. In addition to adducting the thigh, it flexes and medially rotates the lower leg at the knee joint. It is innervated by the obturator nerve.

Hamstrings

The hamstring muscle group consists of the biceps femoris, semimembranosus, and semitendinosus (Figures 1–26 and 1–27). The *biceps femoris* forms the lateral hamstring and consists of a long and a short head. The long head originates from the ischial tuberosity and distal part of the sacrotuberous ligament. As it runs inferiorly, it receives the short head, which originates from the midfemoral shaft. They both form a common tendon that inserts into the fibular head and lateral collateral ligament. The long head receives its innervation from the tibial part of the sciatic nerve, and the short head is innervated by the common peroneal portion.

The semimembranosus and semitendinosus form the medial hamstring group. The *semimembranosus* takes origin from the ischial tuberosity and runs inferiorly to insert on the posteromedial aspect of the medial tibial condyle, giving off attachments that insert into the medial meniscus. The *semitendinosus* shares a common origin with the biceps femoris long head. It travels inferiorly to insert into the posteromedial aspect of the proximal tibia with the gracilis and sartorius in what is called the *pes anserine tendon*. Both muscles derive their innervation from the tibial portion of the sciatic nerve.

Except for the short head of the biceps, the hamstring muscles are biarticular; therefore, their action at the hip is dependent upon the position of the knee. The hamstrings flex the knee; additionally, the medial and lateral groups impart medial and lateral tibial rotation respectively. As a group, the hamstrings extend the hip joint. This action is much more efficient with the knee extended. The biceps femoris assists lateral hip rotation with the knee extended, and the semitendinosus and semimembranosus assist medial hip rotation. Through their pull on the pelvis, the hamstrings are also important in raising the trunk from a bent-forward position while the knees are extended.

Anterior Thigh

The two muscles originating from the anterior aspect of the pelvis that we need to consider are the sartorius and rectus femoris (Figure 1–30). The *sartorius* takes origin from the anterior superior iliac spine. It then wraps around the inside of the thigh and knee to insert into the pes anserine tendon at the medial aspect of the proximal tibia. It acts to flex, laterally rotate, and abduct the hip joint. It also flexes and medially rotates the lower leg at the knee. It is innervated by the femoral nerve.

The *rectus femoris* is part of the quadriceps muscle group, and the fact that it acts at both knee and hip joints makes it significant. Its straight head originates from the anterior inferior iliac spine, and its reflected head arises from just above the acetabulum. It inserts into the superior aspect of the patella. It acts to flex the hip and extend the knee. Its action at the knee, like that of the hamstrings, is dependent upon the position of the hip joint. For example, optimal stretching of the rectus femoris can only be accomplished with the hip in neutral or extension. This muscle is innervated by the femoral nerve.

Pelvic Floor Muscles

The levator ani and coccygeus are two muscles that form the pelvic diaphragm and, as such, are located in the floor of the pelvis. Their importance lies in the fact that spasm of these muscles due to injury is clinically related to a tender coccyx and the perpetuation of the pain of coccydynia.[47]

The *levator ani* is a complex muscle due to its attachments and variously named parts, the *pubococcygeus*, *puborectalis*, and *iliococcygeus* (Figure 1–31). Generally, the levator ani extends between the pubis anteriorly and the coccyx posteriorly and between the two lateral pelvic walls. It is penetrated by the urethra, anal canal, and female vagina. It inserts into the structures that pierce it, the midline, and the coccyx. It forms the majority of the pelvic diaphragm and acts to support the pelvic viscera, especially the female uterus, and to add voluntary control to continence. It is innervated by the fourth sacral and inferior rectal nerves.

The *coccygeus* is a small muscle forming about one fourth of the pelvic diaphragm. It originates from the ischial spine and fans out to insert into the distal two segments and proximal two segments of the sacrum and coccyx respectively. It functions with the levator ani to afford support to the pelvic viscera. Due to its coccygeal attachment, it may pull the coccyx forward after defecation and parturition. It derives its innervation from the fourth and fifth sacral nerves. As an aside, in animals the iliococcygeus muscle is responsible for tail wagging, and the coccygeus muscle serves to pull the tail down and between the back legs.

The perineal body, a dense nodule of fibrous muscular tissue, is between the anus and urethra in men and the anus and vagina in women. It is sometimes called the central tendon of the perineum; however, it is not tendinous. Several muscles, including the levator ani, meet and interlace here, affording more structural support to the pelvic floor. Between the anus and coccyx is a similar structure called the anococcygeal ligament, which is actually made up of fibromuscular tissue.

ARTICULAR INNERVATION

As the lumbar nerve roots exit the spine, they immediately divide into dorsal and ventral primary rami. The dorsal rami arch dorsally to innervate essentially the structures posterior to the transverse process. This includes the dorsal segmental lumbar muscles, the facet joints, and their ligaments. The ventral primary rami enter the lumbar plexus and supply motor, sensory, and reflex innervation to the lower extremity and structures essentially anterior to the transverse process. Therefore, clinical

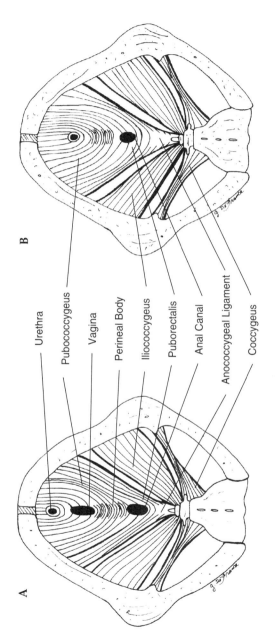

Figure 1–31 Muscles of the pelvic floor, superior aspect. **(A)** Female. **(B)** Male.

Urethra

Pubococcygeus

Vagina

Perineal Body

Iliococcygeus

Puborectalis

Anal Canal

Anococcygeal Ligament

Coccygeus

physical examination tests that assess lower extremity nerve tension signs, muscle strength, and reflex and sensory parameters are actually assessing the ventral primary ramus.

The posterior aspect of the sacroiliac joint is innervated by lateral branches of the L–5 through S-2 posterior primary rami. They form a plexus between the posterior sacroiliac ligament and the interosseous ligament. Anteriorly, the joint is supplied by the L-3 through S-2 nerves.[1,16] Like the temporomandibular joint, the sacroiliac joint is richly supplied with proprioceptors.[48]

The hip joint is innervated by several nerves representing the L-2 through S-1 segments. Branches from the obturator, superior gluteal, and femoral nerves supply the joint. A branch from the nerve to the quadratus femoris also supplies the hip joint.

The pubic symphysis receives articular branches from the obturator nerve, and the sacrococcygeal joint receives its innervation from the lower sacral and coccygeal nerves.

TOPOGRAPHICAL ANATOMY FOR PALPATION

Topographically, the lower back encompasses a vast amount of anatomical territory. We are concerned primarily with the three-joint complex of the pelvis, consisting of the posteriorly paired sacroiliac joints (SIJ) and the anteriorly situated midline pubic symphysis.

Posterior Aspect

On level with the height of the iliac crests is the L4-5 interspinous space (Figure 1–32). The bony PSISs are palpated just deep to the dimples on either side of the lower back. Their size and shape can vary, and detection by palpation can be difficult, especially if a large layer of adipose tissue covers them. The PSISs roughly mark the upper aspect of the SIJ. Situated midway between them is the small S-2 tubercle. The L-5 spinous process is palpated as a small bump between the L-4 spinous process and the S-2 tubercle. Just medial to each PSIS is the area that overlies the SIJ, covered by the thick interosseous sacroiliac ligaments (Figure 1–33). At this level, the joint is about 3 cm deep and is inaccessible to direct palpation. However, SIJ movement can be detected by monitoring the movements that occur between the PSIS and S-2 tubercle.

The iliolumbar ligaments lie extremely deep and are difficult to palpate unless they become painful. The fibers arising from the L-4 and L-5 transverse processes are accessible at their origin and iliac crest insertion.[49]

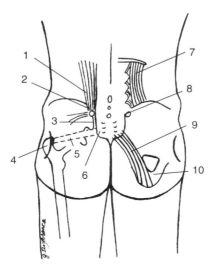

Figure 1–32 Palpation landmarks, posterior aspect. **(1)** Sacrospinalis tendon insertion, **(2)** small origin of gluteus medius muscle, **(3)** posterior inferior iliac spine, **(4)** greater trochanter, **(5)** piriformis muscle, **(6)** inferior lateral angle of the sacrum, **(7)** quadratus lumborum muscle, **(8)** posterior superior iliac spine, **(9)** sacrotuberous ligament, and **(10)** ischial tuberosity.

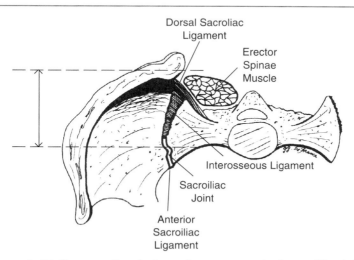

Figure 1–33 Cross-sectional view of upper aspect of sacroiliac joint. Double-headed arrow indicates depth of sacroiliac joint's articular portion. Note interosseous ligament.

Directly cephalad of the PSIS can be felt the tendons of the erector spinae muscle group as they insert into the pelvis. Just lateral to the PSIS is the small origin of the gluteus medius muscle. Approximately 5 to 6 cm inferior and slightly lateral to the PSIS is the posterior inferior iliac spine (PIIS). Just medial to this is the lower aspect of the SIJ, which is the only place where the SIJ can be directly palpated. Inferior and medial to the lower part of the SIJ can be palpated the bony, nonarticular inferior lateral angle of the sacrum. The sacral cornua and interposed sacral hiatus can be felt in the midline on the most inferior part of the sacrum. The ischial tuberosity is easily found at the level of the gluteal fold in the mass of the buttocks. An important structure to identify and palpate is the sacrotuberous ligament. It can be found by following its course between the ischial tuberosity and sacrum. It feels similar to a firm, taut cord. Often, with pelvic joint dysfunction, the sacrotuberous ligament palpates as unduly tense and tender.

The piriformis muscle is best palpated with the patient prone, the knee flexed to 90 degrees, and the thigh internally rotated by pulling the bent leg laterally. This places a stretch on the piriformis. The muscle lies on line with the superior tip of the greater trochanter and the sacrum. It can be palpated at the intersection of two lines: one connecting the PSIS and the greater trochanter, and the other connecting the anterior superior iliac spine (ASIS) and lower pole to the coccyx.[49] It lies deep to the gluteus maximus and may be difficult to feel. However, piriformis spasm is identified as a taut, tender band of muscle in the sciatic notch.

The coccyx is palpated within the confines of the upper aspect of the gluteal cleft. The most effective way to palpate the coccyx is through the rectum. With the patient in the lateral decubitus position, a lubricated, gloved index finger is slowly inserted into the rectum after the external and internal anal sphincters have relaxed. The coccyx can then be palpated between the index finger internally and the thumb externally. However, much information can be obtained via external palpation. For hygienic reasons, a gloved finger should still be used to palpate the coccyx deep in the gluteal cleft. Gentle pressure and patient relaxation combine to allow an effective examination. Surprisingly, most of the coccyx can be felt through the soft tissues of the region.

Lateral Aspect

With the patient in a side-lying position, palpation of the laterally placed structures can be performed. The greater trochanter palpates as a bony mass in the anterior part of the hollow area visible on the lateral aspect of the hip region. The sciatic nerve is palpated midway between the greater trochanter and the ischial tuberosity, with the hip flexed. The bulge of muscle just above and posterior to the greater trochanter consists of the gluteus medius and gluteus minimus. By following a line of palpation from the greater trochanter to the iliac crest, one can locate these muscles. The gluteus minimus lies deep. The origin of the gluteus medius that is just inferior to the crest of the ilium is easily appreciated. The tensor fascia lata is seen as a bulge of muscle just inferior and lateral to the ASIS. The iliotibial tract is a thick band of connective tissue forming a longitudinally running crease in the lateral aspect of the thigh. This is best seen if the patient is supine and asked to raise the straight leg off the table just a few inches.

Anterior Aspect

The ASIS is the prominent bony point that is easily palpated from the front (Figure 1–34). The examiner's thumbs are allowed to contact the ASISs while the hands encircle the iliac crests. The inguinal ligament can be followed by the thumbs medially to the pubic tubercles, small bumps of bone palpable through the mons pubis. The midline symphysis pubis is palpated as a definite sulcus. With the patient supine and the thigh ab-

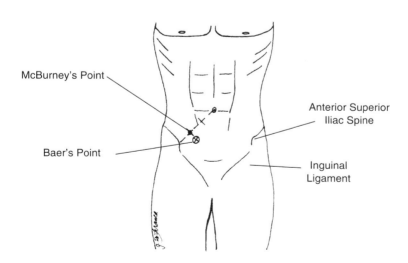

Figure 1–34 Palpation Landmarks, Anterior Aspect

ducted as in the Patrick-Fabere test position, a prominent cord of tendon can be felt extending from the pubic symphysis toward the middle of the thigh. This represents the adductor longus muscle. Medial to and just below the ASIS, the iliacus muscle can be palpated by pressing the fingers inward and laterally.

The psoas muscle can be palpated carefully with the patient in the supine position (Figure 1–35). The palmar aspects of the fingertips contact the skin just lateral to the rectus abdominis muscle at the level of the ASIS and are pressed carefully but firmly in a deep and medial direction. The patient is then asked just barely to raise the straight leg off the table, thus contracting the psoas and allowing its muscle belly to rise up to the examiner's fingers. It should feel mildly taut and painless.

The joining of the middle and lateral thirds of a line connecting the ASIS and the umbilicus marks McBurney's point. Just below this is Baer's sacroiliac point (Figure 1–34). Patients with sacroiliac joint problems often display tenderness here upon palpation, occasionally causing them to complain of abdominal wall soreness in their history. Bourdillion mentions this point as being tender in SIJ infections and strains.[50] The sacral promontory can be palpated in slender people just inferior and deep to the umbilicus by using gentle but increasing pressure until the hard, bony landmark is felt.

CONGENITAL ANOMALIES AND VARIANTS

The transitional areas of the spine are "ontogenetically restless"[51] and therefore are areas where congenital anomalies commonly manifest. The lumbosacral and pelvic areas constitute fertile ground for such occurrences. Likewise, these areas are common sites of painful functional disturbances. Since manual methods entail tests of movement and meticulous palpation of anatomic structures, the influence of anomalous anatomy in clinical assessment needs to be regarded.

The sacrum can appear with a number of different variations. Solonen observed variable widths of the sacrum's lateral aspect in 30 specimens.[16] Only 5 cases (16%) were symmetrical. The left side was wider in 19 cases. Schmorl and Junghanns write of variations in sacral ala height.[51] A lumbarized first sacral segment and sacralized fifth lumbar segment are common occurrences. The L-5 segment can be transitional and can form an adventitious or accessory joint with the sacrum either unilaterally or bilaterally. A large, spatulated transverse process of L-5 can articulate with the ilium through a pseudoarthrosis or fuse with it. In some cases, these accessory articulations may need manual methods directed at them.

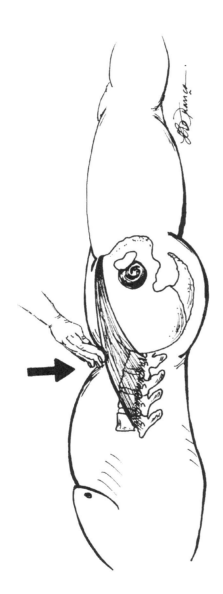

Figure 1–35 Psoas Muscle Palpation

The sacroiliac joint is associated with accessory joint formations in approximately 30% of cases.[52] Trotter[53] noted a higher incidence of accessory joints in whites than blacks. Ehara et al[54] observed accessory sacroiliac joints in 16% of dried specimens and 13% of pelvic CT scans of 100 patients. The sacral articular facets of the accessory joints are located on the posterior surface of the sacrum just lateral to the second sacral foramen. The iliac facets are usually found on the medial aspect of the PSIS. Less frequently, they occur as small bony projections from the iliac tuberosity just medial to the PSIS.[54] It is not definite whether the accessory joints are congenital or acquired. Trotter[52,53] and Seligman[55] report a substantial increase in occurrence of accessory joints with age, indicating they are acquired. Hadley noted arthritic changes in these accessory joints and thus thought they could be a potential source of low back pain.[56] However, as with any other joint, radiographic evidence of osteoarthritis does not correlate well with subjective complaints. Arthritic or not, anomalous joints can be a cause of pain and need to be attended to.

Knife-clasp syndrome can be present where an enlarged L-5 spinous process is associated with spina bifida occulta of the first sacral segment.[57] In Fong's disease, or iliac horns, exostoses are on the posterior aspect of the ilia.[58] In 1850, Hohl first reported sacral agenesis or caudal regression in which the sacrum and sometimes lower lumbar segments were missing.[59] The iliac artery may create an anomalous bony arch called the paraglenoid sulcus, which, if large enough, may confuse palpatory findings.[60] Muecke and Currarino[61] report on congenital widening of the pubic symphysis and its association with genitourinary anomalies. The iliolumbar and sacrotuberous ligaments may calcify unilaterally or bilaterally as isolated variants.

Of what clinical significance are anomalous changes? As far as the body is concerned, the anomalous structure has been part of the normal anatomic inventory since birth. The mere presence of an anomalous structure constitutes shaky evidence on which to blame the patient's presenting symptoms. It is common to observe in clinical practice nearly every type of congenital anomaly known to exist "silently" in asymptomatic individuals, including accessory articulations or pseudoarthroses. Nevertheless, these are potential sites of dysfunction and can be the predominant cause of a patient's low back pain. Commonly observed radiographic evidence of sclerosis in these anomalous joints signifies movement and subsequent wear. Being joints, they are apt to become dysfunctional and painful and need to be examined.

If such is the case, gentle mobilizations directed specifically at the anomalous joint can provide great relief. But standard techniques of mobilization and manipulation of the pelvic joints tend to affect the anomalous joints too. More commonly, however, it is the neighboring joints and tissues, not the anomaly, that create the problem. The anomalous segment can become symptomatic in trying to compensate for dysfunctional neighboring segments. On the other hand, dysfunctional neighboring segments themselves can be causing the pain, but often the anomaly is blamed by mere presence.

Chapter Review Questions

- Name the six categories of articulations found in the pelvic region.
- Describe the differences between the sacral and iliac facets of the sacroiliac joint.
- How is a child's SIJ different from an adult's SIJ?
- Why is the SIJ considered a true diarthrosis?
- What is the significance of the anteversion of both the acetabulum and the femoral head?
- What is the significance of the thoracolumbar fascia? What are the three ways it can stabilize the lumbar spine during flexion?
- Describe Bogduk's elucidation of the lumbar muscular anatomy and how it differed from prior descriptions.
- What important structures can potentially link lumbopelvic and knee function?
- Of what clinical importance are anomalous anatomical variants?

REFERENCES

1. Warwick R, Williams P. *Gray's Anatomy.* Philadelphia, Pa: WB Saunders; 1973.
2. Heylings DJA. Supraspinous and interspinous ligaments of the human lumbar spine. *J Anat.* 1978;125:127.
3. Shellshear JL, Macintosh NWG. The transverse process of the fifth lumbar vertebra. In: Shellshear JL, Macintosh NWG, eds. *Surveys of Anatomical Fields.* Sydney, Australia: Grahame; 1949:21–32.
4. Kapandji IA. *The Physiology of the Joints. Vol 3. The Trunk and the Vertebral Column.* New York, NY: Churchill Livingstone; 1974.
5. Luk KDK, Ho HC, Leong JCY. The iliolumbar ligament. *J Bone Joint Surg.* 1986;68B:197–200.
6. Bowen V, Cassidy JD. Macroscopic and microscopic anatomy of the sacroiliac joint from embryonic life until the eighth decade. *Spine.* 1981;6:620–628.

7. Lynch FW. The pelvic articulations during pregnancy, labour and puerperium: an x-ray study. *Surg Gynecol Obstet.* 1920;30:575.

8. Bellamy N, Park W, Rooney PJ. What do we know about the sacroiliac joint? *Semin Arthritis Rheum.* 1983;12:282–313.

9. Von Luschka H. Die anatomie des Menschen in Rucksicht auf die bedurfnisse der praktischen heilkunde. *N Laupp Tubinger.* 1863;2:89.

10. Albee FH. A study of the anatomy and the clinical importance of the sacroiliac joint. *JAMA.* 1909;53:1273–1276.

11. Brooke R. The sacroiliac joint. *J Anat.* 1924;58:299–305.

12. Sashin D. A critical analysis of the anatomy and the pathological changes of the sacroiliac joint. *J Bone Joint Surg.* 1930;12:891–910.

13. Schunke GB. The anatomy and development of the sacroiliac joint in man. *Anat Rec.* 1938;72:313–331.

14. Illi FW. *The Vertebral Column: Life-Line of the Body.* Lombard, Ill: National College of Chiropractic; 1951.

15. Weisl H. The articular surfaces of the sacroiliac joint and their relation to the movements of the sacrum. *Acta Anat.* 1954;22:1–14.

16. Solonen KA. The sacroiliac joint in light of anatomical, roentgenological and clinical studies. *Acta Orthop Scand.* 1957;27:1–127.

17. Delmas A. Jonction sacro-iliaque et statique du corps. *Rev Rhumatisme.* 1950;9:475–581.

18. Sandoz RW. Structural and functional pathologies of the pelvic ring. *Ann Swiss Chiro Assoc.* 1981;7:101–160.

19. Freeman MD, Fox D, Richards T. The superior intracapsular ligament of the sacroiliac joint: presumptive evidence for confirmation of Illi's ligament. *J Manipulative Physiol Ther.* 1990;13:384–390.

20. Colachis SC, Warden RE, Becthal CO, et al. Movement of the sacroiliac joint in the adult male. *Arch Phys Med Rehabil.* 1963;44:490–498.

21. Vleeming A, Poll-Goudzwaard AL, Stoeckart R, van Wingerden JP, Snijders CJ. The posterior layer of the thoracolumbar fascia: its function in load transfer from spine to legs. *Spine.* 1995;20:753–758.

22. Bogduk N, Macintosh JE. The applied anatomy of the thoracolumbar fascia. *Spine.* 1984;9:164–170.

23. Gracovetsky S, Farfan HF, Lamy C. A mathematical model of the lumbar spine using an optimal system to control muscles and ligaments. *Orthop Clin North Am.* 1977;8:135–153.

24. Gracovetsky S, Farfan HF, Helleur C. The abdominal mechanism. *Spine.* 1985;10:317–324.

25. Gracovetsky S, Farfan HF, Lamy C. The mechanism of the lumbar spine. *Spine.* 1981;6:249–262.

26. Hukins DW, Aspden RM, Hickey DS. Thoracolumbar fascia can increase the efficiency of the erector spinae muscles. *Clin Biomech.* 1990;5:30–34.

27. Bogduk N, Twomey LT. *Clinical Anatomy of the Lumbar Spine.* New York, NY: Churchill Livingstone; 1987.

28. Macintosh JE, Bogduk N. The biomechanics of the thoracolumbar fascia. *Clin Biomech.* 1987;2:78–83.

29. Bogduk N. A reappraisal of the anatomy of the human lumbar erector spinae. *J Anat.* 1980;131:525–540.

30. Bogduk N. The myotomes of the human multifidus. *J Anat.* 1983;136:148–149.
31. Macintosh JE, Bogduk N. The qualitative biomechanics of the lumbar back muscles. *J Anat.* 1985;142:218.
32. Macintosh JE, Bogduk N. The detailed biomechanics of the lumbar multifidus. *Spine.* 1986;1:205–213.
33. Bogduk N, Wilson AS, Tynan W. The human dorsal rami. *J Anat.* 1982;134:383–397.
34. Macintosh JE, Valencia F, Bogduk N, Munro RR. The morphology of the lumbar multifidus muscles. *Clin Biomech.* 1986;1:196–204.
35. Donisch EW, Basmajian JV. Electromyography of deep back muscles in man. *Am J Anat.* 1972;133:25–36.
36. Travell JG, Simons DG. *Myofascial Pain and Dysfunction: The Trigger Point Manual.* Vol 2. Baltimore, Md: Williams & Wilkins; 1992.
37. Kendall FP, McCreary EK. *Muscles: Testing and Function.* 3rd ed. Baltimore, Md: Williams & Wilkins; 1983.
38. Rab GT, Chao EYS, Stauffer RN. Muscle force analysis of the lumbar spine. *Orthop Clin North Am.* 1977;8:193–199.
39. Knapp ME. Exercises for lower motor neuron lesions. In: Basmajian JV, ed. *Therapeutic Exercise.* 3rd ed. Baltimore, Md: Williams & Wilkins; 1978:349–374.
40. Basmajian JV, Deluca CJ. *Muscles Alive.* 5th ed. Baltimore, Md: Williams & Wilkins; 1985.
41. Simons DH. Functions of the quadratus lumborum muscle and relation of its myofascial trigger points to low back pain. In: Pain abstracts, Second World Congress on Pain; August 27 to September 1, 1978; Montreal, Canada. Vol 1:245.
42. Sola AE, Kuitert JH. Quadratus lumborum myofascitis. *Northwest Med.* 1954;53:1003–1005.
43. Waters RL, Morris JM. Electrical activity of muscle of the trunk during walking. *J Anat.* 1972;111:191.
44. Kapandji IA. *The Physiology of the Joints.* Vol 2. New York, NY: Churchill Livingstone; 1974.
45. Kendall HO, Kendall FP, Wadsworth GE. *Muscles: Testing and Function.* 2nd ed. Baltimore, Md: Williams & Wilkins; 1971.
46. Simons DG. Myofascial pain syndrome due to trigger points. In: Int Rehabil Med Assoc Monogr Ser No 1; November 1987:27.
47. Lewit K. *Manipulative Therapy in Rehabilitation of the Locomotor System.* Boston, Mass: Butterworths; 1985.
48. Otter R. A review study of differing opinions expressed in the literature. *Eur J Chiro.* 1985;33:221–242.
49. Dvorak J, Dvorak V. *Manual Medicine: Diagnostics.* New York, NY: Thieme-Stratton, Inc; 1984.
50. Bourdillion JF, Day EA. *Spinal Manipulation.* 4th ed. Norfolk, Conn: Appleton & Lange; 1987.
51. Schmorl G, Junghanns H. *The Human Spine in Health and Disease.* 2nd ed. New York, NY: Grune & Stratton; 1971.
52. Trotter M. Accessory sacroiliac articulations. *Am J Phys Anthropol.* 1937;22:247–261.
53. Trotter M. A common variation in the sacroiliac region. *J Bone Joint Surg.* 1940;22:283–299.

54. Ehara S, El-Khoury G, Bergman RA. The accessory sacroiliac joint: a common anatomic variant. *Am J Radiol.* April 1988;150:857–859.

55. Seligman SB. Articulatio sacroiliaca accessoria. *Anat Anz.* 1935;79:225–241.

56. Hadley AL. Accessory sacroiliac articulations with arthritic changes. *Radiology.* 1950;55:403–409.

57. Starr WA. Spina bifida occulta and engagement of the fifth lumbar spinous process. *Clin Orthop.* 1971;8:71.

58. Fong EE. Iliac horns (symmetrical bilateral central posterior iliac processes): case report. *Radiology.* 1946;47:517.

59. Hohl AF. *Die Gerburten Missgestalteter, Kranker und Tooter.* Verlag der Buchhandlung des Waisenhauses; 1850.

60. Grieve GP. *Modern Manual Therapy of the Vertebral Column.* New York, NY: Churchill Livingstone; 1986.

61. Muecke EC, Currarino G. Congenital widening of the pubic symphysis. *Am J Roentgen, Radium Ther Nuc Med.* 1968;013:179–185.

Chapter 2

Function

It is dangerous to arrogate to oneself the opinion that what one cannot explain does not exist.

—Steindler[1]

Chapter Objectives

- to discuss the functional mechanics of the pelvic joints
- to explain dynamics of the standing posture and gravitational effects thereof
- to describe the various components of gait and how gait relates to pelvic function
- to discuss menstrual and pregnancy changes that affect the pelvic joints
- to explain the mechanics of lifting as it relates to pelvic function
- to review the literature concerning pelvic joint function

In our knowledge of sacroiliac joint function, two things are certain: (1) the sacroiliac joints are considered diarthrodial and therefore do move; (2) the exact character of this movement is controversial. The pelvic ring is made up of a three-joint complex analogous to a spinal motion segment (Figure 2–1). The sacroiliac joints and pubic symphysis function in concert to yield suppleness to the pelvis. This kinematic chain of joints also includes the hip joint, the lumbosacral junction, and the sacrococcygeal joint.

Dempster,[2] the first kinesiologist, was the initial person to apply the engineering concept of links to the human body; he defined a link as the

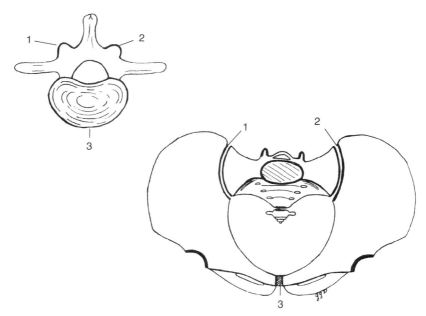

Figure 2–1 The pelvis as a three-joint complex. **(1, 2)** The paired posterior lumbar facet joints are analogous to the paired sacroiliac joints. **(3)** The lumbar interverte-bral disc is analogous to the anteriorly placed pubic symphysis.

distance between adjacent joint axes. A mechanical system of links is termed a *kinematic chain*,[2] and it can be open or closed. Open kinematic chains occur when the peripheral link is free and are the most frequently found systems in the body. For example, the peripheral ends of the limbs are free to move without affecting more proximal joints directly. However, Brunnstrom[2] states that the rib cage and pelvis are the only closed kine-matic chains in the body. In a closed kinematic chain, movement occurs such that all links in the system are affected interdependently. Theoreti-cally, biomechanical stresses can be spread among members of the chain, thereby linking them in function as well as dysfunction. The lumbosacral, sacroiliac, pubic symphysis, and hip joints are linked biomechanically. A problem at one can create compensatory changes in another. As such, hip, lumbar, and sacroiliac joint problems commonly occur together. In addi-tion, a dysfunctional joint on one side may force the opposite side joint to compensate in a painful manner.

Due to their placement between the trunk and lower extremities, and due to the large forces they must sustain, the pelvic joints and their related structures are susceptible to injury and subsequent dysfunction. These can have far-reaching effects in the locomotor system. Therefore, an awareness concerning their role in locomotor disturbances needs to be developed.

Undoubtedly, more research needs to be done to sift through the available information and separate fact from conjecture and error. As pointed out by Grieve,[3] experimental errors due to (1) the use of cadavers for study, (2) attempts to measure joint motion in tightly coapted joints during weight bearing, and (3) failure to put the sacroiliac joints through a full range of motion need to be considered in making conclusions about the scientific evidence before us.

SACROILIAC JOINT

Movement does occur in the sacroiliac joint and pubic symphysis. Although small, and in some instances imperceptible, this movement plays an important role in the overall functioning of the pelvis and lower back. The pelvic joints act to afford shock absorbency and pliability to the pelvis itself.

The symmetrical motion of nutation and the asymmetrical motion of antagonistic iliac rotations at the sacroiliac joints seem to be the more accepted movements and the ones most commonly worked with clinically. Controversy still exists as to the exact axis or axes of rotation found in sacroiliac joint motion. The adaptive movements the pelvis makes in response to postural changes are important to consider. Loss of these movements via dysfunction will make it difficult for the patient to perform normal daily activities. More emphasis is commonly placed on the sagittal plane movements of the ilia, that is, flexion and extension, sacral nutation/counternutation, and the dynamic pelvic changes made during different postures when examining for and treating sacroiliac joint dysfunction.

The sacrum and ilia can move in relation to each other either symmetrically or asymmetrically. Relating these movements to our patients' daily activities and injuries may help us better understand their problems. Symmetrical motions occur when the sacrum moves correspondingly to both ilia simultaneously, as, for example, during nutation or counternutation. Both ilia can move simultaneously in relation to the sacrum in a symmetrical fashion. An example is simultaneous flexion or extension of both ilia on the sacrum.

Asymmetrical motion entails twisting and bending motions of the sacrum in between the ilia or antagonistic movements of the ilia in relation to each other and the sacrum: for example, posterior rotation of the right ilium on the sacrum with anterior rotation of the left ilium.

Symmetrical Motion

Sacral Nutation/Counternutation

During the process of going from supine to standing or during forward bending of the trunk, the sacrum nods or nutates forward and downward between the ilia, with the iliac crests approximating and the ischial tuberosities separating.[4] During nutation, the sacral base moves anteriorly and inferiorly and the sacral apex moves posteriorly, with motion being checked by the sacrotuberous and sacrospinous ligaments. During trunk extension or when going from standing to the supine position, the opposite motions, or counternutation, occur. This explains why a dysfunctional sacroiliac joint that is unable to accommodate to these dynamic postural alterations may provoke pain when a patient attempts to arise from bed or a sitting position. Janse[5] and Illi[6,7] further assume that during flexion the sacrum nutates on one side and counternutates on the other side so that the sacrum torques in between the ilia. In other words, in addition to nutating, the sacrum torques or twists.

Iliac Motion

Walcher[8] demonstrated symmetrical pelvic motion by hyperflexing and hyperextending the hips; flexion increased the pelvic outlet, and extension increased the pelvic inlet.

Gillet and Liekens[9] observed symmetrical pelvic motion via palpation, whereby when someone was sitting, the ischial tuberosities separated slightly, broadening the pelvic base, while the iliac crests approximated each other (Figure 2–2A). Kapandji[10] discusses this same mechanism of motion when the pelvis assumes the sitting posture.

Mennell[11] states that the distance between the posterior superior iliac spines increases by one quarter to three quarters of an inch as the iliac crests separate during the transition from the sitting to the prone position. Similarly, Gillet and Liekens[9] observed the iliac crests to separate and the ischial tuberosities to approximate upon standing, while the reverse occurred on sitting (Figure 2–2B). If the pelvis is unable to perform these adaptive movements to postural change due to dysfunction, a person will experience difficulty in rising from or getting into a seated position. In fact, this is a very common occurrence in sacroiliac joint dysfunction; patients often complain of pain upon rising from a chair. It is not sitting itself that hurts them, but the actual act of arising.

Sturesson et al[12] observed the ilia to rotate posteriorly when the subject moved from supine to sitting or standing. The iliac crests were also noted to approximate each other consistently when going from the supine to sit-

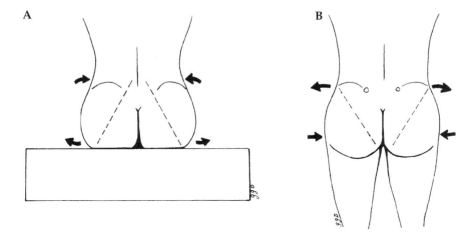

Figure 2–2 Changes in pelvic shape. **(A)** During sitting. **(B)** During standing.

ting posture, thus corroborating the findings of Mennell and Gillet and Liekens in that regard.

Strachan et al[13] observed spinal traction and compression to cause sacral extension and flexion respectively.

Asymmetrical Motion

Asymmetrical or antagonistic motion occurs at the sacroiliac joints such that the sacrum moves in relation to the ilia, or the ilia move opposite to one another in relation to the sacrum.[6,7,9,13–15]

Sacral Motion Relative to the Ilia

Gillet and Liekens comment that "the sacrum flexes easily from side to side, the base usually moving farther than the apex. It is usually passive in its movements, being influenced either by the lumbars if the force comes from above, or by the ilia if it comes from below."[9(p9)] The sacrum tends to follow the lumbar spine during trunk motion.[13,15] It also seems to act like a typical lumbar motion segment in that it displays characteristics of coupled motion.[13,15] Rotation of the lumbar spine causes ipsilateral rotation of the sacrum coupled with contralateral lateral flexion of the sacrum.[14] Lateral flexion of the lumbar spine is associated with ipsilateral lateral flexion of the sacrum coupled with minimal and inconsistent sacral rotation.[13]

Gillet and Liekens[9] speak of sacral rotation occurring between the ilia while the patient is being examined in the sitting position. For example, when left rotation (positive-theta y-axis rotation) is imparted to the trunk while the patient is seated, the thoracolumbar region sways to the right, causing the entire lumbar spine to lean right. This induces a right lateral bending (positive-theta z-axis rotation) to the sacrum. Meanwhile, the sacrum rotates with the lumbar spine, turning left (positive-theta y-axis rotation). In addition, the right iliac crest moves laterally and anteriorly, while the left iliac crest moves medially and posteriorly, but minimally. Figure 2–3 demonstrates the ability of the sacrum to rotate between the ilia, as visualized on a CT scan.

Gillet and Liekens[9] similarly describe sacral motion occurring between the ilia in response to lateral flexion localized strongly to the lumbar spine. When the patient is sitting, the left shoulder is pressed strongly toward the right hip to bend the lumbar spine to the left (Figure 2–4). The sacrum can be observed to follow the sway of the lumbar convexity and to tilt to the right (positive-theta z-axis rotation) between the two ilia. The two ilia slant toward the right side, mimicking a leaning letter "M," with the two vertical lines of the letter representing the ilia.

The Ilia's Motion Relative to Each Other and to the Sacrum

Antagonistic movements of the ilia have been described and will be related here in the context of an examination procedure described by Gillet and Liekens.[9] These authors have used a "leg-raising" test extensively to accentuate gait parameters in order to study sacroiliac joint motion. This is represented graphically in Figures 2–5 and 2–6. Figure 2–6A shows the right sacroiliac joint in neutral position. Gillet and Liekens observed that when a subject stood and raised the right bent knee, for example, the right ilium rotated backward (negative-theta x-axis rotation) so that the posterior superior iliac spine was palpated to move posteriorly and inferiorly in relation to the second sacral tubercle (Figures 2–5 and 2–6B). This movement is termed *flexion of the right sacroiliac joint.*

If the right posterior superior iliac spine and sacral tubercle were still palpated and the subject was asked to raise the left leg, a different motion was perceived at the right sacroiliac joint. When the left ilium reached its end range of motion with the sacrum, further raising of the left leg caused the sacrum to move in relation to the weight-bearing right ilium. For example, as the left knee was raised higher, the left ilium leveraged the sacrum posteriorly and inferiorly relative to the right ilium (Figures 2–5 and 2–6C). This motion is termed *extension of the right sacroiliac joint.* Gillet and Liekens mention that this latter motion of the sacrum relative to the

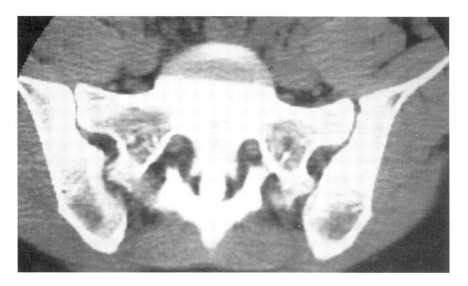

Figure 2–3 CT Scan Showing Sacral Rotation About Its Long Axis. *Source:* Reprinted from *Chiropractic Management of Spine-Related Disorders* by M.I. Gatterman, ed., p. 121, with permission of Williams & Wilkins, © 1990.

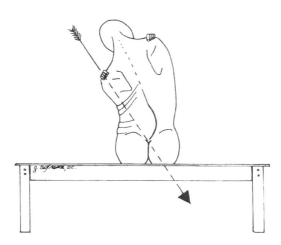

Figure 2–4 Lateral Flexion Localized to the Lumbar Spine

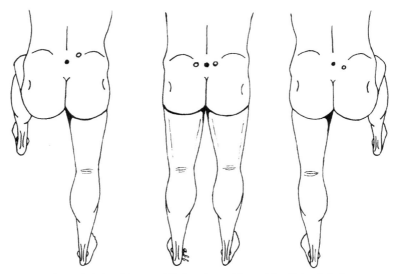

Figure 2–5 Knee-Raising Test and Palpation of Sacroiliac Joint Motion

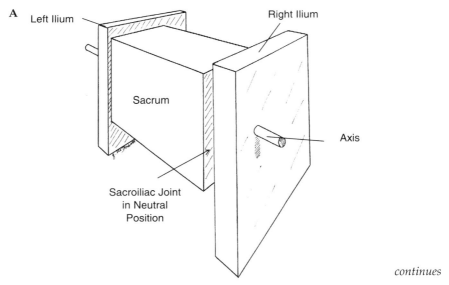

continues

Figure 2–6 Graphic representation of sacroiliac joint motion. **(A)** Right sacroiliac joint in neutral position. **(B)** Motion during right knee raising or flexion of the right sacroiliac joint. **(C)** Motion during left knee raising or extension of the right sacroiliac joint.

Figure 2–6 continued

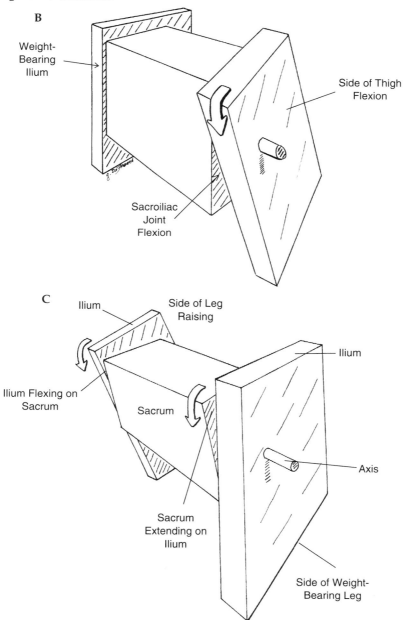

B

Weight-
Bearing
Ilium

Side of Thigh
Flexion

Sacroiliac
Joint
Flexion

C

Ilium

Side of Leg
Raising

Ilium

Ilium Flexing on
Sacrum

Sacrum

Axis

Sacrum
Extending on
Ilium

Side of Weight-
Bearing Leg

weight-bearing ilium does not seem to follow the sacroiliac surface contour and is probably due to joint gapping. Frigerio et al[16] and Wilder et al[17] discuss the possibility of sufficient sacroiliac joint separation being able to occur to allow for joint translation.

The extension motion at the sacroiliac joint mentioned previously is commonly found missing. This is most likely due to the predominant postures that most people assume daily in modern society and a neglect of proper stretching and exercise. Extension of the hip and sacroiliac joints is not often performed in the daily activities of the sedentary person. How many people, especially our patients, fully extend the hip and sacroiliac joints once in a day? Consequently, the body accommodates to more flexion activities at the expense of losing extension ability at these joints.

Sandoz describes the motion between the ilium on the side of the elevated thigh, the sacrum in the middle, and the ilium on the side of stance as a "chain type of movement in which one bone pulls along the next one when the end of articular excursion is reached."[18(p150)] Commenting on the findings of Gillet and Liekens, Sandoz[18] states that at the end of movement in the leg-raising test, the sacrum is nutated on the side of the flexed thigh and counternutated on the side of weight bearing. He also mentions that further thigh flexion causes the pelvis to rotate posteriorly en masse on the stance leg at the hip joint.

Axes of Rotation

As can be seen from the foregoing discussion, there are many opinions relating to sacroiliac joint function. The long-lasting controversy as to pelvic motion is still unsettled. The difficulty in understanding and assessing this joint arises from its complex anatomy and ability to move in a symmetric and asymmetric fashion. Indeed, Sandoz's comments are apropos:

> It would sometimes be more appropriate to speak of resiliency or suppleness of the pelvis, which implies micro-movement instead of perceptible movement of the sacroiliac joints, owing to the relative thickness of the articular cartilages of the sacroiliac joints (twice as thick on the sacral side than on the iliac side), movement probably consists more often of compression in some parts of the articular space and distraction in others rather than actual gliding of the articular surfaces. The summation of such types of movement in both sacroiliac joints and in the symphysis pubis can certainly result in an appreciable degree of pelvic torsion.[18(p109)]

It seems that the gliding motions occur more often in younger, more supple pelvises and in pelvises of women who are pregnant. With aging, motion probably occurs more through the joint compression/distraction action that Sandoz speaks of.

Various axes of rotation for the sacroiliac joint have been proposed by several researchers. Most authorities describe the major movement occurring around a transverse axis through the S-2 segment as one of rotation. Farabeuf[19] places the axis of rotation posterior to the sacroiliac joint facet surface within the interosseous (axial ligament) ligament (Figure 2–7A).

Bonnaire, as described by Kapandji,[10] locates the axis within the sacroiliac joint, midway between the cranial and caudal segments at Bonnaire's tubercle (Figure 2–7B). Weisl[4] describes the axis of rotation as 5 to 10 cm directly below the sacral promontory (Figure 2–7C). In addition, he describes a linear or translatory motion of the sacrum along an axis in the caudal segment of the sacroiliac joint (Figure 2–7D). This may be why the lower joint's excursions seem smaller than those of the upper joint during clinical assessment.

Lavignolle et al[20] applied torque and linear forces to the ilia while the sacrum was fixed. He noted the axis of rotation to be located far anterior to the sacroiliac joint, nearer the pubic symphysis. Mitchell et al[21] describe many axes of rotation, including two horizontal sacral, two horizontal iliac, and two oblique or diagonal axes. They also make the distinction between sacroiliac and iliosacral motion, depending on whether motion is initiated from the trunk or lower limbs respectively.

Egund et al[22] describe a transverse axis of rotation for nutation through the iliac tuberosity on level with the S-2 tubercle. Pitkin and Pheasant[15] found a similar axis but describe it as passing through the body of S-2; they also describe a transverse axis occurring in the pubic symphysis with antagonistic iliac movements.

Wilder et al[17] conclude that rotation cannot occur solely around any one of the previously proposed axes of rotation due to the considerable variation they found between specimens. Any rotation found would include translation, which would tighten the supporting ligaments and function as a shock-absorbing mechanism.

PUBIC SYMPHYSIS

The pubic symphysis contributes to the functional stability of the pelvic ring, and disruption of its integrity can affect sacroiliac joint function. The functional interdependence of the pubic symphysis and the sacroiliac joint is discussed by Harris and Murray.[23] They mention how abnormal pubic

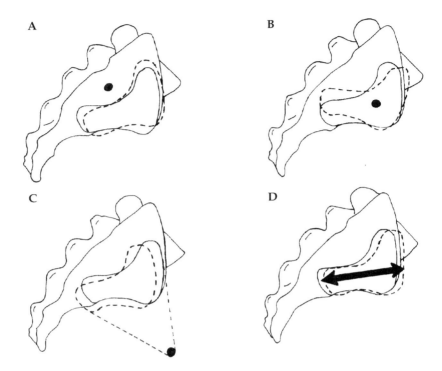

Figure 2–7 Axes of motion at the sacroiliac joint. **(A)** Farabeuf's. **(B)** Bonnaire's. **(C)** and **(D)** Weisl's.

symphysis motion may lead to problems at one or both sacroiliac joints. They state that a width at the pubic symphysis of 10 mm is the upper limit of normal, yet one athlete they examined had a 15-mm cleft with only slight instability present. They also feel that sacroiliac instability could lead to pubic symphysis problems.

The pubic symphysis is powerfully held together by stout ligaments enabling the anterior pelvis to be "spring-loading" under considerable tension, thus stabilizing the pelvic ring.[24] Traumatic disruption of this tension destabilizes the pelvis so that structural integrity is lost. For instance, if the pubic symphysis is disrupted, the pelvic ring springs apart, sacroiliac joint instability occurs, and the sacrum subluxates anteriorly into the pelvis. Pauwels[25] mentions that the pubic symphysis is under predominantly tensile, rather than compressive, forces. In contrast, Kapandji[10] explains how the pelvic force vectors converge on the pubic symphysis.

Sandoz[18] explains how both kinds of forces can act simultaneously, with tensile forces at the pubic symphysis predominating in the recumbent posture but reduced during standing due to their transmission via the femora.

Luschka[26] and Schlenzka[27] compare the pubic symphysis morphologically to the intervertebral discs. Under normal physiological parameters, the joint displays minimal movement, the precise nature of which has not been conclusively elucidated. Pitkin and Pheasant[15] discuss torsional movements occurring around a transverse axis in the pubic symphysis during antagonistic iliac motions (Figure 2–8). Schunke[28] noted that the ipsilateral pubic bone moved forward in a shearing motion during one-legged stance.

HIP JOINT

It is commonly stated that the large ball-and-socket hip joint sacrifices mobility for stability, owing to its deep-set socket as compared to the shallow glenoid fossa of the shoulder joint. In the physiologic position of standing, the femoral head is only partially covered by the acetabulum.

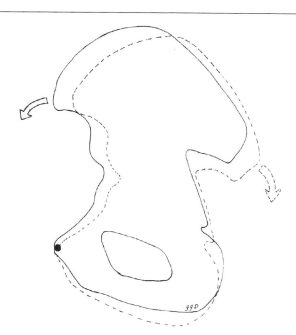

Figure 2–8 Torsional Motion at the Pubic Symphysis

This is due to the anteversion of both the acetabulum and femoral head (Figure 2–9). Consequently, the effective weight-bearing surface area is limited to a small area on the posterosuperior part of the femoral head.

Rotation and translation occur about three axes directed antero-posteriorly, vertically, and transversely from the joint. Translational motion is small and limited to joint play movements. Because many muscles cross both the hip and knee joints, movement at the hip joint is influenced by knee joint position and vice versa. For example, hip flexion is greater with the knee fully flexed due to relaxation of the hamstring muscles. Full hip flexion flattens the lumbar lordosis and can exceed 140 degrees, being stopped by soft tissue approximation.

The hip joint is extended in the standing posture. Most of the major ligamentous support around the hip joint tightens in extension, and therefore the standing position affords considerable stability. As a matter of fact, a person can rest the entire trunk weight on the hip joint ligaments by rolling the pelvis backward, extending the hip and mitigating the need for muscular effort.

Hip extension is affected by the amount of knee flexion present due to tightening of the two-joint rectus femoris muscle. Full flexion of the knee tightens the rectus femoris and therefore limits full hip extension. However, with the knee straight (extended), hip extension can occur to about 20 degrees, being limited by the strong iliofemoral ligament. Hip extension also increases the lumbar lordosis by tilting the pelvic anteriorly. Forceful hip extension imparts a torque force through the sacroiliac joint via the iliofemoral ligament, a situation that becomes useful when one is attempting to manipulate the sacroiliac joint during examination and therapeutic maneuvers.

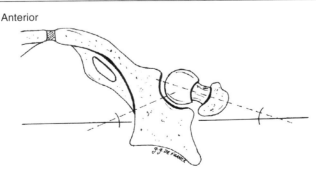

Figure 2–9 Transverse section through femoroacetabular joint. Note anteversion of both the acetabulum and femoral neck.

Because the hip joints are placed laterally in relation to the body's center of gravity, the hip abductor muscles apply considerable forces to the upper femur to help stabilize the pelvis during one-legged stance. The weight-bearing load at the hip joint is approximately equal to the body weight minus the weight of the lower extremities plus the force generated by the contraction of the hip abductors. This can amount to a considerable force approaching three times the body weight.[29] During the stance phase in gait, the ipsilateral hip abductors contract to prevent the pelvis from tilting down on the opposite side (Figure 2–10A). However, during ambulation, the compressive force exerted across the joint due to hip abductor contraction can add considerably to the joint reactive force. With hip abductor weakness, the patient leans toward or even over the involved hip, thus obviating the need for hip abductor contraction to prevent pelvic tilting (Figure 2–10B). The same mechanism occurs with a painful hip. By leaning over the hip joint, the patient reduces the need for the hip abductors to contract. The consequent reduction in joint compression as a result of diminished abductor contraction force lessens the pain response. Thus, in situations of a painful hip or hip abductor weakness, the patient will tend to lean toward the problematic side.

STANDING POSTURE AND GRAVITY

Before we consider the effects of gravitational forces on the pelvis during standing, we need to contemplate the positional relationship between the joints involved (Figure 2–11). The hip joint is situated anterior, inferior, and lateral to the sacroiliac joint by about 2 in. The weight of the trunk being borne by the sacrum is transferred across the sacroiliac joints and along the ilia to meet the ground reactive forces from the lower extremities at the hip joints (Figure 2–12). The weight of the trunk forces the sacrum to nutate forward so that the promontory moves anteriorly and inferiorly and the sacral apex moves posteriorly and superiorly. This movement, or tendency to move, is countered by the anterior sacroiliac ligaments and large, powerful check ligaments: the sacrotuberous and sacrospinous ligaments.

The center of gravity is behind the axis of the hip joint. Consequently, with the weight of the pelvis and trunk, and with the ground reactive force being transmitted up from the femoral heads, the pelvis tends to tip posteriorly on the femoral heads. With the sacrum simultaneously being nutated anteriorly due to the weight of the trunk, a relative accentuation of nutation at the sacroiliac joint occurs. Essentially, the innominates are

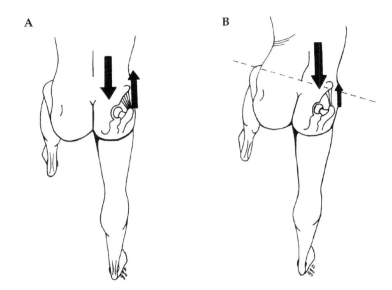

Figure 2–10 Sagittal-plane stability of pelvis in one-legged stance. **(A)** Downward-pointing arrow represents trunk weight borne by femoral head. Upward arrow represents hip abductor muscle contraction creating joint reaction force at hip joint. **(B)** Leaning of trunk over painful hip lessens the hip abductor contraction force needed to stabilize unilateral stance.

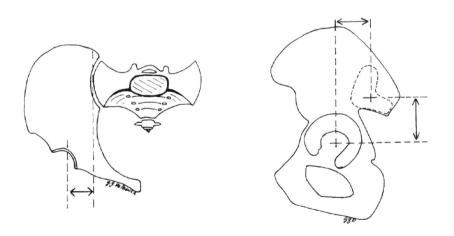

Figure 2–11 Spatial Relationship of Sacroiliac and Hip Joints

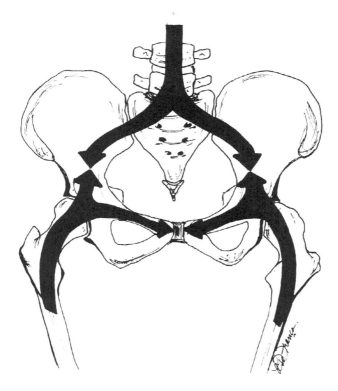

Figure 2–12 Forces from the Spine and Lower Extremities Converging on the Pelvis. *Source:* Adapted from *The Physiology of the Joints*, Vol. 3, by I.A. Kapandji, p. 57, with permission of Churchill Livingstone, © 1974.

forced into posterior rotation while the interposed sacrum is simultaneously forced into anterior rotation (Figure 2–13).

In one-legged stance, the weight-bearing femur imparts a cephalad shear force at the pubic symphysis (Figure 2–14). If an instability were to exist at the pubic symphysis, the pubic bone ipsilateral to the side of weight bearing would shift cephalad.

Due to the offset relationship between the hip and sacroiliac joints, one can appreciate the torsional forces occurring at the sacroiliac joint during one-legged stance, and consequently the discomfort that a patient with sacroiliac joint dysfunction can experience during such a stance. In fact, clinically patients with sacroiliac joint dysfunction typically have difficulty bearing weight on the affected side.

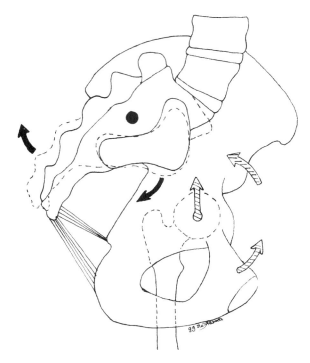

Figure 2–13 Weight-bearing forces acting through the hip and sacroiliac joints. Note that the innominate is tilted posteriorly while the sacrum tilts anteriorly simultaneously. *Source:* Adapted from *The Physiology of the Joints*, Vol. 3, by I.A. Kapandji, p. 71, with permission of Churchill Livingstone, © 1974.

Upon forward trunk flexion, a lumbopelvic rhythm is noted in which the first 60 degrees of flexion is accomplished by flattening of the lumbar lordosis while the pelvis is restrained by the pull of the hamstrings.[30,31] This is followed by an additional 25 degrees of flexion at the hip joints.[30] When full flexion is reached, the erector spinae muscles relax fully.[32] At this point, the sacrum is noted to sink deeper between the ilia as the iliac crests approximate.[4] Gitelman[33] mentions a test used by Grice to monitor this lumbopelvic rhythm. By palpating the posterior superior iliac spine with the index or middle finger and simultaneously palpating the sacral apex with the thumb tip of the same hand, one should observe them to separate up to ½ in during forward trunk flexion if the lumbopelvic rhythm is normal (Figure 2–15). During trunk extension from the forward flexed position, the above events reverse. A similar test can be performed

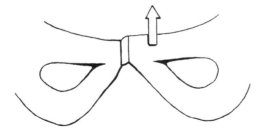

Figure 2–14 Shear Stress at Pubic Symphysis During Unilateral Stance

with the patient seated. In either case, if a posterior superior iliac spine is already noted to be lower than the other side and is observed to move cephalad and surpass its mate during trunk flexion, a positive Piedallu's sign is said to exist. This is indicative of sacroiliac joint restriction on that side as the ilium is carried forward with the flexing sacrum and lumbar spine.

MOTIONS DURING GAIT

Pelvic motions during gait occur in a rhythmic fashion. In addition to the linear progression of the body's center of mass during walking, the pelvis displays superior-inferior oscillations, lateral translations, and rotational movements (Figures 2–16 and 2–17). Illi[6] believes that the sacroiliac joints function to dampen these torsional movements before they are transferred to the lumbar spine. He feels that during gait, the lumbar spine should remain fairly stable and not partake in the rhythmic oscillations to any great extent. He thinks that when it does, the lumbar spine is more prone to scoliotic deformities and degenerative changes as a result of compensation.

During the swing phase of gait, the entire pelvis rotates anteriorly in the horizontal plane on the side of the advancing limb.[34] The gluteus medius on the weight-bearing side contracts to stabilize the pelvis in the horizontal plane. Using cineradiographic techniques, Illi[7] showed that at heel strike the weight-bearing ilium moves posteriorly while the sacrum nutates on that side. Concomitantly, the ipsilateral L-5 transverse process is pulled posteriorly. At midstance, the pelvis sways toward the weight-bearing limb, and the posterior iliac rotation starts to reverse toward neutral and progresses to anterior rotation as the limb is carried into extension for toe-off. The sacral base on that side also reverses from a nutated posi-

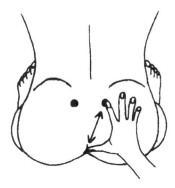

Figure 2–15 Standing-forward flexion test viewed while looking down on person bending forward. Note separation of finger contacts.

tion (anterior-inferior) at heel strike to one of counternutation (posterior-superior) at toe-off as the body moves over the weight-bearing leg. The process is repeated on the opposite side.

SACRAL MOTION WITH RESPIRATION

Sacral motion occurring with the respiratory cycle and the primary respiratory mechanism, ie, the craniosacral rhythm, has been postulated by workers in the chiropractic and osteopathic fields.[35–38] DeJarnette[35] and Sutherland[36] mention how the sacrum inherently nutates and counternutates in a cyclic rhythm. This cyclic nutation-counternutation motion occurs as part of the craniosacral rhythm proposed by Sutherland[36] at a frequency of 8 to 12 cycles per second[37] and is independent of the respiratory cycle. Inhalation is also associated with counternutation, whereas nutation occurs with exhalation. The point is that these movements may be facilitated during manual treatment with respiratory assistance.

MENSTRUAL AND PREGNANCY-INDUCED CHANGES

Brooke[14] states that sacroiliac joint mobility increases by as much as 250% during pregnancy, and Colachis et al[39] and Chamberlain[40] state that increased mobility due to relaxed pelvic and lumbar ligaments is also seen during menstruation. Sandoz[18] mentions that Maignal[41] observed lumbar hypermobility during pregnancy. Young[42] observed that pregnancy is associated with relaxation of the pubic symphysis and sacroiliac joint liga-

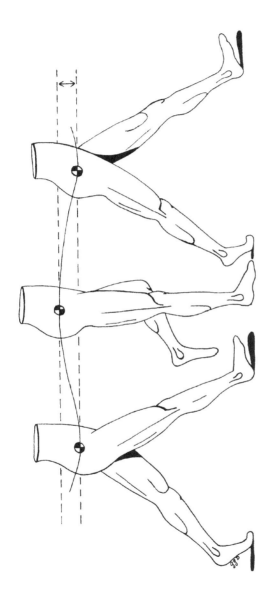

Figure 2–16 Rhythmic Vertical Oscillations of the Pelvis During the Gait Cycle

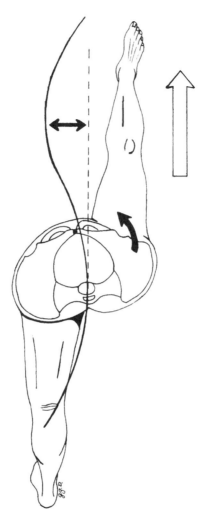

Figure 2–17 Rhythmic Rotational and Lateral Sway Movements of the Pelvis During the Gait Cycle

ments, indicated by a variable degree of interpubic widening. He also recognized that the symphyseal space gradually widened up to the third trimester of pregnancy but did not substantially increase during the last 2 months, and that it took 3 to 6 months for the pubic symphysis to return to the prepregnant state.

Relaxin, a polypeptide hormone resembling insulin, is believed to be responsible for the softening or relaxation of the pelvic ligaments and uterine cervix to facilitate parturition.[43] It is found early in pregnancy and diminishes rapidly after parturition. As a consequence to relaxin secretion, the pelvis demonstrates amplified physiologic movements. Sandoz makes the following comments:

> Pregnancy, delivery, and especially the puerperium constitute privileged moments since physiological intra-pelvic movements are greatly amplified and become more accessible to investigation. As the functional derangements of this period of life represent nothing more than physiological processes that have exceeded the boundaries of the norm, one can, by deduction, imagine rather well what is bound to happen under physiological conditions and is more difficult to investigate because of the small amplitude of pelvic movements.[18(p101)]

Thus, a physiologic instability of pregnancy commonly occurs, what Young[42] terms "pelvic arthropathy of pregnancy," of which he identifies two types. In one type, hypermobility exists at both the pubic symphysis and sacroiliac joint; the other involves only the sacroiliac joints. The more common of the two is the latter. Commonly seen during pregnancy is the characteristic waddling gait secondary to the physiologic instability of the pelvis. This finding indicates the importance of the pelvic joints in gait mechanics.

Pregnancy and the postpartum period are vulnerable times for a woman's pelvic joints. Bending, twisting, and the added tasks of caring for a child put her at risk for sacroiliac joint problems. On the other hand, prudent judgment and care are a must when using manual techniques on pregnant women so as not to intrude on this physiologically vulnerable area.

Most interesting are the cyclic changes that the pelvic joints also manifest during menstruation. It is very common to find sacroiliac joint pain in women near and during the time of their menstrual periods. Even more interesting is the relief gained by women from menstrual discomforts when the pelvic joints are treated for dysfunction.

LIFTING MECHANICS

The lifting of objects results in substantial forces being generated by the musculature in the hip and low back region. Being situated between the trunk and lower extremities, the pelvis itself must withstand tremendous loads during lifting maneuvers. McGill[44] demonstrated how the area of the sacroiliac joint can be subjected to high loads with moderate sagittal-plane lifts. Lifting a 50-lb weight has been shown to exert over 1400 lb of force at the sacroiliac joint region (Figure 2–18). This is due to the force generated by erector spinae muscles and their attachments to the sacrum and ilium. Lifting, however, requires extension not only of the trunk but also extension at the hip joint. The low back muscle mass cannot generate enough strength to lift heavy loads. On the other hand, the hip extensors (gluteus maximus, hamstrings) constitute a large muscle mass that is capable of generating an extensive contraction force. The problem is transferring this force to the lumbar spine without overloading the low back musculature. In an excellent discussion on low back anatomy and its relationship to lifting, Bogduk and Twomey[45] describe the important role played by the low back and hip muscles, the posterior ligaments, and thoracolumbar fascia in this regard.

Various theories try to explain how the low back functions during lifting, but they are not yet fully proven. One involves the role of the abdominal muscles[46] and their ability to create enough intra-abdominal pressure to support the trunk anteriorly. However, as Bogduk and Twomey[45] point out, data from studies concerning this theory do not correlate well with the relationship between intra-abdominal pressure, disc pressure, back muscle activity, and lumbar spine loads.

Another theory involves the use of the posterior ligament system and its ability to sustain higher tensile loads than the muscular system. Bogduk and Twomey summarize:

> The essence of this theory is that the power of lifting stems from the hip extensors. The back muscles do not provide the power. They are relatively too small to lift large weights. During lifting, the lumbar spine acts passively, and is kept flexed to allow the power of the hip extensors to be transmitted through its posterior ligaments. As the spine approaches the upright position, the moment exerted by the lifted weight is reduced, and the back muscles are capable, at last, of continuing the lift.[45(p90)]

Bogduk and Twomey[45] add that somewhere along the way, the force generated for the lift must be transferred from the ligament system to the muscular system. They go on to explain how the thoracolumbar fascia functions to add "dynamic" support to the passive posterior ligament system. (Refer to the discussion on the thoracolumbar fascia in Chapter 1.) Even though this theory seems to explain the mechanisms involved with a heavy lift better than the intra-abdominal pressure theory, it too needs to be experimentally validated.

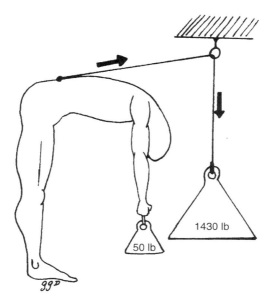

Figure 2–18 Force of Muscle Contraction Exerted Near Sacroiliac Joint

LITERATURE REVIEW OF PELVIC JOINT MOTION

Hippocrates believed that the sacroiliac joint was immobile, but he suggested that movement occurred during pregnancy.[47] In the 17th century, Pare[47] confirmed sacroiliac joint movement during pregnancy, and de Diemerbroeck[48] demonstrated sacroiliac joint motion occurring outside of pregnancy. Walcher[8] published a most controversial paper in the late 1800s that created an uproar in the obstetrical profession at that time. Through palpation and anatomical measurements, he demonstrated how the pelvic diameters could be modified by changes in body position. Thus was "born" the Walcher's position: bilateral hip hyperextension while supine. This was shown to cause anterior innominate rotation and subsequent opening of the pelvic inlet. Ashmore[49] was one of the first to quantify sacroiliac joint motion. She observed changes in the distance between the two posterior superior iliac spines as a consequence of changes in body positioning. She noticed the distance to be greater during standing than during forward trunk bending. A while later, Mennell[50] noticed similar changes as a person went from the seated to prone posture. This is discussed below. Colachis et al[39] failed to confirm changes in distance between the posterior superior iliac spines as a result of changes in body positioning, but clinical experience supports Mennell's findings.

In 1920, Halladay[51] noted movement occurring in the sacroiliac joints and pubic symphysis simultaneously. Using cadaveric specimens, he observed that both sacroiliac joints could move independently of the pubic symphysis but that unilateral sacroiliac joint movement was associated with pubic symphysis motion. On forced sacral rotation, he noted ipsilateral posterior iliac rotation and upward and forward motion of the ipsilateral pubic ramus at the symphysis joint. These movements were presumed to occur during walking. Halladay also observed sacroiliac joint motion to be markedly reduced in specimens over 50 years old.

In 1924, Brooke[14] described sacral movements as gliding and rotatory in nature. Although small, the gliding motion occurred in cephalad, caudal, and posterior directions. However, Brooke stated that the rotatory motion was more important. He described how the sacral articular surface formed a prominent lip at the middle segment, creating a pivot point for interlocking mechanism rotation to take place. He recognized the antagonistic torsional movements of the ilia about the symphysis pubis that Pitkin and Pheasant describe[15] (Figure 2–8). Brooke was of the opinion that such torsional movements occurred during walking. He also observed compensatory hypermobility in the lumbosacral joint when the sacroiliac joint was ankylosed. Could this be why we commonly see L-5 joint and disc problems with sacroiliac problems? Why is it that a normally strong and resilient structure such as the intervertebral disc decompensates prematurely and succumbs to degenerative changes?

In 1930, Siskin[52] studied 29-year-old specimens within 48 hours of death and noted an average rotation of 4 degrees occurring between the sacrum and ilium.

Pitkin and Pheasant[15] observed changes in iliac position when comparing normal stance with stances involving the right and left foot alternately standing on a 1.5-in block. Their conclusions were as follows:

1. Except for flexion and extension, all trunk motions normally caused unpaired antagonistic iliac movements about a transverse axis passing through the symphysis pubis—a fact that we can use to our advantage when we want to mobilize the pubic symphysis.

2. Sacral flexion and extension occurred, with the ilium being fixed into position.

3. Antagonistic iliac movements were associated with sacral lateral flexion and rotation.

Interestingly, Pitkin and Pheasant mention that sacroiliac joint asymmetry is related to hand and eye dominance. Bellamy et al[47] suggest that this could mean that the sacroiliac joints are important in the overall acquisition of stereoscopic vision. This demonstrates the all-important interdependence of the locomotor and nervous systems. A possibility raised by the suggestion of Bellamy et al is that sacroiliac joint morphology and function may be influenced by handedness and eye dominance.

In 1938, Strachan et al[13] used cadaveric specimens with one ilium immobilized in a concrete block. Steel pins were placed into the sacrum and ilium for reference points. Qualitative data on sacroiliac joint motion in response to trunk motion were recorded. The authors made the following observations:

1. The sacrum followed the trunk in flexion and extension relative to the immobilized ilium.
2. The sacrum followed the lumbars in ipsilateral rotation and side bending.
3. With rotation, there was a coupled contralateral side bending of the sacrum.
4. With lateral flexion, there was minimal coupled rotation of the sacrum and an inconsistency as to its direction.

A year later, Strachan et al[53] commented that sacral movements were gliding in nature and occurred more easily in flexion, extension, cephalad, and caudal directions. However, they seemed more difficult in lateral flexion and rotation.

In 1951, Illi[6,7] observed sacroiliac joint motion during a variety of experiments. He embedded small lead cubes on either side of the sacroiliac joints for radiographic index points of measure. He then fixed iron pipes into both acetabuli of cadaver pelvises to substitute for femurs and moved them alternately as in gait. Upon X-raying the apparatus, he was able to visualize sacroiliac joint motion. On direct observation, he described a gyrating sacral motion between the ilia such that the sacral base scribed an almost horizontal figure eight as it moved "obliquely up and down and concurrently anteriorly and posteriorly."[6(p13)] He believed that the function of the sacroiliac joint was to dampen rhythmic torsional movements of the pelvis during gait to spare the lumbar spine from excess compensatory movements. In trying to support his belief, he used cineradiography to observe sacroiliac joint and lumbar motion during gait on living subjects walking on a treadmill. He in fact noticed compensatory lumbar movements in response to dysfunctional sacroiliac joint motion. He noted that a dynamic compensatory lumbar scoliosis occurred, with the convexity being contralateral to the side of unilateral sacroiliac joint blockage. He surmised that the lumbar spine would develop a permanent scoliotic deformity as a consequence to prolonged exposure to such compensation. In addition, he suggested that sacroiliac joint dysfunction led to compensatory stress at the hip joints which, if of long standing, could lead to coxarthrosis. Illi's observations direct us to contemplate the importance of sacroiliac joint dysfunction in possibly causing lumbar spine pathomechanics. Clinically, we often observe lumbar spine joint problems that occur secondary to pelvic joint dysfunctions. Illi's research also raises the question of the importance of assessing younger people's pelvises to prevent future lumbar problems that might be a consequence of poor pelvic function.

In 1952, Simkins[54] believed that the sacrum rotated in the sagittal plane about a transverse axis situated at the union of the second and third sacral segments. He studied lateral X-rays of living subjects during trunk flexion and extension with a grid coordinate system placed at the level of the sacroiliac joint's supposed transverse axis. He reported an 8-degree average sacral range of motion.

In 1955, Weisl[4] used X-rays to measure sacral motion in living subjects as they assumed various degrees of hip and trunk flexion and extension. He stated that angular displacement of the sacrum (translational motion coupled with rotation about an axis) occurred more frequently than pure translational or rotational motions. The greatest motion seemed to have occurred when the subjects changed from the recumbent to the standing position. The sacral promontory was observed to nod or "nutate" anteroinferiorly by an average of 5.6 mm around an axis 5 to 10 cm directly below the promontory. He also described a translational motion along an axis in the caudal segment of the joint. Two other studies by Egund et al[22] and Reynolds[55] using stereoscopic radiography characterized sacral movement as angular.

In 1963, Colachis et al[39] used a very innovative way to assess iliac motion. They embedded Kirschner pins into the posterior superior iliac spines of subjects and measured changes between them in relation to nine different body positions. They found the greatest movement to occur during forward bending while standing. They also confirmed Weisl's work.

In 1968, Gillet and Liekens[9] described various types of motion through extensive palpatory observations. Sandoz mentioned that Gillet's work

> has brought considerable clarification on the question of direction of sacro-iliac movement, by showing that the latter varies with the type of movement that is performed by a subject, in other words, according to the direction in which the physical forces act upon the sacrum, the innominates or both.[18(p106)]

Gillet's assessment of the pelvis was discussed earlier.

In 1974, Frigerio et al[16] used stereoradiographic techniques to document 15.5 to 26 mm of movement between the innominates and the sacrum. In

1989, Sturesson et al[12] used similar techniques to assess sacroiliac joint motion during physiologic movements in symptomatic and asymptomatic subjects. They noted consistent, although minute, motion about a transverse axis. They also found no difference in motion patterns between symptomatic and asymptomatic subjects. However, they assessed motion in only one plane of movement that does not fully represent total sacroiliac joint function.

In 1980, Wilder et al[17] studied 11 fresh pelvic bones and commented that the sacroiliac joint functions as a shock absorber due to the energy-absorbing capacity of the ligaments associated with the joint. This energy-dampening effect may function to protect the lumbar spine and hip joints from unwarranted mechanical stress.

In 1983, Oonishi et al[56] stated that upon loading, the pelvis as a whole is displaced backward while the pubic ramus moves upward.

In 1987, Miller et al[57] studied the load displacement behavior of eight sacroiliac joints. They noticed small amounts of sacroiliac joint motion when both ilia were fixed in position. However, with just one ilium fixed, they observed rotational and translational movements to be three to five times greater.

Also in 1987, McGill[44] studied the load effects of lumbar extensor muscle contraction on the sacroiliac joint region. He found that with a sagittal-plane lift of 50 lb, a force of 1430 lb was generated at the attachment sites of the lumbar extensor muscles near the sacroiliac joint (Figure 2–18). Most of the force was generated by the longissimus thoracis and iliocostalis parts of the erector spinae. Excessive loads produced by lumbar extensor muscle contraction, even when lifting moderate weights, can place the sacroiliac joint region under an extreme load because of the muscle attachments near the sacroiliac joint. The implication is that lumbar extension movements, even under light and moderate loads, can adversely affect the sacroiliac joint. McGill states that this situation is more likely to create muscular insertional strains than joint disorders. However, taking into account that the sacroiliac joint is a mobile articulation, especially in the sagittal plane, it is quite conceivable that extreme loads applied via contraction of regionally attached muscles could cause injury resulting in joint dysfunction.

In 1991, Vukicevic et al[58] studied mobility and deformation patterns of physiologically loaded pelvic specimens, using holographic techniques. They observed a downward translation and a forward and backward tilting of the sacrum to occur through a range of 2 to 7 mm (1/16 to 1/4 in). The axis of rotation was found to be consistent with Weisl's 5 to 8 cm (2 to 3 in) below the sacral promontory. Interestingly, removal of the sacrotuberous and sacrospinous ligaments had no bearing on pelvic and sacral deformation patterns. However, when the interosseous ligament was divided, a substantial change was noted in pelvic motion. The sacrum became wedged between the ilia, demonstrating little movement. The results in this study did not support Bowen and Cassidy's[59] contention that joint surface configuration is important in determining joint function. The results of Vukicevic et al indicate that sacroiliac joint motion is mainly determined by the sacroiliac interosseous ligament. They also noted that during the broad range of applied loads, the sacroiliac joint surfaces were never discovered to be in tight coaptation.

Chapter Review Questions

- What are the different types of SIJ movements?
- Why does a patient with a painful hip joint limp by leaning over the side of pain?
- What is the spatial relationship between the SIJ and hip joint?
- What are the SIJs' function and motions during gait?
- What is meant by "physiologic arthropathy of pregnancy"?
- What occurs at the pubic symphysis and SIJs during one-legged stance?
- Describe what occurs at the SIJs during Gillet's leg-raising test.

REFERENCES

1. Steindler A. *Ilio-Psoas*. Springfield, Ill: Charles C Thomas, Publisher; 1962.
2. Gowitzke BA, Milner M. *Scientific Bases of Human Movement*. 3rd ed. Baltimore, Md: Williams & Wilkins; 1988.
3. Grieve GP. Lumbopelvic rhythm and mechanical dysfunction of the sacroiliac joint. *Physiotherapy.* 1981;67:171–173.
4. Weisl H. The movements of the sacroiliac joint. *Acta Anat.* 1955;23:80–91.
5. Janse J. The clinical biomechanics of the sacroiliac mechanism. *J Am Chiro Assoc.* 1978;12:1–8.
6. Illi FW. *The Vertebral Column: Life-Line of the Body.* Lombard, Ill: National College of Chiropractic; 1951.
7. Illi FW. *Highlights of 45 Years of Experience and 35 Years of Research.* Geneva: Institute for the Study of the Statics and Dynamics of the Human Body; 1971.
8. Walcher G. Die Conjugata eines engen Beckens ist keine konstante Grosse, sondern lasst sich durch die Korperhaltung der Tragerin verandern. *Centralblatt für Gynakologie.* 1889;51:892–893.
9. Gillet H, Liekens M. *Belgian Chiropractic Research Notes.* 7th ed. Brussels: Motion Palpation Institute; 1968.

10. Kapandji IA. *The Physiology of the Joints. Vol 3. The Trunk and the Vertebral Column.* New York, NY: Churchill Livingstone; 1974.

11. Mennell JM. *Back Pain: Diagnosis and Treatment Using Manipulative Technique.* Boston, Mass: Little, Brown & Co; 1960.

12. Sturesson B, Selvik G, Uden A. Movements of the sacroiliac joints: a Roentgen stereophotogrammetric analysis. *Spine.* 1989;14:162–165.

13. Strachan WF, et al. A study of the mechanics of the sacroiliac joint. *J Am Osteopath Assoc.* 1938;37:576–578.

14. Brooke R. The sacroiliac joint. *J Anat.* 1924;58:299.

15. Pitkin HC, Pheasant HC. Sacrarthrogenic telalgia. *J Bone Joint Surg.* 1936;18:365–374.

16. Frigerio NA, Stowe RR, Hower JW. Movement of the sacroiliac joint. *Clin Orthop.* 1974;100:370–377.

17. Wilder DG, Pope MH, Frymoyer JW. The functional topography of the sacroiliac joint. *Spine.* 1980;5:575–579.

18. Sandoz RW. Structural and functional pathologies of the pelvic ring. *Ann Swiss Chiro Assoc.* 1981;7:101–160.

19. Farabeuf LH. Sur l'anatomie et la physiologie des articulations sacroiliaques avant et après la symphyseatomie. *Ann Gynec Obstet.* 1894;41:407–420.

20. Lavignolle B, Vital JM, Senegas J, et al. An approach to the functional anatomy of the sacroiliac joints in vivo. *Anat Clin.* 1983;5:169–176.

21. Mitchell FL, Moran PS, Pruzzo NA. *An Evaluation and Treatment Manual of Osteopathic Muscle Energy Procedures.* Manchester, Mo: Mitchell, Moran & Pruzzo Associates; 1979.

22. Egund N, et al. Movements in the sacroiliac joints demonstrated with roentgen stereophotogrammetry. *Acta Radiol (Diagn).* 1978;19:833–846.

23. Harris NH, Murray RO. Lesions of the symphysis in athletes. *Br Med J.* 1974;4:211–214.

24. Steindler A. *Kinesiology of the Human Body under Normal and Pathological Conditions.* 3rd ed. Springfield, Ill: Charles C Thomas, Publisher; 1970.

25. Pauwels F. *Gesammelte Abhandlungen zur functionellen Des Bewegungsapparates.* Berlin: Springer-Verlag; 1965.

26. Luschka H. *Die Halbgelenke des Menschlichen.* Berlin: Kooprs; 1858.

27. Schlenzka W. Die Besonderheiten der Iliosakralgelenke. *Munich Med Wschr.* 1980;122.

28. Schunke GB. The anatomy and development of the sacroiliac joint in man. *Anat Rec.* 1938;72:313–331.

29. Kessler RM, Hertling D. *Management of Common Musculoskeletal Disorders.* Philadelphia, Pa: Harper & Row; 1983.

30. White AA, Panjabi MM. *Clinical Biomechanics of the Spine.* Philadelphia, Pa: JB Lippincott Co; 1978.

31. Carlsoo S. The static muscle load in different work positions: an electromyographic study. *Ergonomics.* 1961;4:193–211.

32. Farfan HF. Function of erectores spinae in flexion of the trunk. *Lancet.* 1951;260:133.

33. Gitelman R. A chiropractic approach to biomechanical disorders of the lumbar spine and pelvis. In Haldeman S, ed. *Modern Developments in the Principles and Practice of Chiropractic.* New York, NY: Appleton-Century-Crofts; 1980: 297–330.

34. Schafer RC. *Clinical Biomechanics: Musculoskeletal Actions and Reactions.* Baltimore, Md: Williams & Wilkins; 1983.

35. DeJarnette MB. *Sacroccipital Technique.* Nebraska City, Neb: Major Bertrand DeJarnette; 1979.

36. Sutherland WA. *The Cranial Bowl*. Mankato, Minn: Free Press Co; 1939.

37. Upledger JE, Vredevoogd MFA. *Craniosacral Therapy*. Seattle, Wash: Eastland Press; 1983.

38. Magoun HI. *Osteopathy in the Cranial Field*. Kirksville, Mo: Journal Printing Co; 1966.

39. Colachis SC, Warden RE, Becthal CO, et al. Movement of the sacroiliac joint in the adult male. *Arch Phys Med Rehabil*. 1963;44:490–498.

40. Chamberlain WE. The symphysis pubis in the roentgen examination of the sacroiliac joint. *Am J Roentgenol*. 1930;24:621–625.

41. Maignal D. *An Investigation of Possible Segmental Instability in Pre-Parturating Women*. Bournemouth, England: AECC; 1973–1974. Thesis.

42. Young J. Relaxation of the pelvic joints in pregnancy: pelvic arthropathy of pregnancy. *J Obstet Gynec Br Empire*. 1940;47:493–524.

43. Ganong WF. Physiology of reproduction. In Pernoll ML, Benson RC, eds. *Current Obstetric and Gynecologic Diagnosis and Treatment*. 6th ed. Norwalk, Conn: Appleton & Lange; 1987:109–126.

44. McGill SM. A biomechanical perspective of sacro-iliac pain. *Clin Biomech*. 1987;2:145–151.

45. Bogduk N, Twomey LT. The lumbar muscles and their fascia. In: Bogduk N, Twomey LT, eds. *Clinical Anatomy of the Lumbar Spine*. New York, NY: Churchill Livingstone; 1987; 72–91.

46. Bartelink DL. The role of abdominal pressure in relieving the pressure on the lumbar intervertebral disc. *J Bone Joint Surg* Br. 1957;39B:718–725.

47. Bellamy N, Park W, Rooney PJ. What do we know about the sacroiliac joint? *Semin Arthritis Rheum*. 1983;12:282–305.

48. de Diemerbroeck I; Salmon W, trans. *The Anatomy of Human Bodies*. London: Brewster; 1689.

49. Ashmore E. *Osteopathic Mechanics*. Kirksville, Mo: Journal Printing Co; 1915.

50. Mennell J. The science and art of joint manipulation. In: *The Spinal Column*. Vol 2. Philadelphia, Pa: Blakiston Co; 1952.

51. Halladay HV. *Applied Anatomy of the Spine*. Kirksville, Mo: JF Janisch; 1920.

52. Siskin D. A critical analysis of the anatomy and the pathological changes of the sacroiliac joints. *J Bone Joint Surg*. 1930;12:891–910.

53. Strachan WF, et al. Applied anatomy of the pelvis and perineum. *J Am Osteopath Assoc*. 1939;38:359–360.

54. Simkins CS. *Anatomy and Significance of the Sacroiliac Joint*. Colorado Springs, Colo: American Academy of Osteopathy Yearbook; 1952.

55. Reynolds HM. Three-dimensional kinematics in the pelvic girdle. *J Am Osteopath Assoc*. 1980;80:277–280.

56. Oonishi H, Isha H, Hasegawa T. Mechanical analysis of the human pelvis and its application to the artificial hip joint by means of the three dimensional finite element method. *J Biomech*. 1983;16:427–444.

57. Miller JAA, Schultz AB, Anderson GBJ. Load displacement behavior of sacroiliac joints. *J Orthop Res*. 1987;5:92–101.

58. Vukicevic S, Marusic A, Stavljenic A, et al. Holographic analysis of the human pelvis. *Spine*. 1991;16:209–213.

59. Bowen V, Cassidy JD. Macroscopic and microscopic anatomy of the sacroiliac joint from embryonic life until the eighth decade. *Spine*. 1981;6:620–628.

Chapter 3

Clinical Assessment: The History

Linda J. Levine and George G. DeFranca

Chapter Objectives

- to discuss the importance of the history in relation to making a diagnosis
- to differentiate mechanical versus organic lesions from the history
- to discuss the types of questions to be asked during the history taking
- to discuss pain location and character
- to discuss referred pain and its differentiation from radicular pain
- to discuss clues from the history that would identify the type of tissue injured
- to discuss differential diagnosis categories

According to Grieve, "Modern psychology teaches that man 'is prepared to what he is going to see,' recognizing what he already knows and virtually what he is seeking."[1(p235)] How can we remain objective and allow new clinical evidence to gain entry to our minds when they are cluttered with preconceived notions of how things should be? To experience each patient clinically as new and fresh is clearly difficult but at least something to strive for.

Furthermore, when dealing with functional disturbances of the locomotor system, it is best to shift one's focus of assessment from structural pathology to functional pathology. This does not relieve one of the obligation to search for and rule out structural or organic pathology. But in the majority of painful musculoskeletal conditions encountered in clinical practice, dysfunction of the moving parts and related soft tissues is found to be at fault.

CASE HISTORIES

In this chapter, case histories are used to illustrate pertinent aspects of the clinical history in patients with problems in the following areas: sacroiliac joint, pubic symphysis, hip joint, and coccyx. Pain diagrams and, in one case, a visual analog scale, accompany the case histories. The visual analog scale is a 100-mm line that represents a pain spectrum ranging from *none* to *excruciating pain*. Patients are asked to estimate their pain level by placing a mark on the line. The visual analog scale has been found to be more sensitive in quantifying pain intensity than mere verbal descriptors.[2-4] The pain drawing is simply an outline of the body on which patients draw in the location of their pain. It has been shown to be very useful in identifying certain conditions.[5]

Sacroiliac Joint

Case History 1

A 34-year-old woman, 3 months postpartum, presented with severe "hip" and leg pain of 3 weeks' duration after she attempted to move a refrigerator in order to sweep behind it. She said that in so doing, she had twisted her trunk and felt a "catch" (here she pointed to her sacroiliac joint region). The pain was sharp and localized to the left sacroiliac joint and buttock, with occasional radiation into the proximal posterior thigh. Trunk bending and twisting to the left hurt her. Walking and climbing stairs were difficult, as any weight bearing caused jabs of pain. The act of rising from a chair was most difficult, although sitting itself was not. She was able to sleep at night, but at times she would experience her pain upon turning over in bed. Flexing her left knee upon her chest seemed to alleviate the pain for a short period of time. She felt limited in her ability to do normal housework without pain. In the last few days before clinical presentation, she had noticed that her entire left leg felt "heavy" and her calf region felt sore. She denied any bowel or bladder problems, although she admitted to moderate exacerbation of her pain upon performing a bowel movement (see Figure 3–1).

Questions for Thought

- Where is the pain located?
- What aggravates/alleviates the pain?
- Is this an "organic" or a "mechanical" problem? (See below.)
- What about the fact that this woman was recently pregnant?

The above case history illustrates a classic clinical presentation of a sacroiliac joint problem. Generally, pain from sacroiliac lesions can be re-

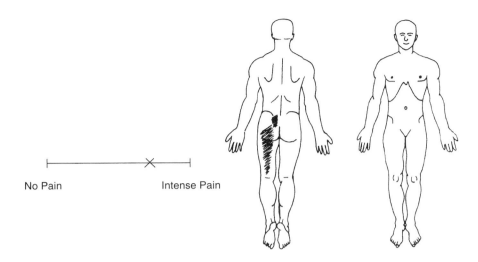

No Pain   Intense Pain

Figure 3–1 Case History 1: Pain Diagram and Visual Analog Scale

ferred to the buttock or haunch area and posterior proximal thigh ("high sciatica") (Figure 3–2). Stoddard[6] mentions that sacroiliac joint pain is always unilateral and never central, whereas disc and lumbosacral pain may be central or unilateral. Hackett[7] mentions that upper-pole sacroiliac joint lesions refer pain posterolaterally and that lower-pole lesions refer pain to the posterior thigh and calf absolutely.

Sacroiliac joint pain can radiate to the groin, anterior thigh, and even the posterior calf and foot.[8] It is experienced as a deep, dull, achy feeling, and the leg is described as heavy or tired. Using joint blocks and provocation injections, Fortin et al[9,10] tried to determine sacroiliac joint pain referral patterns in asymptomatic volunteers. They found that the sacroiliac joint referred pain 3 cm lateral and 10 cm caudal to the PSIS and that a pain diagram depicting this pattern was very accurate in identifying sacroiliac joint problems. The pain was described as achy, numb, paresthetic, and pressurelike. Schwarzer et al[11] noted that groin pain was the only sacroiliac joint referred pain that responded to joint blocks.

Weight bearing on the affected side can bring jabs of pain. However, continued walking may bring relief as the joint "loosens up." Patients often state that lying on the back and flexing the thigh up onto the chest helps. Getting in and out of the sitting posture is usually troublesome. Rolling over in bed at night often causes twinges of pain in the joint.

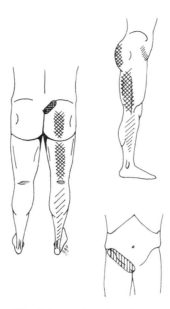

Figure 3–2 Area of sacroiliac joint pain referral. Most common areas of referred pain are cross-hatched.

Commonly, a history of falling on the buttocks is related. Forceful trunk twisting or pushing movements can create sacroiliac joint problems by leveraging large amounts of force to the sacroiliac joint via the lower extremities and trunk. Stepping off a curb or into a hole unexpectedly commonly injures the hip, sacroiliac joint, and lumbar spine. Recent pregnancy tends to put women at risk for suffering sacroiliac joint problems, and this should be asked about in the history.

Pubic Symphysis

Case History 2

A 21-year-old hockey goalie presented with pubic and right proximal adductor pain when, after attempting to block a puck with his right leg, he slipped and hyperabducted his thigh, feeling pain in what he described as below his bladder area. He said it felt as if he had a bladder infection because of his "bladder pain." Several hours later, he experienced an achy pain extending into the proximal medial thighs. He found it difficult to walk upstairs and lie on his abdomen. Putting one shoe on at a time by crossing his leg in a sign-of-four position hurt him. Lying on his back and keeping his thighs adducted afforded him relief. Urination was unaffected (see Figure 3–3).

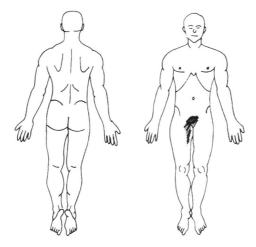

Figure 3–3 Case History 2

Questions for Thought

- Where is the pain located?
- How is this case different from the previous one?
- What do you suppose the mechanism of injury was?
- Why would relaxing the thigh in adduction give this patient relief?

Pubic symphysis dysfunction can occur with sacroiliac joint dysfunction, but activities involving strong and prolonged hip adduction, ie, hockey and other skating/skiing sports, tend more to stress the pubic symphysis. Sudden forced hip abduction, as in performing gymnastic or accidental "splits," tends to foster pubic symphysis joint problems, as in the case above. Athletes who suffer repeated groin "pulls," especially hurdlers, soccer players, and race walkers, should be examined for pubic symphysis and sacroiliac joint problems. Howse[12] states that shear forces are imparted to the pubic symphysis in soccer players and race walkers. Bicyclists who slip off the pedals and fall astride the frame injure the pubic symphysis. Pubic symphysis joint pain is also experienced by women who have recently given birth. This usually subsides after parturition but can remain as a dull, localized ache over the joint. Unilateral weight bearing exacerbates the pain, as does initiating leg movements while seated or lying down. Pain from the pubic symphysis can be experienced locally or referred into the lower abdomen or inner proximal thighs (Figure 3–4).

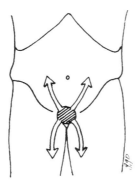

Figure 3–4 Pubic Symphysis Pain Referral Pattern

Patients guard themselves from pain by keeping their thighs from abducting too much.

One must keep in mind the functional interdependence exhibited by the sacroiliac joints and pubic symphysis, mentioned by Harris and Murray.[13] Symptomatic pubic symphysis problems occur in a small percentage of cases when compared to the number of sacroiliac joint problems seen. Most often, treatment directed just at normalizing sacroiliac joint function alleviates the pubic symphysis problem. This is most likely because many manipulations and stretches directed at the sacroiliac joint also physically affect the pubic symphysis.

Hip Joint

Case History 3

A 53-year-old housewife presented with right groin pain and stiffness after gardening for hours while in a crouched position on her hands and knees. She found it painful to stand erect and walk the next morning. She could flex her hip to put on socks, but it hurt her and she could not fully straighten it when lying flat. The front of her thigh ached and felt tight. Her groin pain was described as deep and achy. Sitting did not bother her, but bending did. No back pain was present (Figure 3–5).

Questions for Thought

- Where is this patient's pain felt?
- Is age a factor in this history?
- Why could she not stand erect or straighten her thigh while supine?

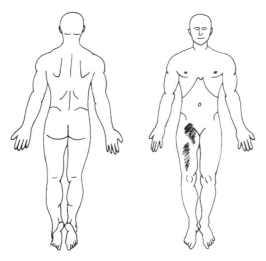

Figure 3–5 Case History 3

Pain from the femoroacetabular or hip joint is often experienced in the groin and anterior thigh, especially in osteoarthritis (Figure 3–6). Referral to the knee is not uncommon, since the knee and the hip share the same innervation levels, L-3 through S-1. Pediatric knee complaints warrant attention directed at the hip, since knee pain is a common presentation for hip problems in children. Offierski and MacNab[14] discuss the hip-spine syndrome and mention how osteoarthritises of the hip and lumbar spine often occur concurrently. The clinical picture can reflect either hip or lumbar involvement predominantly or both simultaneously, causing much confusion. Mid and lower lumbar levels and the sacroiliac joint can refer pain to the hip region. Therefore, hip joint pain necessitates the examination of lumbar and sacroiliac regions in addition to the hip area.

Besides direct trauma from falls on the hip joint, a common presentation of hip joint problems is a late middle-aged or older individual suffering from chronic hip or groin pain of gradual onset. Such is the presentation of an osteoarthritic hip joint. Acute exacerbations typically occur after prolonged sitting postures in which the joint tends to stiffen painfully. Upon arising or attempting some activity afterward, the patient notices a tight soreness that can progress into a dull ache that radiates from the groin into the anterior thigh. Typically, the patient demonstrates his or her painful area by rubbing the hand from the proximal to distal anterior thigh. Unaccustomed activities, such as long walks at a vacation resort, springtime

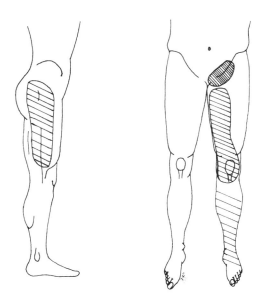

Figure 3–6 Hip Joint Pain Referral Pattern

gardening and housework, or sprinting for first base at the annual company picnic, can easily trigger pain and stiffness in such a hip joint.

Walking can be difficult, and stairs may have to be negotiated one at a time. Hip flexor spasm may create a bent-forward gait when the involved hip is bearing weight. The person usually leans or lurches over the involved side during gait to reduce pain, as explained in Chapter 2. A past history of congenital dislocation, Legg-Calvé-Perthes disease, infection, or serious trauma should be asked about. These conditions can create biomechanical problems long after the disorder is healed.

Sacrococcygeal Joint

Case History 4

Three months ago, a 42-year-old man slipped on a loose stairway rug and slid down three stairs on his buttocks. He felt pain in his "tailbone" that was severe and prevented him from arising. He was taken to the local hospital, where examination findings, including X-rays, were negative for fracture. His pain had subsided slightly since its onset, but he still found it difficult to sit up straight, especially on hard surfaces. His pain was local to his tailbone, but he also said his lower back ached. He said he was aware of a constant tension around his anus, and defecation was painful at times (Figure 3–7).

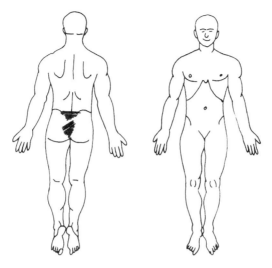

Figure 3–7 Case History 4

Questions for Thought

- Where is this patient's pain felt?
- What is the cause for the tension around the anus?
- What would be an indication of a more serious injury to deeper tissues, eg, the rectum?
- How reliable are radiographs in this situation?

Coccygeal pain, or coccydynia, is extremely uncomfortable and can follow direct trauma, parturition, or joint problems in the lumbosacral and sacroiliac joints. It can be local to the coccyx, usually the tip, or can spread to the buttocks and even the lower back. The coccyx can be injured directly from a fall or sitting down hard, which can result in sacrococcygeal joint dysfunction and resultant pain. Reflex spasm of the pelvic floor muscles occurs and can perpetuate the pain. Traumatic periosteal bruising can also occur after direct trauma.

However, very commonly people present without a history of direct trauma and have a painful coccyx. Often they have a prior onset of lower back pain and even sciatica. Lower lumbar disc protrusions or lumbosacral or sacroiliac joint disorders can refer pain to the coccyx. Often patients with lower back problems who do not complain of coccydynia demonstrate tenderness at the tip of the coccyx on examination.

Patients with coccydynia find it difficult to sit. They tend to lean forward or onto one buttock. Rising from a chair is difficult, and they usually find comfort in sitting on a pillow. Bowel movements can be painful, especially if constipation is a feature. Dyspareunia may also be associated with coccydynia.

The coccyx can be the site of referred pain from trigger points in the pelvic floor muscles yet itself be nontender. The levator ani and coccygeus muscles are commonly at fault. Stiff, painful movements can be found at the sacrococcygeal joint on examination.

X-ray evidence of displacement should not be held as pathognomonic evidence of a coccygeal problem, since growth anomalies and deviations are common.

Coccydynia is thought to occur mostly in women and to be of psychogenic origin. It occurs in men but with less frequency. For the most part, it is not psychogenic. The labeling of chronic coccydynia as psychogenic is most likely due to inadequate understanding of functional problems and referred pain phenomena. Manual methods applied to this area are usually successful in alleviating pain. However, patients in pain for more than 1 year tend to be treatment resistant.

THE HISTORY: LISTEN!

William Osler once said, "Listen, Doctor, your patient is telling you the diagnosis." Nowhere in the examining process is listening more important than the initial history. It is said that God gave us two ears to listen and one mouth to speak with and that we should use them in that proportion. Ideally, the patient should leave the initial consultation saying, "That doctor actually listened and understood me!" This instills rapport and confidence in the doctor-patient relationship. Anyone can listen, but many do not "hear" the spoken message.

In order to hear and facilitate the flow of information from patient to doctor, active listening techniques should be used. This entails the provision of an environment that allows the patient's thoughts and feelings to be expressed and heard. Active listening draws the person out to allow verbalization of his or her story. Interjecting phrases or acknowledgments such as "hmmm," "I see," "I understand," or "what else?" prompts the patient to self-disclose further. Nonverbal cues such as head nodding or just plain silence coupled with an interested look are powerful communicators of "I am interested, I am listening, what else?" Repeating or paraphrasing what the patient says allows the doctor to verify his or her understanding of the problem and further establishes this in the patient's mind.

Obviously, control of the situation must be exerted by the doctor to prevent the patient from rambling on with impertinent information.

To foster trust and self-disclosure in the doctor-patient relationship, doctors must display empathy, congruency, and a positive regard for the patient[15] (Exhibit 3–1). They must be empathic to sense and appreciate the patient's internal reality. They must be congruent by having their actions and language mirror their emotions and opinions. Most important, by showing a positive regard for the patient, they demonstrate an acceptance of him or her as a person.

QUESTIONS TO KEEP IN MIND DURING THE HISTORY

The clinical assessment of a patient begins with the history. Strict attention must be given to its content. Listening with intent, the clinician should consider several important questions. What tissue is involved? More appropriately, multiple tissues should be thought of because people rarely injure a single joint in isolation without trauma to or reaction from the adjacent supportive soft tissues, ie, muscles, ligaments, nerves. Additionally, the primary function of the tissues involved should be understood and kept in mind: joints move freely, muscles contract, ligaments check motion, and nerves conduct impulses. All this should occur painlessly. Ask yourself if you think you are dealing with problems of the locomotor system's "hardware" (bones, joints) or "software" (soft tissues).

Is the lesion organic or mechanical in nature? Is an active inflammation or pathology causing the patient's symptoms? Are there signs and symptoms of systemic disease? How and when did the condition start? What makes it feel better or worse? Where is the pain located? Is the pain referred, radicular, myofascial, or articular? How do postures, movements, rest, and time modulate pain? A mental appraisal should be made of the possible structures that can cause pain locally as well as structures that are distant and can refer pain to the region in question.

In addition to information regarding the patient's presenting concern, questions should be asked about past medical history, and a systems re-

---

Exhibit 3–1 Providing Proper Atmosphere for the History

- *Empathy:* Try to enter the patient's world.
- *Congruency:* Your thoughts and actions must correlate.
- *Positive Regard:* Acknowledge the patient as another person.

view should be performed. Any prior treatment and its efficacy should also be asked about. The patient's occupation should be taken into account, as well as recreational activities. Let us now look more closely at these questions.

Mechanical Versus Organic Lesion?

An important question to keep in mind during the history and throughout the physical examination is whether the patient's presenting problem is organic or mechanical. Most of the time, this question can be answered by the history alone. Obviously, we must know and be familiar with what we are listening for. The following case history illustrates the presentation of an organic disease masquerading as a back problem:

Case History 5

A 68-year-old man presented with coccyx pain of 3 months' duration. He admitted that he had fallen 6 months earlier, but stated that it was his hip that had hurt him then. He said his pain was different now. He described his pain as vague in location, deep, and almost inside his tailbone. He pointed to the tip of his coccyx. Nothing he did seemed to aggravate or alleviate his pain. He stated that it felt sore and achy and was always there. Neither lying down, movements, nor postures could alter his symptom. He denied bowel or bladder problems, yet said he was prone to anal fissures with rectal bleeding. Reproduction of pain could not be accomplished during the examination, which included firm pressures directly on the coccyx and around the area the patient was pointing to.

Questions for Thought

- What things make you think of an organic etiology?
- What is the significance of this patient's age?
- How is his pain description suspect for a nonmechanical lesion?
- What structures can create pain in this particular location?
- Why do you think his coccyx hurt him but direct pressures on it during the examination did not?
- What makes the prior sacroiliac joint case history sound more mechanical in etiology than this one?

One can gain insight as to whether a lesion is mechanical or organic by asking how the pain reacts to rest and movement (Exhibit 3–2). Rest alleviates and movement exacerbates mechanical lesions of musculoskeletal origin. It is important to ascertain which movements in particular increase the patient's pain. Pain that is not relieved by rest or altered by posture or

Exhibit 3–2 Mechanical Versus Organic Lesion

	Mechanical	*Organic*
Rest	Decreased pain	No change/increased
Movement	Increased pain	No change

movements is suspect for organic or inflammatory etiology, as is the case in the above example. Pain that is deep and poorly localized usually comes from deeper tissues or is referred from some other structures. As in this case history, if pain provocation cannot be achieved on examination, suspicion should be raised as to the lesion's etiology. It is most likely referred pain from a distant structure or pain arising from a deeper tissue rather than being of local origin. The above patient was referred for diagnostic workup to rule out organic disease. A digital rectal examination was negative, but upon anoscopic visualization of the rectal mucosa, a raw-looking lesion was biopsied that later proved to be cancerous. Another red flag in the history was that the patient was over 50 years old, an age group in which cancer and organic disease are more prevalent.

Onset of Pain?

Pain can be of recent onset or long-standing. It can be or not be associated with trauma. Trauma can affect any of the tissues listed in Exhibit 3–3 and can have extrinsic or intrinsic causes. Extrinsic trauma is the more commonly recognized trauma and entails an externally delivered force causing injury to the body. However, just as important, a person can become injured or trigger a dysfunctional response via intrinsic trauma to the locomotor system with an unguarded movement. Often a patient is unable to offer a mechanism of injury to explain his or her pain from this type of trauma. This can be frustrating for the patient as well as embarrassing because it raises fears of being viewed as a malingerer or hypochondriac. The experienced clinician recognizes the ease with which musculoskeletal structures can become painful and dysfunctional. Mennell says of intrinsic trauma that "an unguarded movement superimposed on a joint that is going through a normal voluntary movement can and does produce painful dysfunction and must be appreciated before anyone can look at manipulative techniques in diagnosis and treatment with an open mind."[16(p167)] At times, the intrinsic trauma is subtle, not obvious to the doctor or patient, yet can manifest itself with very outstanding symptoms. Nevertheless, a thorough history taken with deliberate listening can often

Exhibit 3–3 Tissues of Musculoskeletal System and Pathologies That Affect Them

Tissue	Pathology
Bone/periosteum	Trauma
Hyaline cartilage	Inflammation
Synovial capsule	Metabolic disease
Ligaments	Neoplasia
Muscles/tendons/sheaths	Congenital
Intra-articular menisci	
Bursae	

incriminate an awkward or unguarded movement that is associated with the pain.

Listening to a patient's descriptive explanation of his or her pain onset can be revealing. The statement that "I felt a catch in my back" or "my back locked up" is suggestive of joint dysfunction. The same can be said of a "pop" sound emanating from the vicinity of the sacroiliac joint during stooping or lifting. Persistent clicking can indicate hypermobility. A pulling or tearing sensation occurring while lifting an object implies muscle injury.

Often the pain onset is delayed and is not coincident with the related act causing the pain. This makes it hard for patients to make the association between the mechanism of injury and the pain. However, they usually make the following remarks: "This may sound silly, but do you think it could be from…?" or "I don't know if this means anything, but…." These statements are usually followed by astute observations by the patient that may sound erroneous to the uninitiated but make good sense to the experienced clinician used to dealing with the many faces of clinical presentations.

Insidious onset suggests organic disease, but joint and muscle dysfunctions can occur without any apparent cause. It is a common frustration of patients to be unable to relate a mechanism of injury to their pains. Recent pregnancy is often associated with pelvic joint dysfunction. The predominant posture that individuals assume during the day may play an important role in their pain. Periods of extreme psychological duress commonly trigger latent muscle and joint dysfunctions. Nontraumatic acute onset of joint pain often heralds the existence of an inflammatory process, such as gout or rheumatoid arthritis. Chronic pain of insidious onset with a progressive and unrelenting nature is often ominous.

Night Pain?

Night pain is commonly, although not invariably, associated with neo-plasia and inflammatory conditions. Patients with bone tumors commonly state that they sleep best while upright in a chair, since their pain worsens shortly after they become recumbent.

However, patients with mechanical lesions can be painfully awakened from sleep upon rolling over or changing positions at night. It is best to ask, then, if movement during their sleep hurts them or if the pain itself wakes them up. Myofascial trigger points in the gluteus medius and minimus muscles can become active in the side-lying posture, making sleep difficult. Recumbency affords relief from gravity's compressive forces but induces translational forces that affect the musculoskeletal structures differently. Ligamentous pain from nocturnal postural over-load can result, especially in tissues that are already biomechanically com-promised or inflamed. However, this pain starts bothering patients after they have been recumbent for awhile. Patients with inflammatory condi-tions usually feel stiffer after a period of rest.

Morning Stiffness?

Patients with spondyloarthropathy typically have a hard time early in the morning, awakening with stiffness and pain. This may take several hours to diminish. At times they cannot wait to get out of bed because of the ache that plagues them. Chronic diarrhea and sacroiliac pain, espe-cially if bilateral, should alert one to investigate for inflammatory bowel disease and associated sacroiliitis. Abdominal pain, fever, and weight loss are other associated symptoms in inflammatory bowel disease. Osteoar-thritis usually presents with morning stiffness in the lower back or hips, but unlike spondyloarthropathy, it typically diminishes after a short while, usually 30 minutes, once the patient is up and about.

Continued Symptoms and Compensatory Reactions?

When listening to patients with pelvic joint or muscle disorders, it is important to remember how the body tends to compensate for its prob-lems. As mentioned in Chapter 2, compensatory reactions resulting from or causing pelvic joint disorders can confuse the clinical picture. A hint that the clinician is dealing with a compensation rather than a primary biomechanical fault is the recurrence of the compensatory reaction after seemingly appropriate treatment. The body also tends to adapt with compensatory reactions when a joint or muscle problem is of long standing. Another possibility is that prior treatment was aimed at the site of referred pain and not the problem itself. Lack of improvement, therefore, demands continued and astute assessment for remote conditions causing continued painful compensatory reactions.

Fever and/or Weight Loss?

The presence of systemic signs of disease should be asked about, including fever, nausea, weight loss, and fatigue. Infectious and neoplastic disease should be suspected and ruled out.

Visceral Disease?

Questions directed toward function of the genitourinary or gastrointestinal systems must be asked, since lower back pain can be caused by disease involving them. Colicky pain incriminates a hollow viscus. Flank pain radiating to the groin and genitals signifies kidney and ureteral disease. Frequency of urination with nocturia, frequency and ineffectual urge to urinate along with perineal, rectal, and/or sacral pain indicate prostate disease. Monthly back pain in women associated with their menstrual cycle can be from dysmenorrhea or endometriosis.

Occupation? Posture?

Inquiry into the individual's occupation and its related demands should include questions on sustained postures, repetitive movements, exertional activities, and even job satisfaction and stress. Prolonged periods of sitting place the pelvic and hip joints at risk for dysfunction. A painful crisis is often precipitated after a period of prolonged posturing, either sitting or standing. As stated in Chapter 2, a pelvis that is unable to adapt dynamically to changes in posture will ultimately reveal itself with pain and dysfunction. This usually occurs after prolonged postural abuse. Patients should also be questioned as to the age and quality of their mattresses. Patients sleeping with poor mattress support typically awaken with a stiff and sore back that gradually loosens up after an hour of being up and about. A mattress that is too firm can be just as bad as one that sags.

Pain Location and Character?

Anyone experienced with treating musculoskeletal lesions using manual methods is very aware of the regularity with which the locomotor system manifests its problems in peculiar and mutable ways. Textbook presentations are almost an exception rather than the rule. Joint and soft tissue dysfunctions are not "aware" of the appropriateness of a classic presentation. This is especially so for patients' descriptions of pain, complete with their local and referred patterns. Owing to segmental overlap, pain superimposition from dissimilar tissues, and the overlapping territories of dermatomes, sclerotomes, and myotomes, one cannot diagnose the level of lesion with great confidence by virtue of knowing the pain pattern alone. The situation gains more perplexity when one considers that soft tissue and bony anomalies are common, especially around the pelvis, that post- and prefixed plexuses occur, and that dermatomal territories are neurophysiologic entities that change size depending on cord facilitation.[17]

Pain production and its perception are in-depth topics, and such a discourse is outside the scope of this book. However, the clinician must fully be aware of pain and its referring tendencies to understand the sundry clinical presentations that are possible. A painful lesion is not concerned with our concepts and theories of how it ought to present clinically. Rigid thinking about how pain patterns ought to be, and clinging to the security of what is known or thought to be known in this regard aid in classifying a pain presentation under a presumed diagnosis, but do not help practitioners to look objectively at the evidence before them. Knowing a person's pain pattern will get one in the "ballpark," but a more exacting assessment is needed to "play the game."

Pain and referred pain from either neural or non-neural tissues are peculiarities of the central nervous system. It is known that pain can be experienced in a limb that no longer exists (so-called phantom limb pain) and in an area that has been anesthetized.[18] Harman[19] showed how saline injections into paraspinal ligaments caused referred pain to be experienced in amputees as if the phantom limb were still intact. From the above, it can be seen that pain does not inhabit the very tissues or locale where it is felt. It is a neurophysiologic phenomenon that is "all in the head," occurring centrally.

The skin, deep tissues, and viscera are the three main groups of pain-sensitive structures encountered clinically (Figure 3–8). Lesions of the deep tissues and viscera account for most of the clinically relevant pain discussed here. The deep soft tissues and the superficial skin are innervated differently, with the latter receiving numerous receptors for localization purposes and the former being sparsely populated in that regard. The pain-sensing function of the skin must be able to locate accurately any offending stimulus in order to initiate the appropriate withdrawal mechanisms effectively. Therefore, increased nociceptor density and rapid conduction velocities predominate in the neurophysiologic organization of the skin.

Nociception from deep tissues differs, probably due to different survival priorities. Where reflex withdrawal from a painful stimulus is impractical in addition to being impossible, immobilization from nociceptive input seems to be the rule, and reflexogenic muscle spasm is used. Accurate stimulus localization and rapid conduction of stimulus information are not critical. Hence, a patient is less apt to localize accurately a lesion in the deep somatic tissues, notably joints and related soft tissues, than a more superficial lesion. This is evidenced by a patient's roughly designating the area of pain using the whole hand, in contrast to a discriminating pointing finger.

Whereas pain from skin and superficial lesions is sharp and well localized, that from deep somatic tissues is dull, achy, and diffuse. The achy articular pain of osteoarthritis is a prime example. The deep somatic tissues include articulations and their related soft tissues, ie, capsules and ligaments. Joint capsules and ligaments are richly supplied with nociceptors, especially the former. Extremes in a joint's range of motion and intense pressure will stress these structures and incite pain from them

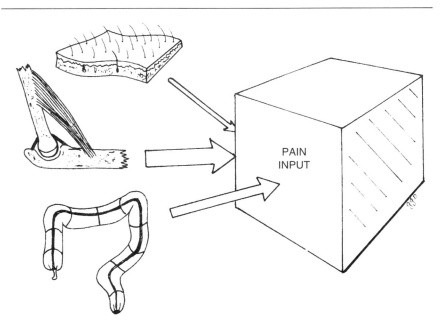

Figure 3–8 Three Main Sources of Pain Input: Skin, Tissues, and Viscera

if they are involved. Interestingly, Floyd et al[20] and Iggo et al[21] have shown that inflamed joints require only slight movements well within the normal range of motion and minimal pressures to instigate pain responses.

Generally, different types of pain are perceived when dissimilar musculoskeletal tissues are injured, yet more often than not, a generic presentation is seen for a variety of tissues and sites of lesion. For example, just as the deltoid region is a generic referral site for problems in the lower cervical spine, glenohumeral joint, myofascial trigger points, bursitis, and even thoracic viscera, the hip area seems to be a similar district for referred pain from the thoracolumbar spine, lumbar spine, sacroiliac joints, hip joint, trigger points, bursitis, and pelvic viscera (Figure 3–9).

Referred Pain?

That pain from deep somatic tissues is frequently experienced at a distance far removed from the site of tissue irritation is well known but not commonly recognized. Painful sites continue to be massaged, manipulated, stimulated with physical therapy modalities, injected, iced, and heated, even though the pain may be referred from some other site. Consequently, these therapeutic modalities may either temporarily relieve or be ineffective in reducing the pain. It behooves us to understand and appreci-

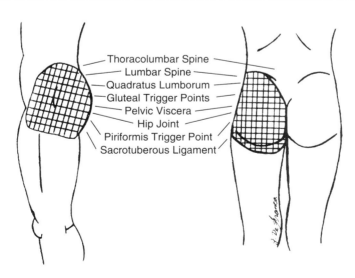

Figure 3–9 Generic Site of Pain Referral to the Hip Region

ate the referral of pain from deep somatic tissues, since these structures are very commonly affected by dysfunction and injury, eliciting painful syndromes that cause patients to seek our help.

Referred pain in this instance pertains to pain perceived at a site different from the site of non-neural tissue irritation. Irritation of neural tissue, in particular nerve roots, displays itself in the form of "root" or radicular pain. However, referred pain from non-neural tissues occurs twice as commonly as radicular pain.[8] The confusion comes from not realizing that pain can be referred or projected from non-neural and neural tissues alike and that referred pain does not always imply nerve irritation from mechanical deformation by anatomical structures, the so-called "pinched-nerve" syndrome. On the contrary, evidence now suggests that abnormal neurophysiology is more likely to be the culprit in referred pain.[1]

Dermatomes are territories of skin representing nerve segmental levels (Figure 3–10). In comparison, sclerotomes represent the segmental nerve supply to the deep soft tissues and bone, and myotomes represent the segmental nerve level to muscles. Referred pain from deep non-neural soft tissues, usually referred to as *sclerotomic*, is usually described as deep, dull, achy, and diffuse and can be accompanied by autonomic concomitants, ie, sweating, pallor, nausea, bradycardia, and hypotension.[18] Patients commonly use the descriptive term *toothache* when addressing such pain. Referred pain from low back, pelvic, and hip structures commonly travels into the lower extremity, usually staying above the knee. More distal radiation can occur, but this is more common in nerve root lesions.

Distant pain referral from non-neural tissue stimulation has been demonstrated by various investigators. This referred pain is a result of irritated nerve endings in injured or dysfunctional tissues projecting nociception centrally, where it is interpreted as coming from some other site. In 1938, Kellgren[22] injected hypertonic saline solution into muscle tissue and observed referred pain phenomena. Six years later, Inman and Saunders[23] and Campbell and Parsons[24] investigated referred pain responses from non-neural structures and also demonstrated distant pain referral. In 1954, Feinstein et al[25] injected hypertonic saline solution into the interspinous tissues and observed segmentally arranged patterns of referred pain differing from dermatomes. These nondermatomal territories were termed *sclerotomes* and in some instances differed considerably from dermatomal distribution (Figures 3–11 and 3–12). Hockaday and Whitty[26] in 1967, and McCall et al[27] in 1979, commented on the variability of these referred pain patterns. McCall et al[27] showed how injection of both intracapsular and extracapsular structures of the upper and lower lumbar segments demon-

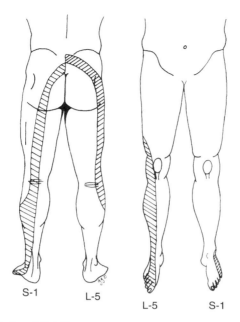

S-1   L-5

L-5   S-1

Figure 3–10 L-5 and S-1 Dermatomes

strated overlap of the referred pain patterns, especially over the iliac crest and inguinal regions.

Injection of the lumbar facet joints themselves has been shown to cause low back and referred leg pain[28,29] and other investigators are of the opinion that facet joints are capable of causing referred leg pain in addition to low back pain.[30–32] The sacroiliac joint has been known to refer pain to the posterior thigh, groin, calf, and even foot.[8–11] Grieve[1] refers to Kellgren's[33] observation of pain radiating to the heel after saline injection of the sacroiliac joint. According to Bourdillion and Day, "It is reasonable to suggest that on confronting a patient in severe pain of sciatic distribution, the first thought should be 'sacroiliac' not 'disc,' even if only because of the statistical probability."[34(p230)]

Dvorak and Dvorak[35] cite references describing pain referred to the lower abdomen and inner proximal thighs after infiltration of the pubic symphysis with an irritant. Pain referred to the groin, testicles, and lower abdomen can be a feature in lumbar and sacroiliac joint problems, but organic pathology needs to be ruled out. Baer[36] describes a painful abdomi-

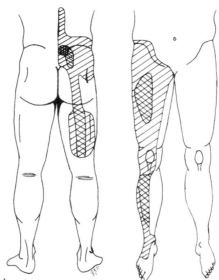

Figure 3–11 L-5 Sclerotome

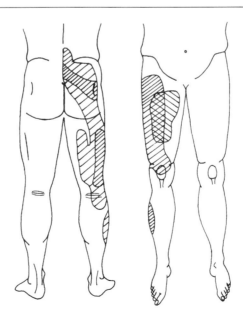

Figure 3–12 S-1 Sclerotome

nal point associated at times with sacroiliac joint lesions (see Chapter 1, Figure 1–34). Named after him, it is located just lateral to and below the umbilicus. Bourdillion and Day describe it as being "in the right iliac fossa just medial to McBurney's appendix point."[34(p20)] Pain in and around the sacroiliac joint region is not invariably sacroiliac in origin. Maigne[37] describes how thoracolumbar joint dysfunction caused pain in the lumbosacral, sacroiliac, and iliac crest areas in 40% of a group of low back pain patients. Manipulation of the thoracolumbar region alleviated the lower back pain.

Tenderness, or augmented sensitivity to palpation of the skin, subcutaneous tissues, or deep tissues, is commonly referred, either locally or at great distances, in response to lumbar and pelvic locomotor dysfunctions. It represents a type of referred pain. As mentioned before, painful periosteal points at the posterior and anterior superior iliac spines, greater trochanters, and fibular heads are common sites of referred tenderness that often respond immediately to manipulation of proximal spinal and pelvic segments.[35,38] Muscles sharing the same segmental innervation of the involved segment often palpate as tender.

Cutaneous zones of secondary hyperalgesia are seen in skin sites sharing the same segmental innervation as irritated viscera. Head[39] carefully mapped these zones (Head's zones) in patients suffering from various visceral diseases. These zones approximate dermatomal territories, extend around the trunk and into the extremities, and can be objectively observed. They roughly overlap the areas of referred pain from viscera.

Visceral pain can be referred to the lower back and pelvis (Figure 3–13). Viscerogenic referred pain tends to have a periodicity to it, although not invariably. A hollow viscus that is attempting to expel its contents under pressure creates pain that quickly rises in 20 to 30 seconds, has a duration of 1 to 2 minutes, and recedes only to recur again in minutes.[40] Back and leg pains are rarely the only symptoms of visceral disease. Manifestations of visceral dysfunction are usually apparent; however, it is important to keep in mind that visceral disease can masquerade as low back and pelvic joint disorders.

As can be seen, the body's response to a painful stimulus is complex, since the nervous system mediates a variety of responses involving multiple tissues. This is manifested by subtle changes observable in the different tissues innervated by the segment involved. Lewit[38] mentions how a painful stimulus causes reactions in the various tissue served by the related segment in the form of cutaneous hyperalgesic zones, muscle spasms, painful periosteal points, joint dysfunction, and possibly some level of organ dysfunction. In other words, the tissues served by the same

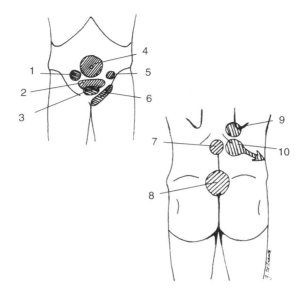

Figure 3–13 Visceral pain referral patterns. **(1)** Appendix, **(2)** large bowel, **(3)** urinary bladder, **(4)** small bowel, **(5)** ovary, **(6)** ureter, **(7)** pancreas, **(8)** uterus, rectum, prostate, **(9)** gallbladder, **(10)** kidney.

neurologic "circuit" as the involved segment will experience reflexogenic effects on some level.

Radicular Pain?

Radicular or "root" pain is a type of referred pain consequent to nerve root irritation. Radicular pain is described as shooting, lancinating, burning, sharp, and even sickening. It is more easily localized by the patient as compared to referred pain from deep somatic tissues. See Exhibit 3–4 for a comparison of radicular and referred pain from non-neural tissues. At times radicular pain comes on after a delay of several seconds following movement of a vertebral segment, akin to shaking a hornet's nest and witnessing the buzzing storm shortly after. It is usually more severe distally in the limb. Its course typically coincides with the nerve root's distribution, ie, the sciatic nerve in the posterior aspect of the thigh and leg. However, it is not always a continuous line of pain from proximal to distal. A shooting, traveling sensation accompanying coughing, sneezing, and a Valsalva maneuver is commonly associated with root involvement. How-

Exhibit 3–4 Non-Neural Versus Neural Referred Pain

Non-Neural	*Neural*
Dull, achy	Sharp, lancinating
Diffuse	Able to locate
Can be posterolateral	Usually pain along nerve
No sensory loss	Can have sensory loss
No motor loss	Can have motor loss
No reflex loss	Can have reflex loss
No nerve tension signs	Nerve tension signs

ever, these procedures transmit forces that stress joints and deep somatic tissues, including the sacroiliac joints, especially if they are inflamed. In addition, venous pressure is increased by coughing, leading to engorgement and possible nociceptor stimulation.

Interestingly, some investigators have observed that direct nerve root pressure is not painful and that only when an existing inflammation is present does pain occur with compression.[41–43] Grieve[1] references Triano and Luttges,[44] who point out that (1) severe nerve pain is not invariably due to nerve root compression, irritation, or inflammation; (2) root trespass causing referred pain is not necessarily severe; and (3) somatic nerve root compression need not be painful, and the same can be said for proven bony or soft tissue trespass.

Leg pain with low back pain usually leads to the mistaken conclusion that nerve root compression is at fault. Actually, most leg pain syndromes are referred and not radicular in etiology as was shown by a study involving over 1200 low back pain cases.[7] O'Brien[45] states that nerve root compression accounts for less than 10% of the total problem. In discussing sacroiliac pain referral, nerve root compression is not a viable etiology due to the anatomical relationship between the joint and the nerve roots.[46] This fact, combined with the unappreciated phenomenon of referred pain from non-neural tissues, has led orthodox practitioners to overlook the sacroiliac joint as causing low back and leg pain.

To further confuse the situation, radicular and referred pain syndromes can coexist. Radicular lesions usually manifest with neurologic signs of involvement, such as hypesthesia, hyporeflexia, and myoparesis to some degree. Nerve tension signs, eg, a positive straight-leg–raising test, are commonly present and help to differentiate neural from non-neural referred pain. Leg pain associated with "hard neurological" signs of loss leads one to suspect radicular involvement; otherwise, the pain may be referred from non-neural tissues.

CLUES IN THE HISTORY TO THE TYPES OF TISSUES INJURED

In listening to our patients' histories, certain clues can lead us to suspect a particular type of lesion, although we should bear in mind that it is more important for therapeutic and assessment purposes to ascertain how postures, movements, rest, and time modulate pain.

Mennell[16] discusses seven anatomical structures occurring in the musculoskeletal system and cross-matches them with five possible pathological changes that can affect them (Exhibit 3–3). This results in 35 possible diagnoses to consider (7 anatomical structures × 5 pathological changes = 35 possible diagnoses). In reality, the 5 pathological processes do not usually affect all 7 anatomical structures, and Mennell states that a more realistic figure of possible diagnoses is 23. Admittedly, this is not an all-inclusive method, but by cross-matching the anatomical structures with the possible pathological changes that can affect them, an organized approach to a diagnosis can be made. Often, clues in the history arise that incriminate certain tissues more.

Hyaline Cartilage, Menisci, Synovial Membrane

Most patients consult a clinician due to pain. However, on pain response alone, one can rule out hyaline cartilage, intra-articular menisci, and synovial membrane as primary etiologies, since they are devoid of pain fibers. Intra-articular menisci and bursae occur only in select parts of the body, and knowledge of the precise location will aid in incriminating them as painful offenders. Intra-articular menisci are not found in the pelvic region but are found only in the temperomandibular joint, the ulnomeniscotriquetral joint at the wrist, occasionally the radiohumeral joint at the elbow, the knee joint, and the sternoclavicular joint. The pelvic region is also devoid of tendon sheaths, structures occurring at the wrists and ankles.

Even though hyaline cartilage is incapable of producing pain in and of itself, the complaint of a "grinding" noise, known clinically as *crepitus*, can indicate the degree of articular cartilage wear. A fine sandpaper gritting sound connotes minimal attrition, whereas coarse crepitus denotes advanced changes. This is usually not a typical feature in the history of a patient with pelvic joint dysfunction, let alone hip problems, but is more commonly seen in advanced coxarthrosis.

The synovium reacts to injury by secreting synovial fluid. It is only a few cells thick and is devoid of nociceptors. However, pain fibers are found nearby between the synovium and capsule. Synovitis causes a slow swelling over a period of hours, and the patient typically comments on noticing the joint swelling or pain the next day. On the other hand, hemarthrosis creates pain and swelling in minutes due to the higher-pressure arterial system's hemorrhaging into the joint. Hence, the time of onset of joint swelling and pain can lead the practitioner to suspect either synovitis or hemarthrosis.

Bursae

Bursae do occur in and around various pelvic structures. Bursitis is rarely a primary condition and is more commonly a reaction to some other problem. It can also be a harbinger of systemic disease of the collagen-vascular type. Commonly, true bursal involvement causes considerable tenderness, swelling, warmth, and possibly discoloration in a known anatomical location of a bursa. Most movements are arrested, and direct pressure hurts. The painful locale and swelling must coincide with the known anatomic location of a bursa for the practitioner to entertain a diagnosis of bursitis. This may seem to be an obvious point, but the bursa is a commonly incriminated structure because of the practitioner's willingness to please the patient with a diagnosis. So, too, the diagnosis of arthritis, another vague and useless descriptor. Referred pain from trigger points in the quadratus lumborum and gluteus minimus and lumbar and sacroiliac joint problems commonly masquerade as trochanteric or ischial bursitis to the uninitiated by virtue of their pain distribution.

Common sites for bursitis about the pelvis are the greater trochanter, ischial tuberosity, and psoas tendon anterior to the hip joint (Figure 3–14). Other bursal locations exist and can potentially be a site for bursitis (Exhibit 3–5). A history lacking direct trauma or overuse as possible etiologies in bursitis should alert the clinician to the likelihood of a collagen-vascular disorder or gout.

Bone, Periosteum

Bone tissue itself is insensitive to pain, but the periosteum and endosteum are pain sensitive. The periosteum is very sensitive to pain and is usually injured directly, ie, by direct trauma, fracture, or sustained pressure. The pain is sharp and intense, as anyone who bangs his bare shin on a low coffee table knows. A history devoid of traumatic etiology should lead to a suspicion of pathology. A space-occupying lesion or pressure-building infection within bone creates a deep, boring endosteal pain that is progressive and sometimes throbbing in nature. Night pain and resting pain are ominous symptoms usually associated with pathology.

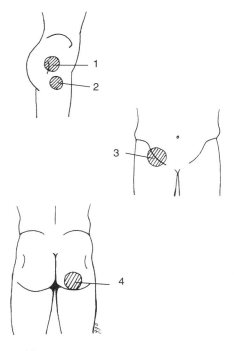

Figure 3–14 Sites of bursitis around the hip. **(1)** Trochanteric bursa, **(2)** gluteofemoral bursa between gluteus maximus and vastus lateralis, **(3)** iliopectineal bursa under the psoas major tendon, **(4)** ischial bursa. See also Exhibit 3–5.

More commonly, bony insertion sites are described as sore or as having a "bruised" feeling. Patients often describe such sensations occurring at their spinous processes, posterior superior iliac spine, greater trochanter, and bony rim of the iliac crest. This is frequently a referred tenderness phenomenon. More often, patients are aware of these painful periosteal points only when they are touched. Interestingly, some painful periosteal points are representative of certain joint or muscle problems. For example, the fibular head is often painful in short, tense hamstrings. The pubic tubercle is often painful in pubic symphysis, sacroiliac joint, and hip adductor muscle problems. The iliac crest is usually tender with thoracolumbar joint dysfunction and quadratus lumborum and gluteal muscle problems. Hip joint problems are associated with a painful greater trochanter. The posterior superior iliac spine is often tender in a number of problems and is not specific for any.

Exhibit 3–5 Lesser-Known Bursal Locations

Bursae are located between the following structures:
- gluteus medius tendon and greater trochanter
- gluteus minimus tendon and greater trochanter
- obturator externus tendon and hip joint capsule
- obturator internus tendon and lesser sciatic notch
- quadratus femoris tendon and lesser trochanter

Joint Capsules

Joint capsules are very sensitive to pain and, if they lie deep to the body surface, yield a dull, achy articular discomfort often associated with referred pain phenomena. The same can be said for the deep periarticular ligaments. Pain is elicited by motion stretching the capsule, ie, close-packing movements, or specific movements performed to place maximum tension in isolated ligaments. Sustained stress applied to ligaments is often associated with a burning discomfort after a latent period of up to 30 seconds. This is usually encountered in hypermobility states and situations of postural overload.

Muscle

Muscle is made up of three types of tissue: fleshy belly, tendon, and fascia. Certain locations in the body entail tendon sheaths as an added component to the musculotendinous unit. However, these are not found in and around the pelvis and hip regions. Kellgren[22] noted that fascial pain induced by hypertonic saline injections was described as sharply localized, whereas pain from muscle injection was diffuse and tended to refer in apparent spinal segmental patterns different from the segmental innervation of the skin. Grieve[47] mentions that an "oppressive weary ache" is usually an attribute of limb and vertebral muscle pains seemingly secondary to spinal joint problems. Muscle lesions are usually associated with overload, sudden pulls, sustained activities, or direct trauma. Patients may state they felt something "tear" or "pull." Contracting or stretching the muscle with various movements hurts. Postexercise soreness is also a common complaint, usually worse the second day after the activity.

Muscles act as loyal, ever-obedient servants of the nervous system, the master that governs their every action. Their response to injury and dysfunction is reflex, a response to the nervous system's directives. Muscle spasm is generally thought to be painful, yet it is commonplace to locate clinically muscle spasm that is not. Barring direct trauma, referred tenderness, or referred pain, muscle spasm is usually experienced as tightness and not as pain. Reflex muscle spasm in response to joint or deep somatic tissue trauma is protective in nature, and some investigators feel it has little to do with pain.[48]

Myofascial pain is an important and common cause of discomfort arising from the musculoskeletal system. Travell and Simons' myofascial trigger points typically refer pain distally from the involved trigger point. The pain is usually experienced as deep, dull, and achy and does not follow a simple segmental pattern.[49] The referred pain does not invariably follow dermatomal, myotomal, or sclerotomal distributions. It is referred in specific patterns peculiar to each muscle. For example, the gluteus minimus muscle refers pain down the lateral or posterior thigh and leg, mimicking a radicular problem (Figure 3–15).

Myofascial pain can occur with rest or motion. Many times, patients are aware only of the referred pain and not of the location of the inciting trig-

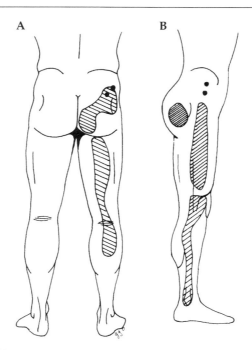

Figure 3–15 Gluteus minimus trigger point pain referral pattern. **(A)** Posterior portion of muscle. **(B)** Anterior portion.

ger point. The important point is that trigger points regularly refer pain in patterns characteristic for each muscle and that this can be, and often is, at a distance from the trigger point.

Nerve Root

Sharp, lancinating pain is usually associated with nerve involvement. So-called "root" pain is described as severe, sickening in nature, tending to follow a nerve root distribution, and usually worse distally in the limb. Tingling and numbness may also indicate a possible nerve involvement. See the previous section "Radicular Pain."

Joints

Joints themselves may pop or click. Hypermobility of the pelvic and hip joints is commonly associated with clicking, and patients will comment on a "clunking" noise while walking or getting in and out of a chair. The noise is often painless. A snapping noise about the lateral hip is indicative of a "snapping-hip" syndrome, in which the iliotibial band snaps over the greater trochanter. Joint pain from joint dysfunction is usually sharp and occurs with movement. Rest alleviates the pain, and swelling is typically not a feature. It is often seen in joints after trauma and immobilization. Mennell[16] believes that some of the pain of arthritis is due to joint dysfunction.

Unilateral pain presentation is characteristic of joint dysfunction unless multiple trauma has occurred. Bilateral symptoms, ie, in both sacroiliac joints, without a history of trauma, is more indicative of inflammatory disease, and further questioning as to diarrhea, fever, and other symptoms of systemic disease should be asked.

DIFFERENTIAL DIAGNOSIS

Pain in and around the pelvic region can be caused by a myriad of conditions that demand clinical differentiation. The clinician should possess a framework of differential diagnoses in his or her mind from which to work. When a patient presents with lower back, buttock, and thigh pain, the clinician must decide whether the condition is a mechanical/locomotor condition or an organic/medical disease.

When attempting to diagnose a particular problem, the clinician should attempt to relate the symptom or symptoms to the known principles of anatomy, histology, and physiology. Take, for instance, the following case history:

Case History 6

A 38-year-old woman presented with left lower back pain after lifting her 3-year-old daughter. The pain was located just medial to the posterior superior iliac spine and was of a sharp, jabbing nature. She said she heard and felt a pop sound when she stooped down. The pain radiated into the buttock, felt achy, and was deep and hard to localize exactly. It ached and made her back stiffen with rest for the first 2 days, and moving around at first relieved her. Afterward, rest made it feel better and was not accompanied by stiffness, but bending, getting in and out of her car, and climbing stairs hurt her. She admitted to sleeping well, except for the first night. She admitted to no sphincter problems or bowel or bladder changes (Figure 3–16).

First, looking at the history, the clinician should get an overall feel for the case and summarize it. For instance, the complaint summarized above sounds mechanical in etiology and nature. It seems to be attributable to a lifting injury, alleviates with rest, and worsens with movement.

Next, by visualizing the anatomy in the area, the clinician should attempt to formulate the possible structures involved that could cause the

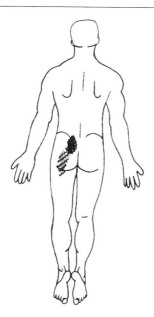

Figure 3–16 Case History 6

patient's symptoms. In addition to the local structures, any tissue, even if remotely distant, that can refer pain into the area in question needs to be considered. In reference to the above example, a number of structures beside the sacroiliac joint can refer pain medial to the posterior superior iliac spine. Lumbar and thoracolumbar facet joints, erector spinae and quadratus lumborum myofascial trigger points, and pelvic viscera are just a few examples.

By visualizing the anatomy in layers going from the outside inward, one can mentally question a list of possible structures. The first layer of anatomy at the pain site includes the skin and subcutaneous structures. Is this referred tenderness, a case of shingles that is pre-eruptive, or a painful lipoma? The next layer is the fascia and superficial muscles. Is this myofascitis or a strain? The next layer is the deeper muscles, ligaments, nerves, and articulations. Is there evidence of deeper myofascial pain, muscle strain, ligament sprain, joint dysfunction, or radicular involvement? Still deeper is the vertebral or pelvic bone involved. Is the pain from osteomyelitis, neoplasia, or fracture? Going still deeper are visceral structures, including the vasculature. Is there visceral disease or vascular compromise that can account for this pain?

As the list of tissues is compiled, the pathologies possibly affecting them should be considered. Does the etiology involve trauma, inflammation, neoplasia, metabolic disease, or functional loss? For example, in this case history the presence of tissue inflammation is suspected by the occurrence of stiffening with rest occurring in the first 2 days. However, as the patient's inflammation subsided, rest afforded her more relief and movements caused her more of a problem, suggesting a mechanical dysfunction.

Once the anatomical structures affected are compiled and are crossmatched with the possible pathologies affecting them, a differential list of diagnoses can be made. The last step is to use the history and physical examination to rule in or out any of the possibilities compiled on the diagnosis list. Examination of the patient in the above case history revealed sacroiliac joint dysfunction, and she resolved completely with manual treatment directed at that joint.

The clinician confronted with lower back pain should first rule out severe disease. Although rare, an emergent medical condition to rule out first when dealing with lower back pain is the cauda equina compression syndrome. Patients should be suspected of having this if they present with back pain, bilateral lower extremity weakness, and bilateral leg pain and numbness, along with saddle paresthesia and loss of sphincter control. If they are suspected of having this condition, an immediate myelogram and, if positive, surgical decompression should be performed, since permanent neurologic loss is imminent.

Next, the presence of organic disease should be ruled out. According to Borenstein and Weisel,[40] patients with medical disease causing their low back pain usually present with symptoms belonging to one of the following groups:

- fever and/or weight loss
- pain at night
- morning stiffness
- acute, localized bone pain from fracture or bone expansion
- visceral pain

Patients belonging to any of the above groups need to be assessed medically for organic disease.

Several categories of etiologies should be foremost in the clinician's mind when he or she confronts a patient with pain in the lower back, pelvic region, and lower extremities. The following categories are only a few that can be used to organize one's thinking process and are adapted from Borenstein and Weisel[40]:

- mechanical
- rheumatologic
- infectious
- neoplastic
- vascular
- visceral
- metabolic/endocrine
- psychologic

Mechanical

Fortunately, mechanical etiologies of back pain are more common than other etiologies. However, they tend to cause pain in similar areas, and a functional physical examination needs to be performed to differentiate among the various conditions. The more common mechanical disorders will be differentiated.

Sacroiliac joint disorders cause pain unilaterally that can extend into the lower extremity, but so do lumbar facet and disc lesions. However, whereas getting in and out of a chair bothers a patient with either a sacroiliac joint dysfunction or a disc syndrome, the act of sitting itself will bother a disc patient more. Coughing, sneezing, and straining at the stool will exacerbate a lumbar disc condition but not a sacroiliac joint problem. Additionally, the disc patient will exhibit an antalgic posture, with much difficulty bending forward. The patient with a sacroiliac joint condition will have difficulty bending forward but can usually be coaxed to bend more than a disc patient. A patient with a lumbar facet syndrome can bend forward without too much difficulty but experiences pain with trunk extension. Additionally, rising from a forward-flexed position can cause a jab of pain ("reversal sign") with a facet syndrome. Also, whereas leg pain tends to remain above the knee in referred pain syndromes from sacroiliac or facet joint problems, it commonly radiates to below the knee in radicular pain syndromes of disc origin.

On examination, signs of neurologic loss of motor, sensory, and reflex functions and nerve tension signs are not present in sacroiliac or facet joint problems, whereas they are in disc conditions. The straight-leg–raising test is usually negative or mildly positive in sacroiliac and facet joint disorders, but strongly positive in disc involvement.

Thoracolumbar joint dysfunction often refers pain to the sacroiliac and buttock regions. However, a painfully restricted thoracolumbar junction with segmental muscle spasm will be evident in the absence of lower lumbar facet or sacroiliac joint signs. Nerve signs will be missing.

Hip joint problems can cause buttock and groin pain, as can sacroiliac joint disorders, but with hip joint problems, joint signs of pain, spasm, and restricted range of motion will be localized to the hip joint. Hip pain can also radiate into the anterior thigh and knee. Hip flexion with adduction will cause groin pain mostly with hip conditions.

The pubic symphysis will refer pain anteriorly to the lower abdomen and inner thighs. Recent pregnancy or prolonged hip adduction activities are commonly associated with the onset of pain. Tenderness over the pubic symphysis, pubic tubercles, and adductor insertions is present, and tension in the inguinal ligament is common.

Osteoarthritis of the lumbar spine and hip joints usually presents in older patients with morning stiffness that only lasts about 30 minutes after being up and around. Stiffness is a major feature on physical examination, and radiographs demonstrate evidence of degenerative joint disease.

In older patients with advanced osteoarthritis and bizarre lower extremity symptoms, one should think of central stenosis. Bilateral numbness, achiness, paresthesias, and weakness are common. Different parameters of neurologic function as well as levels of innervation can be affected between the two lower extremities. Neurogenic claudication can be a feature and is usually relieved by flexing the trunk, as in bending over or sitting. There are no pulse deficits or trophic changes of the lower extremities, as in vascular intermittent claudication. Claudication symptoms of neurologic origin abate more slowly after resting than those of vascular origin. Riding a bike, due to the flexed position of the trunk, is tolerated better by a patient with central stenosis causing neurogenic claudication than by one with vascular claudication. Degenerative changes causing enlarged facet joints and narrowed central canals are evident on a computed tomography (CT) scan.

Stenosis of the lateral canal will present with unilateral symptoms of buttock, thigh, and even leg and foot pain and will look like a posterior facet syndrome. Radiographic evidence of disc narrowing and facet enlargement and CT scan images of a narrowed lateral canal aid in the diagnosis.

Myofascial trigger points of the erector spinae, quadratus lumborum, glutei muscles, and piriformis can cause pain in and about the lower back, buttocks, and lower extremities. However, their pain referral patterns are specific and reproduced on finding the appropriate trigger point. These are discussed in a later chapter.

Coccyx pain often occurs with a history of direct trauma or recent pregnancy. The patient has great difficulty sitting and localizes the pain to the coccyx. Levator ani spasm is present.

Meralgia paresthetica is a nerve entrapment of the lateral femoral cutaneous nerve as it leaves the pelvis under or through the inguinal ligament. The symptoms are pain and paresthesias in the anterolateral thigh. It can be seen in obese or pregnant patients, in whom the inguinal ligament is stressed. Direct trauma to the nerve at its emergence near the anterior superior iliac spine can be a factor.

Rheumatologic

Rheumatologic disorders of importance for our discussion are the seronegative spondyloarthropathies. The characteristic symptom of severe morning stiffness that loosens up after a few hours leads one to suspect an inflammatory arthropathy. The sacroiliac joints are commonly involved, either bilaterally or unilaterally. The absence of the rheumatoid factor and an elevated erythrocyte sedimentation rate (ESR) are also characteristic. This group of inflammatory arthropathies most commonly includes ankylosing spondylitis, Reiter's syndrome, psoriatic arthritis, and enteropathic arthritis.

In ankylosing spondylitis, also known as Marie-Strümpell's disease, the sacroiliitis is usually bilateral, involves young males, and is associated with spinal stiffness. Although all the seronegative spondyloarthropathies can have an elevated HLA-B27, this occurs more commonly in ankylosing spondylitis and Reiter's disease.

Reiter's disease involves the triad of conjunctivitis, urethritis, and arthritis of the lower back and lower extremities. The sacroiliitis is usually unilateral and occurs in young males.

Psoriatic arthritis entails the characteristic psoriatic skin lesions associated with axial skeletal and upper extremity joint pains. Psoriasis usually occurs first but can occur simultaneously with or after the onset of arthritis. Onychodystrophy (onycholysis, ridging, pitting) is commonly present. It affects both males and females equally.

A history of Crohn's disease or ulcerative colitis together with lower extremity arthritis and sacroiliac pain should tip the clinician off to the possibility of enteropathic arthritis. Diarrhea, either bloody or nonbloody, with abdominal pain and cramping that are associated with low back pain, is characteristic. Both sacroiliac joints are usually involved.

Rheumatoid arthritis occurs more commonly in females and involves the cervical spine more commonly than the lower axial skeleton. A symmetric upper or lower extremity arthritis is characteristic with joint pain, redness, and swelling. The rheumatoid factor is usually present in 80% of cases.

Infection

Infection is not a common cause of lower back pain but should enter the differential diagnosis. Osteomyelitis, pyogenic sacroiliitis, and herpes zoster are examples. Fever and malaise are present but are general constitutional signs. Localized tenderness over the involved infection is present. A history of intravenous drug use or urinary tract infection should raise the suspicion of spinal infection.[50] The ESR is almost always elevated, but the white blood count may not be. X-ray findings show up later in the disease process. Definitive diagnosis is accomplished via cultured tissue aspirations.

In herpes zoster (shingles), a burning pain appearing in a segmental distribution is characteristic. Approximately 1 week after the onset of pain, the typical erythematous papular rash that develops into a vesicular rash appears. A prodrome of fever, malaise, and gastrointestinal symptoms occurs before the segmental shooting, burning pain. Difficulty in diagnosis arises when the patient presents in the pre-eruptive phase. However, recognizing the quick onset of a segmental burning pain that does not cross the midline and waiting a short period for the rash to develop will aid in the diagnosis.

Neoplasia

Neoplastic disease should be suspected in a patient with a progressive clinical course that displays night pain and with symptoms that are not relieved by rest or position. The following case history typifies a suspicious lesion:

Case History 7

A 39-year-old man presented with hip and groin pain that had been progressively getting worse over the last 3 months. No history of trauma could be recalled. The patient stated that the pain was constant and kept him up at night. He could not get into a comfortable position. The pain was described as being deep and achy. Walking was difficult. He admitted to feeling hot and tired.

Physical examination of this individual revealed an ill-appearing person displaying a limp favoring the affected limb. Hip range of motion was very painful and limited due to pain, with an empty end-feel. X-rays revealed multiple permeative lucencies throughout the femoral neck and head with extension into the proximal femoral diaphysis. Biopsy revealed a rare aggressive bone cancer. The patient died 3 months later. Needless to say, someone with back pain who has a prior history of cancer should be suspected of having metastatic disease, especially if the back pain is new and of recent onset. Deyo et al[50] comment that a previous history of cancer has a high diagnostic specificity (.98) and that such patients should be considered to have cancer until proven otherwise. However, only one third of patients with an underlying malignant neoplasm have this history.[50]

Aspects in the history that are moderately specific findings are unexplained weight loss, pain of more than 1 month duration, and failure to respond to conservative therapy.[50] Bed rest commonly does not relieve the pain of malignancy. Eighty percent of the patients diagnosed with malignant neoplasms are over the age of 50, a significant factor in the patient's history.

An elevated ESR leads one to suspect organic disease. Imaging studies aid in locating various tumors, but 30% to 50% of bone loss needs to be present before bone destruction can be evidenced by X-ray. A bone scan is a very sensitive but nonspecific test. CT scans and MRIs aid in visualizing the tumor. Definitive diagnosis is achieved through biopsy.

Multiple myeloma is the most common primary bone tumor. It often initially presents as generalized backache and osteoporosis. The classic "punched-out" lytic lesions are often not found. Multiple compression fractures and ill health followed by the presence of Bence Jones protein in the urine help establish the diagnosis. Bone marrow biopsy may be necessary.

Vascular

Abdominal aortic aneurysm is an uncommon source of back pain and usually occurs in white males between the ages of 60 and 70.[51] Lower back pain occurs due to dilatation and compression of adjacent structures or rupture. The back pain is associated with a dull, steady epigastric pain unrelated to posture or meals. On examination, a pulsatile mass may be palpated on level with the umbilicus, with lateral expansion present. Streaks of calcification in the wall of an arteriosclerotic aorta may be seen on X-ray. CT scan or ultrasound examination of the abdomen will visualize the aneurysm.

Arterial occlusion of the aorta at the bifurcation can result in Leriche syndrome, characterized by low back pain, buttock or thigh pain of a claudication type, and impotence.

Visceral Disease

Some visceral organs of the abdomen and pelvis are in close proximity to the spine and pelvic musculoskeletal structures. Visceral disease can cause low back and pelvic pain due to inflammation, expansion, perforation, bleeding, or infection. Direct stimulation of nociceptors can cause local pain, or pain of a referred nature can be felt, often at a distance from the diseased organ.

Visceral pain is not relieved by rest or aggravated by activity. Signs and symptoms of organic disease can usually be found. Pain and tenderness at the costovertebral angle, groin pain, and urinary changes indicate kidney disease. Severe pain that causes the patient constantly to writhe about searching for relief and that starts in the back and radiates to the groin and genitals indicates renal colic and ureteral disease. A urinalysis is most helpful. Groin pain accompanied by a visible or palpable mass that occurred after heavy exertion signifies an inguinal hernia.

Gastrointestinal problems may show altered bowel movements or occult blood with a normal urinalysis. Acute pancreatitis patients classically assume the sitting posture with their knees curled up for relief of their intense epigastric and upper lumbar pain. Bladder infections can cause lower abdominal and sacral pain, with frequency, dysuria, hematuria, and nocturia being the classic presentation.

Prostatic pain can be referred to the perineum, rectum, and sacral regions. Symptoms of nocturia, frequency, incomplete emptying, and ineffectual urge to urinate indicate obstructive disease. Rectal examination and serum prostatic acid phosphatase assay should be performed.

The female organs of reproduction can cause lower back pain. Such pain is invariably associated with other signs of pelvic organ disease. The pain is often sacral as well as lower abdominal. Dysmenorrhea, abnormal uterine bleeding, and infertility indicate the necessity for a gynecologic workup.

Metabolic/Endocrine

Symptoms of lower back pain with bone changes found elsewhere besides the axial skeleton, blood chemistry changes, and systemic changes may indicate endocrine or metabolic disease. Presence or absence of compression fractures after minor incident, radiographic changes of diminished bone mass, and generalized backache in an elderly woman with no abnormal blood chemistry findings indicate osteoporosis. Osteomalacia may be indistinguishable from osteoporosis except for bone biopsy and decreased serum calcium. Hyperparathyroidism is usually associated with hypercalcemia, female predominance, gastrointestinal symptoms, renal colic, and a history of parathyroid tissue removal by surgery.

Diabetes mellitus can present with neurologic disease as a consequence to hyperglycemia. Femoral neuropathy is common, with anterior thigh pain of a burning quality, often worse at night. Increased thirst and polyuria are present. The fasting blood sugar is elevated, and a prior diagnosis of diabetes has often been made.

Psychologic

Patients who have had organic pathology ruled out, do not respond to appropriate care, and display symptom magnification, nonphysiologic pain patterns, and marked dependency on the health care provider need to be evaluated for psychologic overlay of their back pain. Malingering is a rare form of back pain and can be identified by distraction tests and observation of discrepancies between subjective and objective information. Waddell et al[52] use five groups of tests to evaluate for signs of nonorganic disease during the examination: (1) tenderness, (2) simulation tests, (3) distraction tests, (4) regional disturbances, and (5) overreaction to pain. Tenderness as an indicator of nonorganic disease pertains to an excessive pain response to mild stimulation over a wide area of tissue and/or tenderness not related to a specific structure.

Simulation tests simulate a real test that in fact is not being performed. An example is applying cervical axial loading that results in the patient's complaining of low back pain. This response should not occur, serving to raise the suspicion of the examiner to a nonorganic basis of pain.

Distraction tests include rechecking a previously positive finding by distracting the patient with another normally nonpainful maneuver. An example is performing the sitting leg-raise test after the patient responds positively to a supine straight-leg raise. The two should correspond. If the patient reports pain with the straight-leg–raising test and if no pain is elicited with the sitting straight-leg–raising test (Bechterew's test), then a discrepancy is present.

The category of regional disturbances pertains to findings of cogwheel weakness or strength that suddenly gives way on a muscle strength test or findings of sensory disturbances that do not follow neurologic principles.

Overreaction pertains to inappropriate verbal and expressive responses to examination procedures. This includes exaggerated limb withdrawal and painful grimaces.

CONCLUSION

The history is paramount in formulating a diagnosis. Listening to the patient is key. Clues to the etiology are sought. An overall impression of the case should be visualized first. The anatomical structures possibly involved in pain generation should be considered as well as the different pathologic processes that may be operant. A list of possible diagnoses is made, and the differential is narrowed with the physical examination and the use of ancillary procedures such as X-ray and other imaging studies or laboratory diagnosis.

Chapter Review Questions

- What distinguishes a mechanical versus an organic lesion in the history?
- What is intrinsic trauma?
- What is the difference between root or radicular pain and non-neural referred pain?
- What clues in the history indicate the various tissues that can be involved in a musculoskeletal condition?
- Review the mental process used in formulating a differential diagnosis.
- Patients with medical disease causing their lower back pain can be classified into what five groups?
- Name the categories of etiologies the clinician should think of when confronted with a low back pain patient.
- What are the nonorganic signs of disease according to Waddell et al?

REFERENCES

1. Grieve GP. *Modern Manual Therapy of the Vertebral Column.* New York, NY: Churchill Livingstone; 1986.
2. Scott J, Huskisson EC. Graphic representation of pain. *Pain.* 1976;2:175–185.
3. Huskisson EC. Measurement of pain. *Lancet.* 1974;2:1127–1131.
4. Ohnhaus EE, Adler R. Methodological problems in the measurement of pain: a comparison between the verbal rating scale and the visual analog scale. *Pain.* 1975;1:379–384.
5. Uden A, Landin LA. Pain drawing and myelography in sciatic pain. *Clin Orthop.* 1987;216:124–130.
6. Stoddard A. *Manual of Osteopathic Practice.* London: Hutchinson, Long; 1969.
7. Hackett JS. *Joint Ligament Relaxation.* Springfield, Ill: Charles C Thomas, Publisher; 1957.
8. Bernard T, Kirkaldy-Willis W. Recognizing specific characteristics of nonspecific low back pain. *Clin Orthop.* 1987;217:266–280.
9. Fortin JD, Dwyer AP, West S, Pier J. Sacroiliac joint: pain referral maps upon applying a new injection/arthrography technique. Part I: Asymptomatic volunteers. *Spine.* 1994;19:1478–1482.
10. Fortin JD, Aprill CN, Ponthieux B, Pier J. Sacroiliac joint: pain referral maps upon applying a new injection/arthrography technique. Part II: Clinical evaluation. *Spine.* 1994;19:1483–1489.
11. Schwarzer AC, Aprill CN, Bogduk N. The sacroiliac joint in chronic low back pain. *Spine.* 1995;20:31–37.
12. Howse JJG. Osteitis pubis in an Olympic road walker. *Proc R Soc Med.* 1964;57:88.
13. Harris NH, Murray RO. Lesions of the symphysis in athletes. *Br Med J.* 1974;4:211–214.
14. Offierski CM, MacNab I. Hip-spine syndrome. *Spine.* 1983;8:316–321.
15. Rogers C. *Client-Centered Therapy.* Boston, Mass: Houghton Mifflin Co; 1951.
16. Mennell JM. *Joint Pain.* Boston, Mass: Little, Brown & Co; 1964.
17. Kirk EJ, Denney-Brown D. Functional variation in dermatomes in the macaque monkey following dorsal root lesions. *J Comp Neurol.* 1970;139:307–320.
18. Feinstein B. Referred pain from paravertebral structures. In: Buerger AA, Tobis JS, eds. *Approaches to the Validation of Manipulation Therapy.* Springfield, Ill: Charles C Thomas, Publisher; 1977:139–174.
19. Harman JB. The localization of deep pain. *Br Med J.* 1948;1:188–192.
20. Floyd K, Hick VE, Morrison JFB. Mechanosensitive afferent units in the hypogastric nerve of the cat. *J Physiol (Lond).* 1976;259:457.
21. Iggo A, Guilbaud G, Tegner R. Sensory mechanisms in arthritic rat joints. In: Kruger L, Liebeskind JC, eds. *Neural Mechanisms: Advances in Pain Research and Therapy.* Vol 6. New York, NY: Raven Press; 1984.
22. Kellgren JH. Observations on referred pain arising from muscle. *Clin Sci.* 1938;3:175–190.
23. Inman VT, Saunders JB. Referred pain from skeletal structures. *J Nerv Ment Dis.* 1944;99:660–667.
24. Campbell DG, Parsons CM. Referred head pain and its concomitants. *J Nerv Ment Dis.* 1944;99:546–554.

25. Feinstein B, Langton JNK, Jameson RM, Schiller F. Experiments on pain referred from deep somatic tissues. *J Bone Joint Surg.* 1954;36A:981–997.

26. Hockaday JM, Whitty CWM. Patterns of referred pain in the normal subject. *Brain.* 1967;90:481–496.

27. McCall IW, Part WM, O'Brien JP. Induced pain referral from posterior lumbar elements in normal subjects. *Spine.* 1979;4:441–446.

28. Hirsch D, Ingelmark B, Miller M. The anatomical basis for low back pain. *Acta Orthop Scand.* 1963;33:1–17.

29. Mooney V, Robertson J. The facet syndrome. *Clin Orthop.* 1976;115:149–156.

30. Ghormley RK. Low back pain: with special reference to the articular facets. *JAMA.* 1933;101:1773–1777.

31. Hadley LA. Apophyseal subluxation: disturbances in and around the intervertebral foramen causing low back pain. *J Bone Joint Surg.* 1936;18:428.

32. Badgley CE. The articular facets in relation to low back pain and sciatic radiation. *J Bone Joint Surg.* 1941;23:481–496.

33. Kellgren JH. Deep pain sensibility. *Lancet.* 1949;1:943–949.

34. Bourdillion JF, Day EA. *Spinal Manipulation.* 4th ed. Norwalk, Conn: Appleton & Lange; 1987.

35. Dvorak J, Dvorak V. *Manual Medicine: Diagnostics.* New York, NY: Thieme-Stratton, Inc; 1984.

36. Baer WS. Sacroiliac strain. *Bull Johns Hopkins Hosp.* 1917;28:159–163.

37. Maigne R. Low back pain of thoracolumbar origin. *Arch Phys Med Rehabil.* 1980;61:389–395.

38. Lewit K. *Manipulative Therapy in Rehabilitation of the Locomotor System.* Boston, Mass: Butterworths; 1985.

39. Head H. On disturbances of sensation with special reference to the pain of visceral disease. *Brain.* 1893;16:1–133.

40. Borenstein DG, Weisel SW. *Low Back Pain: Medical Diagnosis and Comprehensive Management.* Philadelphia, Pa: WB Saunders; 1989.

41. Frykholm R. The clinical picture. In: Hirsch C, Zotterman Y, eds. *Cervical Pain.* Oxford: Pergamon Press; 1971:5.

42. Lindahl O. Hyperalgesia of the lumbar nerve roots in sciatica. *Acta Orthop Scand.* 1966;37:367–374.

43. Sunderland S. Traumatized nerves, roots, and ganglia: musculo-skeletal factors and neuropathological consequences. In: Korr I, ed. *The Neurologic Mechanisms in Manipulative Therapy.* New York, NY: Plenum Publishing Corp; 1978:137–166.

44. Triano JJ, Luttges MW. Nerve irritation: a possible model of sciatic neuritis. *Spine.* 1982;7:129–136.

45. O'Brien JB. The role of fusion for low back pain. *Orthop Clin North Am.* 1983;14:639–647.

46. Pitkin HC, Pheasant HC. Sacrarthrogenic telalgia. *J Bone Joint Surg.* 1936;18:365–374.

47. Grieve GP. *Common Vertebral Joint Problems.* New York, NY: Churchill Livingstone; 1981.

48. Judovich BD, Nobel GR. Traction therapy: a study of resistance forces. *Am J Surg.* 1957;93:108.

49. Travell JG, Simons DG. *Myofascial Pain and Dysfunction: The Trigger Point Manual.* Baltimore, Md: Williams & Wilkins; 1983.

50. Deyo RA, Rainville J, Kent KL. What can the history and physical examination tell us about low back pain? *JAMA.* 1992;268:760–765.

51. Gore I, Hirst AE Jr. Arteriosclerotic aneurysms of the abdominal aorta: a review. *Prog Cardiovasc Dis.* 1973;16:113–150.

52. Waddell G, McCullogh JA, Kummel E, Venner RM. Non-organic physical signs in low back pain. *Spine.* 1980;5:117–125.

Chapter 4

Clinical Assessment: General Considerations

Chapter Objectives

To discuss the following topics:

- the vertebral subluxation complex
- physical signs of pathologic versus functional disease
- the "Five Nevers" of musculoskeletal diagnosis
- whether a lesion is pelvic or lumbar in origin
- "joint irritability" and its significance
- the examination of range of motion
- joint play/dysfunction and joint signs
- the importance of using joint compression during the examination
- tissue tension testing
- the use of palpation during the examination
- the soft tissue and skin changes seen on examination
- length-strength assessment and movement patterns
- leg-length inequality

The purpose of this chapter is to discuss in general various topics of importance related to examination of the pelvic locomotor complex for functional musculoskeletal disturbances. Chapter 5 discusses the actual examining process more specifically.

Where the history raises suspicions as to the etiology (or etiologies) of a problem, the examination sets out to confirm them. The factors gathered in the history should decide the extent of the examination. One should pay strict attention to the subjective complaints of the patient while at the same time searching for related problems. The examination should be tailored to assess the anatomical and functional integrities of the musculoskeletal system that are suspected to be involved. This is, of course, assuming that visceral and other forms of pathology are ruled out. Joint signs of pain, stiffness, and spasm are looked for and related to where they occur in the available range of motion.

The locomotor system is a complex entity to assess. Osseous structures articulate via kinematically linked joints, and both of these are enveloped by inert and contractile tissues. Meanwhile, the nervous system is carefully "listening," biasing information, and directing function by the millisecond. Joints function to move; muscles contract and generate tension; ligaments restrain. These basic functions should be assessed to ascertain the tissue involved and the dysfunction present. Findings on physical examination can be organized into different categories to aid in making a diagnosis and treatment plan. For example, a patient can be examined to determine which of the five components of the vertebral subluxation complex are involved.

VERTEBRAL SUBLUXATION COMPLEX[1]

Although the terminology is not quite accurate, the concept of the vertebral subluxation complex (VSC) provides a practical model to work with. Unfortunately, terminology can be confusing, with connotations attached to words that do not cross over to other professional disciplines. The word *subluxation* is not used here in its literal sense of a bone out of place. The VSC is a complex, multifaceted clinical entity made up of five basic components that may be singularly, but are usually multiply, operant in a patient's presenting problem, all contributing to the clinical picture:

1. *Neuropathophysiology*[2-4] involves changes, both subjective and objective, that indicate nerve involvement, facilitation, inhibition, or atrophy.
2. *Kinesiopathology*[5-7] involves changes concerned with joint biomechanics, ie, abnormal mobility (hypo- or hypermobility), joint play loss, compensatory reactions, "pathomechanics."
3. *Myopathology*[8-10] concerns reactions of muscle to injury and dysfunction, ie, spasm, weakness, myofascial trigger points, shortening, and inactivation.
4. *Histopathology*[11,12] involves the cellular, vascular, and tissue response to inflammation, ie, edema, lymphedema.
5. *Biochemical response*[13,14] involves the chemical response in the local area of inflammation and the general response (Selye's general

adaptive syndrome)[13] of the body to stress, ie, proinflammatory and anti-inflammatory hormones.

Keeping the VSC in mind, one can identify the specific components that are active in the patient's condition. Most patients have more than one component involved. Aberrant joint mechanics (kinesiopathology) can stimulate arthrokinetic reflexes (neuropathophysiology) that facilitate skeletal muscle contraction, resulting in a guarding spasm (myopathology). Any inflammatory changes contributing to edema and pain (histopathology and biochemical) will most likely be present. A superimposed general adaptive syndrome due to abundant stress factors will affect the entire process through the increased circulation of proinflammatory hormones. These patients are typically stressed and exhibit multiple pain syndromes that inflame for no apparent reason and tend to recur.

Knowing which components are involved aids in formulating a specific therapeutic approach. For example, mechanical joint dysfunction requires mobilization or manipulation; the local inflammatory response requires anti-inflammatory therapy (cryotherapy, electrotherapy, medication); and muscle spasm, trigger points, or shortened muscles can benefit from myofascial therapy, postisometric relaxation, transverse friction, or stretches. Finally, individuals can be counseled concerning their stressful lifestyles and taught such methods of stress reduction as meditation, yoga, aerobic exercise, and biofeedback.

PATHOLOGY

As stated in the previous chapter, certain historical features can lead one to suspect pathology. Similarly, the examination will lend several clues, as will be discussed. The patient generally, but not necessarily, will appear ill. Changing posture will not seem to alleviate the pain, and the examiner may have a difficult time reproducing the presenting symptoms, especially if the pathology is visceral and not affected by movements. The temperature should be taken, along with other vital signs. Systemic illness, infection, and inflammation can raise the body temperature, whereas mechanical problems of the musculoskeletal system do not. The examiner should keep in mind the "irritability" of the painful area (see below). Minor movements that trigger immediate muscle spasm, especially if intense and widespread, should warn of possible pathology. Obviously, swellings and masses should be noted, along with areas of warmth and redness. Regional lymphadenopathy is an important finding of serious disease. In addition, functional disorders, ie, joint dysfunction and myofascial trigger points, and referred pain from non-neural tissues are not associated with "hard" neurologic signs, ie, myoparesis, hypesthesia, and hyporeflexia. Nerve tension signs are similarly absent.

Question for Thought

Does restoring joint mobility with manipulation that alleviates a patient's pain nullify the presence of a pathologic process?

THE "FIVE NEVERS"

Zohn and Mennell[15] mention the "Five Nevers" when discussing generalities of the physical examination:

1. Fluid can never be palpated in a normal synovial joint.
2. The normal joint capsule is never palpable.
3. Normal ligaments are never painful on palpation.
4. Osteoporosis senilis never affects the skull.
5. Osteoporosis senilis never affects the lamina dura around the teeth.

The third "never" is important to bear in mind when palpating the ligaments around the sacroiliac joint and pubic symphysis. Mennell[16] mentions that ligaments are never painful unless traumatized or unless the joint they support is dysfunctional. As joint mobility and inflammation are corrected with treatment, joint ligament tenderness usually abates. This can serve as a general indicator of progress for both clinician and patient.

LUMBAR VERSUS PELVIS

When suspecting pelvic joint dysfunction, it is well to rule out lumbar spine involvement first (Figure 4–1). Look for joint signs (pain and stiffness, local muscle guarding, segmental dysfunction) localizing to the lumbar spine. Lumbar joint dysfunction is associated with a painfully restricted lumbar motion segment. Hard neurologic signs (myoparesis, hyporeflexia, hypesthesia, nerve tension signs) localizing to lumbar levels raise the suspicion of a radicular problem. Keep in mind that thoracolumbar joint dysfunction can create pain in the sacroiliac region[17] (Figure 4–2).

JOINT IRRITABILITY

Regarding joint irritability, the response to examination maneuvers can yield important therapeutic information. A sense of a condition's irritabil-

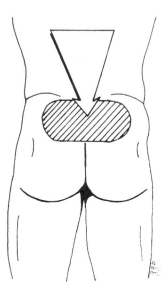

Figure 4–1 Lumbar Localizing Signs

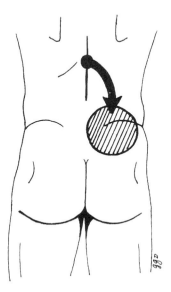

Figure 4–2 Thoracolumbar Joint Pain Referral

ity can also be derived from the history. The degree of joint irritability is determined by (1) the amount of movement needed to provoke pain, (2) the magnitude and amount of symptoms elicited, and (3) the time it takes for the joint to "settle down" to its undisturbed state. Acutely inflamed joints and tissues tend to exacerbate easily and should be handled with extreme care. Attention must be paid to any sudden muscle-guarding response to joint movements. The more irritable the joint condition, the more brisk the muscle guarding. These joints demand care and respect and will revolt with pain and spasm if their "warnings" are not heeded. A vigorous examination will result in painful retribution and further needless suffering. It is better to assess such a situation gently over a few days than to perform a full-scale examination all in one visit. In addition, most provocative tests will be positive in such a highly irritable state, and the clinical picture will appear confusing. Chronic conditions seem less irritable, being able to tolerate more vigorous examination maneuvers.

RANGE OF MOTION

Range-of-motion testing assesses the active, passive, resisted, and joint play movements occurring across joints (Figure 4–3). An adequate appraisal of a joint's functional status cannot be made until all aspects of the range of motion are addressed. Active movement is essentially subjective in that all it tells us is the willingness of the patient to perform the movement and the general area of involvement. Passive movements include physiologic and accessory or joint play movements. Passive physiologic movements are the same as active movements; however, an examiner performs them for the patient. Accessory or joint play movements are involuntary movements also performed by the examiner and are intrinsic to normal joint function. Taking a joint through a passive range of motion provides information as to the integrity of the joint motion and soft tissue restraints (see the section "Selective Tissue Tension" later in this chapter). However, gross range-of-motion testing can be normal in spite of segmental movement abnormalities. For instance, the overall range of motion shared by several joints in a kinematic chain can be normal, yet loss of joint play at one level can be hidden by compensating hypermobile joints at adjacent or distant levels. Thus, specific segmental movement assessment needs to be incorporated to examine accessory movement or joint play function. This is imperative in manual therapy, since manipulative techniques should be based on the loss of accessory or joint play movements. As Grieve states: "There appears no effective substitute for passive movement and palpation as methods of seeking, segment by segment, to provoke or reproduce symptoms reported by patients."[18(p359)]

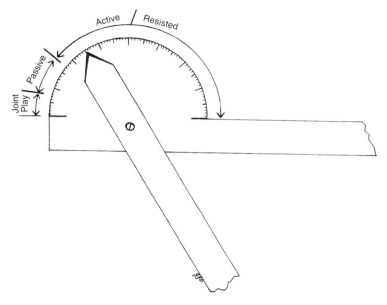

Figure 4–3 Range of Motion

Resisted muscle testing performed at the joint's midrange of motion can be included in range-of-motion testing and is designed to assess neuromuscular, musculotendinous, and tenoperiosteal integrities (see the section "Selective Tissue Tension" later in this chapter). The strength of contraction and the quality of movement are important factors to assess.

When assessing joint range of motion and joint play, the point in the range at which pain commences is important to ascertain. Immediate onset of pain without any resistance from the joint or periarticular structures implies severe pain from active inflammation or unwillingness of the patient to allow the movement to be performed. Pain throughout the range of motion (through-range pain) similarly indicates an actively inflamed joint and one that is constantly painful. Pain onset that is commensurate with resistance at or near the end of a joint's range of motion usually indicates adaptive shortening of the periarticular soft tissues (inert, capsuloligamentous), which is more indicative of a chronic problem.

JOINT PLAY/JOINT DYSFUNCTION

Joint play motion testing assesses the involuntary accessory movement characteristic of all synovial joints. Joint play[16,19] is the small (1/8- to 1/4-

inch) involuntary range of motion that is necessary for all synovial joints to function smoothly during active physiologic movements. Being involuntary, joint play cannot be evaluated by active range-of-motion tests but must be assessed directly by palpating the passive movement characteristics of the joint. Likewise, joint play cannot be restored by exercise, which is an active range-of-motion activity. In fact, exercise may delay recovery if utilized on joints that lack joint play.[6]

Question for Thought

Why is it unwise to exercise a joint that has joint dysfunction?

The loss of joint play is termed *joint dysfunction* and is characterized by painful restriction, impaired function, and pain. Mennell states:

> "This leads to reiteration of the basic truisms, which are too often neglected in practice, that: (1) when a joint is not free to move, the muscles that move it cannot be free to move it, (2) muscles cannot be restored to normal if the joints which they move are not free to move, (3) normal muscle function is dependent on normal joint movement, and (4) impaired muscle function perpetuates and may cause deterioration in abnormal joints.[19(p4)]

What causes joint dysfunction? Usually trauma, both intrinsic and extrinsic, but also disuse, postural indiscretions, and preexisting inflammations or disease. Joint dysfunction can even be a manifestation of viscerosomatic reflex processes (ie, heart-shoulder). Mennell[6] believes that joint dysfunction is the most common cause of osteoarthritic joint pain. Mennell[16] outlines the examining rules for joint play assessment:

1. Both the patient and examiner must be relaxed.
2. One joint and one movement are examined at one time.
3. One facet of the joint being examined is moved upon the other stabilized facet.
4. Movement is compared to that of the joint on the opposite side.
5. No forceful or abnormal movements should be used.
6. The examining movements must be stopped at the onset of pain.
7. Examining movements should not be done in the presence of joint inflammation or disease.

JOINT SIGNS

When one is examining a patient with a probable joint involvement, comparable joint signs[20] in the appropriate joint should be sought. Signs of joint involvement are pain, stiffness, and spasm. Comparable joint signs are those that correlate with the patient's subjective account. The appropriate joint should exhibit these comparable joint signs. For example, a patient with an acute left sacroiliac joint problem may exhibit localized pain and stiffness upon testing of the left sacroiliac joint with passive movements or provocative tests. These are comparable joint signs exhibited by the appropriate joint. However, additional testing may incidentally reveal a positive right Patrick-Fabere test, localizing a possible hip problem. Further hip testing may uncover restricted passive physiologic movements and pain that the patient was not even aware of before the examination. This is not to say that the hip problem has nothing to do with the overall picture of this patient's sacroiliac joint but that it does not correlate with the patient's history. Another example would be finding stiffness of the opposite knee joint in the above-described hypothetical patient. This is not an appropriate joint sign reflective of the patient's history of acute sacroiliac joint pain.

JOINT COMPRESSION WITH PASSIVE TESTING

Often in our search for comparable joint signs, we fall short of reproducing the patient's symptoms. In this instance, meticulous testing of accessory movements throughout the joint's range of motion may bear fruit. In addition, using joint compression while simultaneously testing passive physiologic or accessory movements can be helpful in eliciting the elusive signs and symptoms (Figure 4–4). Maitland[21] considers joint compression an important procedure to add to passive movement testing. He feels that it can reveal subtle, early changes in the friction-free movement of joints due to a joint surface disorder. *Joint surface* here means the structures interposed between the subchondral portions of each bone participating in the articulation. Included is the synovial fluid. Normal hyaline cartilage and synovial fluid are necessary for friction-free movement. Changes in synovial fluid, as seen in osteoarthritis, traumatic arthritis, and rheumatoid arthritis,[22] may have a role in altering its protective action on hyaline cartilage. These changes, as well as early degenerative changes of the articular cartilage, can increase the coefficient of friction—a situation that may be detectable in its early stages by testing passive movements with simultaneous joint compression. Maitland comments:

> Everyone is familiar with the feel of moving a joint which is devoid of all, or nearly all, its hyaline cartilage. Similarly, we would all accept that some of these joints have a rougher feel when moved than others. We should, therefore, be able to accept the

fact that a stage must exist when this change in friction first becomes perceptible on physical examination. It is the early stages in the changes of friction-free movement which...can be assessed by passive movement, and...this assessment can be appreciated earlier if joint compression is utilized during the test movement.[21(p111)]

Compressing a joint when testing passive movements, both physiologic and accessory, can reveal fine crepitus or reproduce the patient's pain where testing without compression could not. Since articular cartilage is devoid of pain fibers, the pain may be from sensitive subchondral bone. According to Maitland,[21] joint compression should be used in three instances:

1. when the patient's symptoms cannot be reproduced with regular testing procedures
2. when the patient experiences pain-through-range testing without joint compression; in this case a comparison should be made with compression-through-range testing, and if the pain response is greater with compression, a joint surface disorder should be suspected
3. when crepitus is present but no symptoms are evident

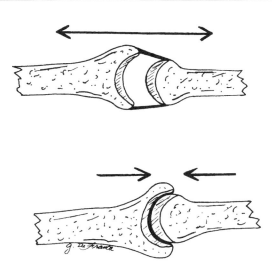

Figure 4–4 Joint Distraction and Compression

SELECTIVE TISSUE TENSION

Cyriax[23] developed a system of assessment aimed at incriminating the type of tissue responsible for a patient's pain. Essentially, it is based on whether the tissue is contractile and how it responds to active, passive, and resisted range-of-motion testing. In addition to muscle, the contractile tissues include those structures affected by the contraction of muscle, ie, tendon and tendon insertions. The noncontractile or inert tissues include the passive elements of the musculoskeletal system, ie, joint capsule, ligaments, bursa, fascia, dura mater, and nerve roots. Passive motion is tested first while observing for pain response and type of end-feel exhibited. Cyriax[23] mentions six end-feels to differentiate among (Exhibit 4–1).

An active motion stresses both contractile and inert tissues and is only a general guide. However, passive motion that is painful in one direction and active motion that is painful in the opposite direction incriminate a contractile tissue, since it is stressed during both contraction and stretching (Figure 4–5). When passive and active motions are painful in the same direction, inert or passive elements are incriminated (Figure 4–6).

A resisted muscle test with the joint held at midrange theoretically stresses mostly the contractile elements and helps to rule out the inert structures. However, one must bear in mind that muscle contraction also creates joint reaction forces. These forces create joint compression and some amount of articular stress. Holding the joint in its neutral range

---

Exhibit 4–1 End-Feels[23]

Bone on Bone	A hard, abrupt cessation of movement, as experienced in passive extension of the normal knee
Soft Tissue	The sensation experienced in passive flexion of the normal knee and hip
Spasm	Twanglike cessation of movement due to muscle spasm guarding a fracture, inflammation, or neoplasia. Always abnormal
Capsular	Hard cessation of movement, as when a leather strap is stretched. Normally felt at the extreme of hip rotation. Abnormal if felt sooner or firmer than usual
Springy Block	A rubbery end to motion, as when a door hits a hard rubber ball stuck between the door and its jamb. Indicates internal derangement, as in a torn knee meniscus
Empty Feeling	More movement seems possible but is quickly arrested by the patient's experience of pain. There is no sense of articular or soft tissue resistance. Always abnormal; usually seen in abscess, neoplasia, bursitis

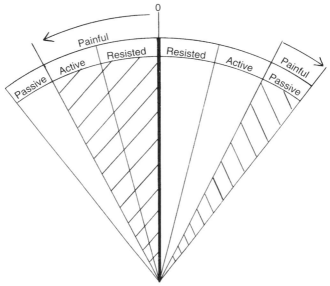

Figure 4–5 Range-of-Motion Pain Response When Contractile Tissue Is Involved

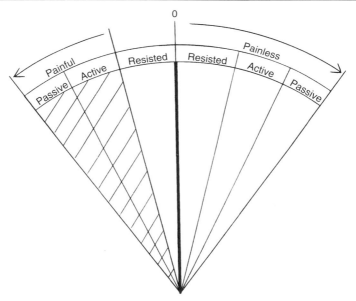

Figure 4–6 Range-of-Motion Pain Response When Passive or Inert Tissues Are Involved

should limit this to some extent. Generally, a strong and painless contraction denotes a normal contractile element. A strong and painful contraction indicates a minor lesion, whereas a weak and painful contraction means a more serious lesion, possibly a breach or tear in the structures contracted. A weak and painless contraction denotes neurologic compromise. It is extremely difficult truly to isolate specific tissues on examination, and therefore selective tissue tension tests should be weighed judiciously.

PALPATION

Grieve states that: "three-quarters of the emphasis, in assessing where to work in mobilizing or manipulating the vertebral column, should perhaps rest on what is found by palpation, following regional active, and passive segmental, tests of movement."[18(p196)]

It seems that palpation is more an art than a science, yet it forms an important cornerstone in the evaluation process of the dysfunctional locomotor apparatus. It is a psychomotor skill that requires patience and experience to develop. Heart and lung auscultation demand nothing less, as do ophthalmoscopic and otoscopic examinations—procedures that demonstrate both error and subjectivity on the part of the examiner. Palpation is the process of using the hands to touch and feel our patients to gain information about tissue texture, temperature, moisture, resistance, movement, size, and position. It is also a powerful tool to assist in the doctor-patient bonding process.

Gillet and Liekens[5] developed a palpatory method for assessing sacroiliac joint motion. A few studies investigating the reliability of this procedure demonstrated mixed findings,[24–26] with reliability ranging from slight to good. Evaluation of the sacroiliac joint's upper aspect was associated with better results. Intraexaminer scores seemed better than those between examiners. Herzog et al[26] comment that their results suggest that Gillet's procedure can be used in the clinical assessment of sacroiliac joint motion because intraexaminer reliability is more important: in most clinical situations, only one examiner is involved in the assessment of the patient. Others contend that palpation is too subjective and yields questionable reliability. A possibility to be considered is that the examination tests themselves may effect changes in the musculoskeletal system, creating confusion and skewed results during experimental study. At present, palpatory assessment maintains a central role in the examination of locomotor dysfunctions. Unfortunately, as in other areas of clinical practice, conclusive data are not available; yet palpation continues to be a widely used procedure, for either empirical or emotional reasons. More studies and better methods will undoubtedly appear to improve our present approach.

Palpation attempts to localize areas of pain and movement restriction and demonstrate to patients that we as clinicians understand their problems. Unfortunately, patients seeking a functional assessment often exclaim that their previous doctor/therapist never even touched them, let alone touched the painful area. From the patient's standpoint, it is critical that the examiner touch the painful area or at least demonstrate to the patient that he or she knows where the patient hurts. It is also important to have the patient say, "That's it! That's my pain! You've found it!" Through palpation and provocative testing, we should try to reproduce the patient's exact symptoms. Sometimes we cannot, especially in cases of referred pain. Many times our palpatory findings are all that we have to go by.

Movement palpation entails feeling the motion of joints, particularly a joint's accessory motion or joint play.[1] Actual motion in the sacroiliac joint is difficult to feel; a sense of pliability seems to be a more accurate description. Since the sacroiliac joint is not moved directly by any particular muscle group, its motion is subsequent to hip or trunk motions while it seemingly "floats" in a range of joint play. In a similar situation, the talus operates independently of any direct muscle control, since it receives no tendinous attachments. Its movements are consequential to movements of the surrounding joints and muscles. In contrast, the sacrum has several trunk and hip muscles attaching to it that indirectly affect its motion. Thus, it seems that the sacrum is dependent on sacroiliac joint play integrity to function painlessly between the ilia.

In motion palpation, it is not so much the motion as the feeling that is important. Fortunately, the body has two sides whose findings can be compared, and this should be taken advantage of in the examination. It has been said that the more lightly one touches, the more one feels. This cannot be overstated.

SOFT TISSUE AND SKIN CHANGES

The skin can yield important clues to locomotor disturbances through close observation and palpation. Signs of overactive physiological functions[27] can be observed. These include changes in skin temperature, sweating, and electrical resistance. Recent problems can manifest with soft, smooth thickenings of the soft tissues (ligaments, muscles, capsules, subcutaneous tissues), whereas tissue thickenings of more chronic conditions feel hard and stringy.[28] The skin can become thickened and tender and take on a "puckered" appearance when it is lifted and squeezed between the fingers—the so-called "peau d'orange" effect.[29] Rolling the skin off the underlying muscle layer will meet with a resistance and tenderness over joint and muscle lesions[6,16,28,30] and can be used as a confirmatory sign of their existence. In slender individuals, if the skin over a problematic sacro-iliac joint is rolled, it will be tender, taut, and possibly slightly thickened.

To perform skin rolling, one pinches the skin between the thumb and fingers on each hand. One holds both thumbs down on the skin tip to tip, and advances them by rolling a fold of skin up over them with the fore- and middle fingers (Figure 4–7).

LENGTH-STRENGTH AND MOVEMENT PATTERNS

In conjunction with range-of-motion testing is the "length-strength" testing of muscles and the observation of key movement patterns. The nervous system directs movements in terms of whole motions and not individual muscle activations.[2] Normal activation sequences have been ob-

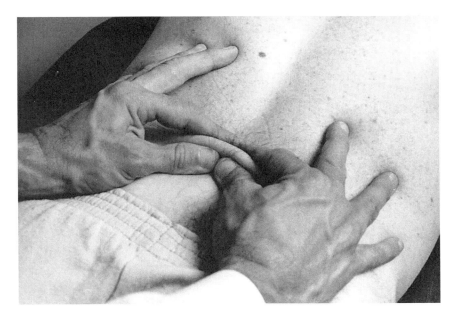

Figure 4–7 Skin Rolling

served for various movements.[31] However, overactivation of antagonists and synergists with resultant inhibition of agonists yields poor movement patterns.

Certain muscles have a predilection to become shortened and tight, as observed by Janda[31] (Exhibit 4–2). He noted that the important postural muscles demonstrate the greatest propensity to shortening, especially in response to poor posture and improper motor patterns.[10,31] Janda[10] states that due to reciprocal inhibition, tight hypertonic muscles inhibit their antagonist muscle groups and cause a *pseudoparesis* ("false weakness"). It is known in the field of neurophysiology that facilitation of an agonistic muscle group is associated with reflex neurologic inhibition of its antagonist (Figure 4–8). For instance, a contraction of the quadriceps will effectively extend the knee joint only if the hamstrings are inhibited from resisting. This phenomenon is "hard-wired" into the system and is reflex based. The same phenomenon is thought to occur when a muscle is shortened and tight (facilitated). The innocent antagonist to this muscle obeys the reflex command of inhibition and "gives in" to the agonist. Often, by just lengthening the shortened and tight muscle, one can note an immediate strengthening response in the previously weak and inhibited muscle. This is because the muscle weakness was functionally induced as a consequence of neurophysiologic processes, ie, reciprocal inhibition mediated via the nervous system, and not loss of neuromuscular control. The process does not entail a true paresis in the usual sense, and thus the term *pseudoparesis* is used.

On the other hand, a tight and shortened muscle will not spontaneously lengthen. It needs a force external to itself to lengthen it. In quoting Ralston, Kendall and McCreary[32] point out that muscles lengthen by the

---

Exhibit 4–2 Common Imbalance of Pelvic Muscles

Shortened/Tight	*Weakened/Inhibited*
Quadratus lumborum	Gluteus maximus
Hamstrings	Gluteus medius
Erector spinae	Gluteus minimus
Psoas	Vasti
Rectus femoris	Rectus abdominis
Tensor fascia lata	
Oblique abdominals	
Piriformis	
Hip adductors	

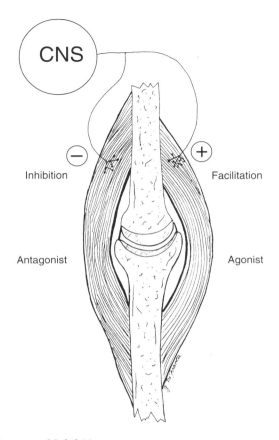

Figure 4–8 Reciprocal Inhibition

pull of antagonistic muscles, gravity, or some other process outside the control of the muscle in question. The lengthening of a shortened muscle is passive, not active. Therefore, shortened muscles tend to remain short unless some extrinsic factor lengthens them. Shortened, tight muscles can overpower any weaker antagonists, either by force or by neurologic inhibition, and create a postural imbalance. If this situation is prolonged, the weaker antagonists can suffer from what Kendall and McCreary call "stretch-weakness."[32] Unfortunately, if the tight, hypertonic muscle state persists, inhibiting antagonist muscles, aberrant movement patterns result that can be habituated by the neuromuscular system. The cerebellum "memorizes" these inappropriate movement patterns, and they become ingrained into the system. The tight muscles adapt and shorten; the weak antagonists weaken more and lengthen. Reeducation of normal movement patterns by remedial exercises and proper proprioceptive input from the periphery can help correct the habituation.

Thus, the adaptive shortening of one group of muscles fostering a stretch-weakness of its antagonists can create postural imbalances altering locomotor function. These imbalances occur in often-observed patterns, as described by Janda.[31] The issue of which of the two above problems is primary, the adaptive shortening or the stretch-weakness, is tantamount to the question of which came first, the chicken or the egg.

Three maneuvers for the lower back region can be used to assess movement pattern quality (see below and Chapter 5). In the prone position, hip extension is performed, and the proper contraction sequence of the hamstring, gluteus maximus, and erector spinae muscles is looked for (see below). The second movement pattern tested is hip abduction in the side-lying position, and the simultaneous contraction of the tensor fascia lata and gluteus medius is looked for. The third movement pattern tested is a trunk curl-up while the patient's feet are cradled to detect lifting off. Lifting up of the feet signifies inappropriate hip flexor recruitment.

In the pelvic region, a few patterns of imbalance seem to predominate. One is the pelvic crossed syndrome: tight and shortened erector spinae and psoas muscles crossed with weak and inhibited abdominal and gluteus maximus muscles[33] (Figure 4–9). The erector spinae and psoas muscles reciprocally inhibit their antagonists, the abdominals and gluteus maximus respectively. An anterior pelvic tilt is usually observed in this situation (see Chapter 5, the section "Posture").

A second common pattern seen about the pelvis includes tight, shortened tensor fascia lata and quadratus lumborum muscles and weak, inhibited glutei minimus and medius muscles. The iliotibial band is usually taut as well. An abnormal movement pattern in this situation entails asynchronous firing of the glutei medius/minimus and tensor fascia lata during hip abduction. Although they usually all contract together during hip abduction, the above imbalance usually results in the tensor fascia lata firing earlier, causing hip flexion. Iliopsoas activity also becomes involved, causing external hip rotation.[31] Tight hip adductor muscles and weak hip abductors often coexist, in which case the patient has a difficult time raising the uppermost leg in the side posture. Just by stretching the adductor muscles to their normal length and tension, the patient is usually able to abduct the leg and thigh more efficiently.

The layer syndrome[33] is another pattern observed and can be visualized posteriorly on postural examination (Figure 4–10; see also Chapter 5). In

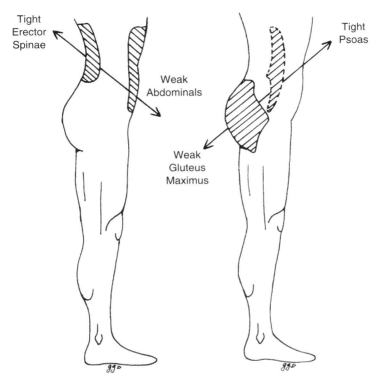

Figure 4–9 Pelvic Crossed Syndrome

this syndrome, areas or layers of weak, inhibited muscles alternate with layers of shortened, tight muscles. For example, from the posterior one can commonly observe tight hamstrings, weak gluteus maximus muscles, tight lumbar erector spinae, weak midthoracic muscles, and tight upper trapezius muscles.

It appears that the muscles with a greater postural importance show more of a tendency to shorten. Those muscles that show a greater tendency for weakness are termed *phasic*.[10] These muscle imbalances are thought to create abnormal movement patterns that can adversely affect the locomotor system. An example can be found in the abovementioned movement pattern of hip extension. Polyelectromyography has shown that the prime movers in order of firing are the hamstrings, gluteus maximus, and erector spinae.[34] In a situation of disturbed muscle function, the gluteus maximus is usually weak, and its contraction is retarded, dimin-

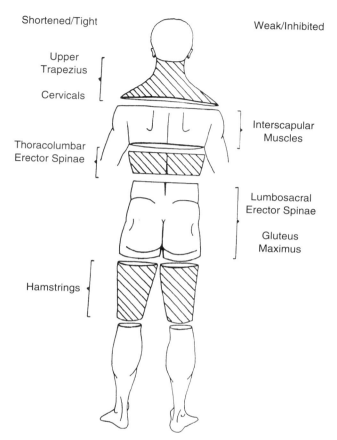

Figure 4–10 Layer syndrome. Muscles listed on the left are often tight and short-ened; those on the right, weak and inhibited.

ished, or even absent, yet the hamstring and erector contractions compen-sate to carry out hip extension. The tight and shortened muscles (ham-strings and erector spinae) seem to activate readily during movements, competing for action at the expense of the inhibited gluteus maximus muscles.

Janda states that "there is now enough evidence that impaired function of muscles occurs in close relationship with development of joint dysfunc-tions which is considered to be the most common cause of painful condi-tions such as low back pain."[35(p199)] Impaired afferent proprioception from dysfunctional joints is thought to cause reflexogenic muscular responses.[36,37] Janda[10] stresses the importance of a properly controlled and coordinated neuromuscular system to the protection and health of the osteoarticular system. Abnormal tensions developed across joints due to muscular imbalances may hasten degenerative changes and foster joint dysfunctions.[10] Interestingly, Radin[38] relates how a shortened muscle's failure to lengthen contributes to degenerative changes in the joint and cartilage.

Length-strength testing is important for gaining a sense of balance of tension across joints. Passively stretching the various muscles about the pelvis during the examination can yield information about muscle distensibility and any adaptive shortening. Muscles of interest about the pelvis include the erector spinae, abdominals, quadratus lumborum, psoas, gluteals, hamstrings, rectus femoris, adductors, and quadriceps. Stretching and strengthening regimes can be formulated for these. In addition, proprioceptive input provided by the clinician or special exercises can re-educate the nervous system to use more appropriate movement patterns. Bullock-Saxton et al[39] showed that use of wobble boards or balance shoes enhanced or "reactivated" gluteus maximus muscle activity and decreased its time to 75% maximum contraction.

Question for Thought

What do you think happens when a person is allowed to exercise when poor movement patterns exist?

LEG-LENGTH INEQUALITY

There is a high correlation between leg-length inequality (LLI) and pelvic obliquity (tilting in the frontal plane) seen on postural examination, yet much debate still exists as to the role of LLI in low back pain.[40] Of patients studied with low back pain, 13% to 22% demonstrated an LLI of ⅜ in (1 cm) compared to about 7% (range 4% to 8%) of asymptomatic adults. Giles[40] states that LLI of 1 cm or more seems to be more prevalent in people with lower back pain than in the asymptomatic population.

There is tremendous debate as to what constitutes a clinically significant LLI (Table 4–1). Rush and Steiner[41] found an LLI of 3/16 in (0.5 cm) or more to relate significantly to the backache of 1000 soldiers studied. Travell and Simons[42] regard ½ in (1.3 cm) as a significant amount of LLI to correct for, even in asymptomatic people as a preventive measure.

Friberg[43] studied LLI in over 1100 subjects, 359 of whom were controls. Chronic low back pain and unilateral chronic hip pain were common in

Table 4–1 Leg-Length Discrepancies Found To Be Significant

Investigator	Leg-Length Discrepancy
Rush, Steiner[41]	3/16 in (0.5 cm)
Friberg[43]	3/16 in (0.5 cm)
Giles[40]	3/8 in (1.0 cm)
Travell, Simons[42]	1/2 in (1.3 cm)

the study group. Her study demonstrated a higher incidence of LLI on the right side (53%) compared to the left (39%). The etiology of the short leg was idiopathic in 92% of the cases, in contrast to known surgical, traumatic, or growth abnormality factors. An LLI of 5 mm or more was found to be significant in 75% of the patients, as compared to 43.5% of the controls. Further, she found a sixfold increased incidence of having an LLI of 15 mm (0.58 in) in a group of subjects with low back pain when compared to those without. Hip pain, hip osteoarthritis, and sciatica were more common on the long-leg side. In writing about the "hip-spine syndrome," Friberg[44] observed both hip pain and sciatica to occur on the same side, which happened to be the long-leg side, 91% of the time. The average LLI in those patients with hip-spine symptoms was 12.8 mm (1/2 in) versus 5.2 mm (1/5 in) in the control group. Friberg found that lift therapy commonly resolved her patients' symptoms, even chronic low back and hip pain.

Measurement

The most commonly used clinical method for measuring LLI entails measuring the distance between the ASIS and the inferior aspect of the ipsilateral medial malleolus. A more functional method is to observe the patient in the standing posture and palpate the relative heights of the anterior and posterior superior iliac spines and iliac crests. If a leg-length discrepancy exists and manifests itself by pelvic obliquity, the needed amount of lift material is placed under the presumed short leg until the pelvis appears level via visual inspection or with the aid of a leveling device (Figure 4–11). This method is more functional in that it tests the patient in the standing position. The patient can also perceive the leveling of the pelvis, and the examiner can observe the initial postural distortions (pelvic obliquity, spinal curvature, trunk contours) self-correct. Travell and Simons[42] feel that this clinical trial method of determining LLI is more accurate than measuring LLI via tape measure while the patient is supine.

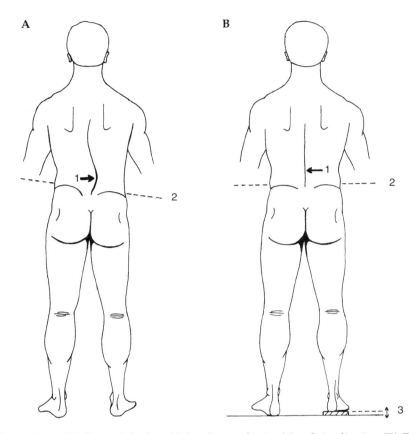

Figure 4–11 (A) Short right leg: **(1)** lumbar scoliosis; **(2)** pelvic oliquity. **(B)** Postural correction after clinical trial of lift placement: **(1)** reduction of functional scoliosis; **(2)** leveling of pelvis; **(3)** height of lift material.

Unfortunately, clinical methods for the assessment of LLI are inaccurate for several reasons. First, accurate palpatory location of subcutaneous bony landmarks is difficult at times, especially in muscular and obese patients, thus affecting the precision of measuring LLI. Second, asymmetry within the pelvis itself, due to either a small hemipelvis or counterrotation of the innominates at the sacroiliac joints, causes a disrelationship between the palpable landmarks, creating error in measuring. These clinical methods are also inadequate because they do not yield information about the position of the sacral base upon which the spine rests or about how the spine reacts to the pelvic obliquity.

As long as their limitations are kept in mind, the clinical methods for determining LLI can be used as simple screening methods. Interestingly, Triano[45] investigated the erector spinae EMG response to LLI and a lift placed under the heel while standing and under the ischium while sitting, observing whether the lifts balanced any asymmetric EMG response noted beforehand. After comparing the EMG results with radiographic findings, he concluded that EMG was a more accurate determinant of lift placement than conventional methods used to assess pelvic and sacral obliquity.

After screening tests identify a leg-length discrepancy, specific radiographic techniques can be used to assess LLI further.[40,46] Radiographic examination allows visualization of how the spine and pelvis biomechanically react to an LLI. It is generally understood that in response to a short leg, the pelvis drops on that side and the lumbar spine exhibits a scoliosis with the convexity to the short-leg side. Janse[47] mentions a basic distortion pattern of the pelvis commonly associated with an LLI, in which the ilium on the short-leg side rotates posteriorly, the sacral base on the same side rotates anteriorly and inferiorly, and L-5 counterrotates on the sacrum, with its transverse process going posteriorly on the side of the posterior innominate.

Bailey and Beckwith[48] studied the spinal postural changes to LLI in over 400 subjects. Results showed that during standing, the ipsilateral innominate and sacral base were lower in 88% and 72% of the cases respectively. However, lumbar scoliosis convexity was ipsilateral (short-leg side) in only 45% of the cases, with 32% being contralateral and 23% showing no deviation.

Radiographs are also needed to visualize any sacral base obliquity. Sacral base unleveling is unusual in low back pain patients in the absence of an LLI.[49] Giles[40] mentions the importance of determining the sacral base obliquity in relation to the LLI. Due to pelvic asymmetries and anomalies within the pelvis, sacral base obliquity may not correspond to the LLI. For example, the sacral base may be level in the presence of an LLI without a resultant lumbar scoliosis. Applying a lift to this patient may then unlevel the sacral base and cause possible lumbar compensations. Travell and Simons[46] mention that an LLI is significant to lumbar spine biomechanics insofar as there exists a sacral base unleveling. They illustrate various combinations of sacral base obliquity and LLI.

Asymmetric joint loading is thought to occur as a result of postural deviations imposed by LLI. Giles[40] has found structural changes in lumbar zygapophyseal joints associated with a 1- to 1.5-cm LLI and has studied the relationship between low back pain and LLI. The changes consisted of articular cartilage and subchondral bone asymmetries at both the lumbosacral level and the apical segment of the scoliosis. Osteophytes and lumbar vertebral wedging were also found.[50] Giles's histological and clinical studies have led him to conclude that patients with an LLI of 1 cm or more and a postural scoliosis should be equilibrated with shoe lifts to lessen the compensatory burden on the lumbar spine and pelvis.[40]

LLI carries with it potent biomechanical consequences and can be considered a potential risk factor for arthritic changes in the hip and spine. For example, LLI is associated with osteoarthritic changes in the hip[43,51,52] and knee[53] joints. Interestingly, these changes were noted more commonly on the longer-leg side. The hip on the long-leg side is in a relative position of adduction, which subsequently reduces the weight-bearing area of the hip joint. As a result, greater joint surface forces are generated, and degenerative changes occur.[53,54] In addition, Morscher[54] noted a marked asymmetry in the EMG response in the low back and hip muscles with an LLI of 3/8 in. The hip abductors on the long-leg side were contracted, causing a higher joint reactive force. This, coupled with the smaller available area of acetabular articulation, contributed to more joint stress on the long-leg side. Vink and Kamphuisen[55] noted an increased EMG activity in the paraspinal muscles contralateral to the LLI. This response was noted in subjects with an LLI as little as 1.5 mm.

Mahar et al[56] demonstrated that the body's weight shifted to the long-leg side and that there was an increased postural sway proportional to the amount of LLI. They stated that their findings support the viewpoint that minor differences in leg length may be biomechanically significant.

Lawrence[57] investigated the effects of LLI on lateral weight distribution. He noted that more weight was carried on the short-leg side when the LLI was small (1 to 4 mm). On the contrary, a larger LLI (more than 6 mm) resulted in weight bearing lateralizing to the longer-leg side. Lawrence surmised that the weight shift to the long-leg side was probably due to righting reflexes and gluteus medius activation to level the pelvis.

Bandy and Sinning[58] used heel lifts to correct 3/16- to 3/8-in LLIs and noticed that sagittal-plane kinetic patterns were improved in the hip, knee, and ankle while the subjects were observed walking and running on a treadmill.

D'Amico et al[59] measured foot function during gait and noted that the stance phase was increased on the long-leg side. In addition, the long-leg side received more weight percussion energy (impact force), which was normalized after heel lift placement.

In an interesting study, DeLacerda and Wikoff[60] demonstrated an increased $\dot{V}O_2$ uptake during a constant workload in subjects with LLI.

Travell and Simons[42,46] mention how LLI is the most common perpetuating factor in quadratus lumborum trigger points, the most overlooked myofascial source of low back pain. They also cite Gross's work[61] that failed to show any help from lifts used to correct 3/15-in LLIs in marathon runners. It is thought that because both feet do not simultaneously touch the ground during running, the lumbar spine does not compensate with a scoliotic curve.[46] However, Bandy and Sinning[58] did demonstrate improvement in gait parameters in runners after lift placement.

From the above, it can be seen that LLI can create compensatory changes to the locomotor system and therefore should be screened for and, if deemed appropriate, corrected. However, joint and muscle dysfunctions should be attended to first and the clinical situation reassessed prior to implementing lift therapy.

An individual with a leg-length deficiency should first be assessed for postural changes and joint/muscle dysfunctions in the locomotor system. The dysfunctions are addressed first in addition to appropriate exercise therapy focusing on lengthening tight muscles and strengthening weak ones. If the patient continues to present with recurrent problems, the LLI is investigated more closely by clinically leveling the patient's pelvis while he or she is standing and then observing for any resulting postural corrections. The patient is left standing on the lift material with weight equally distributed over both feet for 3 minutes. This allows the patient to kinesthetically accommodate to the "corrected" posture. The lift material is then removed from under the short-leg side. Patients invariably notice a kinesthetic difference and comment how the corrected position feels relieving. The height of the lift material is noted, and the pelvis is X-rayed to demonstrate sacral base obliquity and compensatory changes in the spine. X-rays can be taken in the uncorrected and corrected positions to determine how the spine/pelvis compensates to the lift height. Radiographic evidence of sacral base obliquity that is corrected after lift application along with the thoracolumbar segment being placed over the sacrum indicates a favorable response. The patient can then be referred to a competent orthotist for lift therapy.

Chapter Review Questions

- What are some physical signs of pathology?
- Generally, differentiate a typical lumbar problem from one of pelvic origin.
- What important information does a joint's level of "irritability" yield?

- What important factors concerning a joint's range of motion should be considered during a thorough functional examination?
- Discuss joint play and its relation to normal joint motion.
- What is meant by testing "selective tissue tensions"?
- What soft tissue changes are seen in acute versus chronic conditions?
- Which muscles around the pelvis have a tendency to shorten and become tight?
- What is the significance of leg-length inequality in lower back pain?

REFERENCES

1. Faye LJ. *Motion Palpation of the Spine.* Huntington Beach, Calif: Motion Palpation Institute; 1981.
2. Korr IM. The spinal cord as organizer of disease processes: some preliminary perspectives. *J Am Osteopath Assoc.* 1976;76:35–55.
3. Korr IM. The spinal cord as organizer of disease processes III: hyperactivity of sympathetic innervation as a common factor of disease. *J Am Osteopath Assoc.* 1979;4:57–62.
4. Korr IM, ed. *The Neurobiologic Mechanisms in Manipulative Therapy.* New York, NY: Plenum Publishing Corp; 1978.
5. Gillet H, Liekens M. *Belgian Chiropractic Research Notes.* Huntington Beach, Calif: Motion Palpation Institute; 1984.
6. Mennell JM. *Back Pain: Diagnosis and Treatment Using Manipulative Technique.* Boston, Mass: Little, Brown & Co; 1960.
7. Jirout J. Studies on the dynamics of the spine. *Acta Radiol.* 1956;46:55–60.
8. Travell JG, Rinzler SH. The myofascial genesis of pain. *Postgrad Med.* 1952;11:425–434.
9. Korr IM. Proprioceptors in somatic dysfunction. *J Am Osteopath Assoc.* 1975;74:638–650.
10. Janda V. Muscles, central nervous regulation, and back problems. In: Korr IM, ed. *The Neurobiologic Mechanisms in Manipulative Therapy.* New York, NY: Plenum Publishing Corp; 1978:27–41.
11. Cotran RS, Kumar V, Robbins SL. *Pathologic Basis of Disease.* 4th ed. Philadelphia, Pa: WB Saunders; 1989.
12. Salter RB, Simmonds DF, Malcolm BW, et al. The biological effect of continuous passive motion on healing of full-thickness defects in articular cartilage: an experimental study in the rabbit. *J Bone Joint Surg.* 1980;62A:1232–1251.
13. Selye H. *The Stress of Life.* New York, NY: McGraw-Hill Publishing Co; 1956.
14. Levi L. *Stress: Sources, Management, and Prevention.* New York, NY: Liveright; 1967.
15. Zohn DA, Mennell JM. *Musculoskeletal Pain: Diagnosis and Physical Treatment.* Boston, Mass: Little, Brown & Co; 1976.
16. Mennell JM. *The Musculoskeletal System: Differential Diagnosis from Symptoms and Physical Signs.* Gaithersburg, Md: Aspen Publishers, Inc; 1992.

17. Maigne R. Low back pain of thoracolumbar origin. *Arch Phys Med Rehabil.* 1980;61:389–395.

18. Greive GP. *Common Vertebral Joint Problems.* New York, NY: Churchill Livingstone; 1981.

19. Mennell JM. *Joint Pain: Diagnosis and Treatment Using Manipulative Techniques.* Boston, Mass: Little, Brown & Co; 1964.

20. Maitland GD. *Peripheral Manipulation.* 2nd ed. Boston, Mass: Butterworths; 1977.

21. Maitland GD. The importance of adding compression when examining and treating synovial joints. In: Glasgow EF, Twomey LT, Scull ER, Kleynhans AM, eds. *Aspects of Manipulative Therapy.* 2nd ed. New York, NY: Churchill Livingstone; 1985.

22. Broderick PA, Corvese N, Pierik MG, Pike RF, Mariorenzi AL. Exfoliative cytology interpretation of synovial fluid in joint disease. *J Bone Joint Surg.* 1976;58A:396–399.

23. Cyriax J. *Textbook of Orthopaedic Medicine. Vol 1. Diagnosis of Soft Tissue Lesions.* London: Balliere Tindall; 1978.

24. Wiles MR. Reproducibility and inter-examiner correlation of motion palpation findings of the sacroiliac joints. *J Can Chiro Assoc.* 1980;24:59–68.

25. Carmichael JP. Inter- and intra-examiner reliability of palpation of sacroiliac joint dysfunction. *J Manipulative Physiol Ther.* 1987;10:164–171.

26. Herzog W, Read LJ, Conway PJW, Shaw LD, McEwen MC. Reliability of motion palpation procedures to detect sacroiliac joint fixations. *J Manipulative Physiol Ther.* 1989;12:86–92.

27. Glover JR. Characterization of localized back pain. In: Buerger AA, Tobis JS, eds. *Approaches to the Validation of Manipulation Therapy.* Springfield, Ill: Charles C Thomas, Publisher; 1977:175–186.

28. Maitland GD. *Vertebral Manipulation.* 5th ed. Boston, Mass: Butterworths; 1986.

29. Stoddard A. *Manual of Osteopathic Practice.* London: Hutchinson, Long; 1969.

30. Bourdillion JF, Day EA. *Spinal Manipulation.* 4th ed. Norwalk, Conn: Appleton & Lange; 1987.

31. Janda V. *Muscle Function Testing.* Boston, Mass: Butterworths; 1983.

32. Kendall FP, McCreary EK. *Muscles: Testing and Function.* Baltimore, Md: Williams & Wilkins; 1983.

33. Jull GA, Janda V. Muscles and motor control in low back pain: assessment and management. In: Twomey LT, Taylor JR, eds. *Physical Therapy of the Low Back.* New York, NY: Churchill Livingstone; 1987:253–277.

34. Lewit K. *Manipulative Therapy in Rehabilitation of the Locomotor System.* Boston, Mass: Butterworths; 1985.

35. Janda V. Muscle weakness and inhibition (pseudoparesis) in back pain syndromes. In: Greive GP, ed. *Modern Manual Therapy of the Vertebral Column.* New York, NY: Churchill Livingstone; 1986:197–201.

36. Wyke B. Articular neurology: a review. *Physiology.* 1972;58:94–99.

37. Slosberg M. Effects of altered afferent articular input on sensation, proprioception, muscle tone and sympathetic reflex responses. *J Manipulative Physiol Ther.* 1988;11:400–408.

38. Radin EL. Aetiology of osteoarthrosis. *Clin Rheum Dis.* 1976;2:509–522.

39. Bullock-Saxton JE, Janda V, Bullock MI. Reflex activation of gluteal muscles in walking. *Spine.* 1993;18:704–708.

40. Giles LGF. *Anatomical Basis of Low Back Pain.* Baltimore, Md: Williams & Wilkins; 1989.

41. Rush WA, Steiner HA. A study of lower extremity length inequality. *Am J Roentgen Rad Ther.* 1946;56:616–623.

42. Travell JG, Simons DG. *Myofascial Pain and Dysfunction: The Trigger Point Manual.* Vol 1. Baltimore, Md: Williams & Wilkins; 1983.

43. Friberg O. Clinical symptoms and biomechanics of lumbar spine and spine and hip joint in leg length inequality. *Spine.* 1983;3:643–651.

44. Friberg O. Hip-spine syndrome: clinical biomechanics, diagnosis, and conservative treatment. *Manual Med.* 1988;3:144–147.

45. Triano JJ. Objective electromyographic evidence for use and effects of lift therapy. *J Manipulative Physiol Ther.* 1983;6:13–16.

46. Travell JG, Simons DG. *Myofascial Pain and Dysfunction: The Trigger Point Manual.* Vol 2. Baltimore, Md: Williams & Wilkins; 1992.

47. Janse J. *Principles and Practice of Chiropractic.* Lombard, Ill: National College of Chiropractic; 1976.

48. Bailey H, Beckwith D. Short leg and spinal anomalies. *J Am Osteopath Assoc.* 1937;134.

49. Friberg O. The statics of postural pelvic tilt scoliosis: a radiographic study on 288 consecutive chronic LBP patients. *Clin Biomech.* 1987;2:211–219.

50. Giles LGF, Taylor JR. Lumbar spine structural changes associated with leg-length inequality. *Spine.* 1982;7:159–162.

51. Gofton JP, Trueman GE. Studies in osteoarthritis of the hip: Part II. Osteoarthritis of the hip and leg-length disparity. *Can Med Assoc J.* 1971;104:791–799.

52. Krakovits G. Uber die Auswirkung einer Beinverkurzung auf die Statikund Dynamik des Huftgelenkes. *Z Orthop.* 1967;102:418–423.

53. Dixon ASJ, Campbell-Smith S. Long leg arthropathy. *Ann Rheum Dis.* 1969;28:359–365.

54. Morscher E. Etiology and pathophysiology of leg length discrepancies. *Progr Orthop Surg.* 1972;1:9–19.

55. Vink P, Kamphuisen HAC. Leg length inequality, pelvic tilt and lumbar back muscle activity during standing. *Clin Biomech.* 1989;4:115.

56. Mahar RK, Kirby RL, MacLeod DA. Simulated leg-length discrepancy: its effect on mean center-of-pressure position and postural sway. *Arch Phys Med Rehabil.* 1985;66:822–824.

57. Lawrence DJ. Lateralization of weight in the presence of structural short-leg: a preliminary report. *J Manipulative Physiol Ther.* 1984;7:105–108.

58. Bandy WD, Sinning WE. Kinematic effects of heel lift use to correct lower limb length differences. *J Orthop Sports Phys Ther.* 1986;7:173–179.

59. D'Amico JC, Dinowitz HD, Polchaninoff M. Limb length discrepancy: an electrodynographic analysis. *J Am Podiatr Med Assoc.* 1985;75:639.

60. DeLacerda FG, Wikoff OD. Effect of lower extremity asymmetry on the kinematics of gait. *J Orthop Sports Phys Ther.* 1982;3:105–107.

61. Gross RH. Leg length discrepancy in marathon runners. *Am J Sports Med.* 1983;11:121–124.

Chapter 5

Examination

Chapter Objectives

- to provide an overview of the manual functional examination
- to describe the examination of gait and posture
- to discuss palpation, provocative testing, and length/strength tests with the patient standing, sitting, supine, and prone

---

The essential features of the manual functional examination are postural and gait observations; joint range of motion, including joint play assessment; specialized provocative maneuvers; observation for poor locomotor movement patterns; muscle length and strength testing; and observation of soft tissue changes. This is in addition to assessing motor, sensory, reflex, and vascular functions of the region concerned. Assuming that pathology has been ruled out, the main goal of the functional examination is to rule in functional aberrations of the locomotor system. As stated before, serious pathology accounts for only a small percentage of patient presentations. However, the possibility of its presence must be borne in mind.

For our discussion, pathology has been ruled out, yet the patient is still in pain and in need of a functional assessment. Whereas in the subjective part of the examination we are all ears, fully attentive to information being communicated to us by the patient, in the objective examination we are all eyes and hands, looking, feeling, and sensing for dysfunction in the various tissues of the locomotor system that may be involved.

During the examination, short and tight muscles are noted along with their weak, inhibited antagonists. Joint restriction and myofascial trigger points are searched for. These joint and muscle dysfunctions are identified in order to consider an appropriate treatment plan to implement. Certain tests will reproduce the patient's presenting symptoms, whereas others will not. It is important that the examiner reproduce the patient's joint and muscle pains for three reasons: (1) to let the patient know that the exam-

162

iner knows where the pain is, (2) to understand the condition better, and (3) to give the examiner important clues as to how to treat the condition.

Rarely do locomotor disturbances occur in isolation. A clinical case may present clues that will alert the clinician to search for associated or linked dysfunctions. For example, the postural examination may indicate a weak and inhibited gluteus maximus because of atrophy or sagging. The gait examination may link decreased hip extension on that side. Poor hip extension and abduction patterns may be observed further on in the examination. Tight psoas and erector spinae muscles may be associated with the above and may be found together with poor lumbar spine motion on full-trunk flexion. Provocative and function testing may be positive for joint dysfunction in the hip and sacroiliac joints, with accompanying gluteal trigger points being found. When the examination is over, the clinician knows that in addition to manipulating joint dysfunctions, he or she needs to address trigger points; short, overactive muscles; weak, inhibited muscles; and poor movement patterns. The web of dysfunctions and compensations that is spun in so many cases, especially chronic ones, must be analyzed with the understanding that the locomotor system is functionally interdependent. Because of this interdependence, dysfunctions are often linked together in chains, almost predictably so. Chapter 10 discusses this in more depth.

In this chapter, we examine the patient in the standing, sitting, supine, lateral decubitus, and prone positions, paying particular attention to certain salient features that pertain to our discussion of pelvic joint and muscular dysfunctions. This discussion is not meant to represent a comprehensive examination—nor a complete one, for that matter. Furthermore, an attempt has been made to mention the many tests used in examining this area. This is not intended to imply that all of them should be performed at one time. Some tests duplicate each other; however, this can afford further confirmation of findings. No one examination procedure has shown enough sensitivity or specificity to be diagnostic by itself. However, the more physical examination findings that incriminate a particular structure, eg, the sacroiliac joint, the greater the chance of establishing a diagnosis. Griner et al[1] state that the specificity of a diagnosis is enhanced when it is established on a combination of confirmatory tests.

STANDING

Gait

In the initial aspect of the examination, a gait and postural assessment should be made to ascertain any deviations from the normal. It is well to consider that asymmetry is the rule in the human body and that just because something is not the way it is "supposed to be" according to some preconceived norm does not automatically mean that it is the cause of the problem. However, clinical inferences can be made and explored.

During gait, one should note a fluid, rhythmic movement in the pelvis while observing from the anterior, posterior, and lateral perspectives. Gait is conveniently divided up into stance and swing phases, with 60% of the cycle being spent in the former and 40% in the latter. The stance phase is subdivided into heel strike, foot-flat, midstance, and push-off (Figure 5–1). The swing phase is subdivided into acceleration, midswing, and deceleration (Figure 5–2). During the swing phase, one limb swings like a pendulum toward heel strike while the other provides unilateral support. At the instant of heel strike, the opposite rearward leg is still in contact with the ground, creating what is called the double-support or double-stance phase.[2] During running, there is no double-support phase, and the body is literally in flight between steps.

The hip, knee, ankle mortise, and metatarsal-phalangeal joint axes are oriented to allow forward progression in gait. Whereas the hip joint allows motion in multiple directions, the knee, mortise, and metatarsal-phalangeal joints allow movement only in flexion-extension. The movement of forward progression in gait is provided by a thrust in the sagittal plane powered by the calf, quadriceps, and gluteus maximus muscles. As the leg swings through its step, it is functionally shortened by hip and knee flexion and ankle dorsiflexion to allow for ground clearance. The hamstrings act to retard the motion of the swinging leg. Short stride lengths can be seen in painful antalgic conditions of the sacroiliac and hip joints, shortened and tight hamstring and hip flexor muscles, and the elderly.

The astute beach observer is pleasantly aware of the motions the pelvis exhibits during gait. While we walk, the pelvis courses through a sinusoidal oscillating motion in the sagittal plane, as well as deviating laterally as it shifts over the weight-bearing extremity. The center of gravity is displaced about 2 in as it goes from its highest point at unilateral support during midstance to its lowest point during double support. The pelvis and trunk counterrotate in the horizontal plane with respect to each other. The pelvis rotates anteriorly about 40 degrees ("pelvic step") on the side of the advancing limb by turning around the contralateral weight-bearing hip joint via contraction of the internal hip rotators (Figure 5–3). Patients are unable to rotate around a painful and stiff hip during gait and will demonstrate a diminished pelvic step.[2] During the swing phase, the gluteus medius on the stance-leg side contracts to afford horizontal stability of the pelvis. Hip abductor weakness is manifested by a slight drop of the

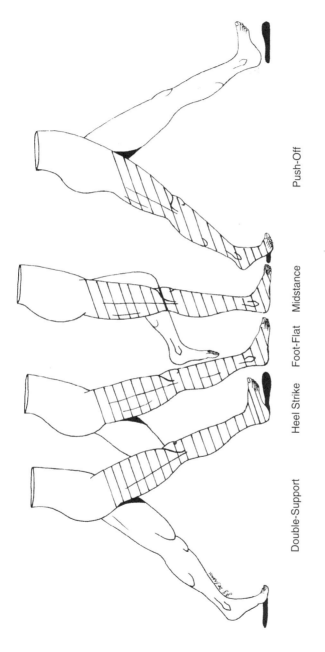

Double-Support   Heel Strike   Foot-Flat   Midstance   Push-Off

Figure 5–1 Stance Phase of Gait

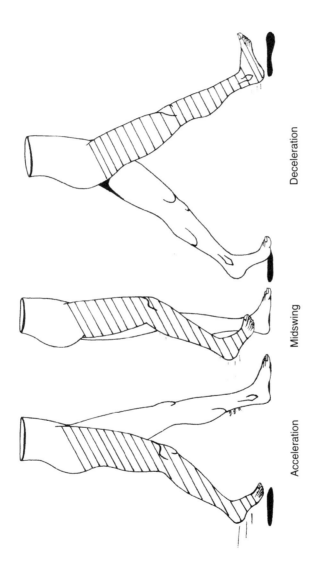

Deceleration   Midswing   Acceleration

Figure 5–2 Swing Phase of Gait

pelvis on the swing-leg side. Additionally, a gluteus medius lurch may be evident (see below).

The pelvis is also noted to deviate laterally about 1 in each way as the body weight is transferred alternately with each step due to the lateral thrust of gait. This movement occurs principally due to the subtalar and hip joints and determines the width of the step.[3] The main muscles responsible for this action are the *retromalleolars* (peroneals) and gluteus medius. During the stance phase, the weight-bearing leg is adducted relative to the

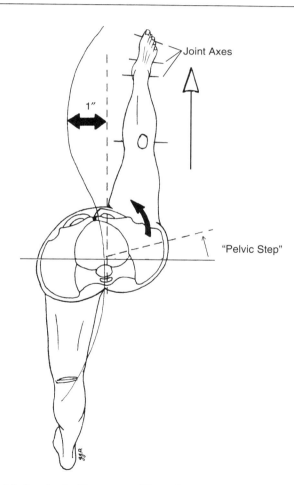

Figure 5–3 Pelvic Motion in the Transverse Plane During Gait

pelvis, and the swing leg is abducted. Disruption of the symmetric lateral sway to each side of the midline may be a sign of sacroiliac and/or hip joint dysfunctions. Interestingly, some studies relate temporal and kinetic gait variables, as measured by a force platform, to have improved after sacroiliac joint manipulation.[4-6] The movements the pelvis makes as a result of the well-orchestrated activity of many muscles and joints help dampen the vertical motion and shock forces generated in gait.

In painful limps, the patient remains on the symptomatic side as little as possible. In addition, the patient will diminish the load applied to the painful limb by trying to "jump" over it using a propulsive force supplied by the good limb and quick upward movements of the upper limbs. The observer gains a sense that the patient tries to walk with a lightness versus a heaviness when weight bearing with the painful side. The trunk is also inclined laterally away from the painful side. Auditory cues alone can betray an abnormal gait, as any good horse trader knows.

Painful hip problems create a limp such that the patient leans over the affected side. As mentioned in Chapter 2, placing the body's center of gravity over the painful hip joint eliminates the need for the usual hip abductor contraction required to stabilize the pelvis in the coronal plane. This tends to lessen the joint reaction force from muscle contraction and therefore diminishes pain.[7] This leaning or lurching is often manifested in hip osteoarthritis and can be a very subtle movement. This lurching to one or both sides is not to be confused with the lurch of a weak gluteus medius. It is similar but occurs for antalgic reasons as opposed to a neuromuscular deficit. That is not to say that a gluteus medius weakness cannot coexist. An inhibited or "pseudoparetic" gluteus medius muscle is often compensated for by an overactive quadratus lumborum muscle. This is evidenced by hip elevation or "hip hiking" seen during gait.

Question for Thought

How would you differentiate a gluteus medius lurch from a painful hip joint gait?

Painful hip conditions, especially chronic ones, are commonly associated with shortened, tight hip flexors that tend to pull the affected hip joint into flexion and the lumbar spine into more lordosis. Consequently, the patient is forced to stoop over into flexion when bearing weight on that leg (Figure 5–4). If both hips are involved, the patient walks with a stooped hip-contracture gait. Weakness of the gluteus maximus results in an extensor gait in which the trunk is extended back when bearing weight on the

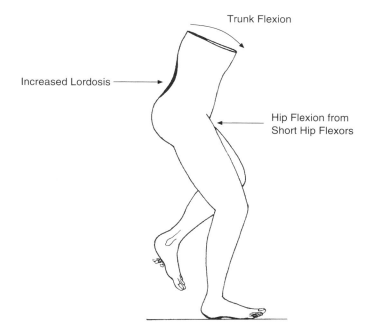

Trunk Flexion

Increased Lordosis

Hip Flexion from
Short Hip Flexors

Figure 5–4 Gait Appearance with Shortened Hip Flexors

affected side (Figure 5–5). Painful stiffness or stiffness alone in the hip joint will result in a lack of lateral sway of the pelvis during the stance phase in gait.[3] Commonly seen in hip problems, especially osteoarthritis, is a toeing-out gait.

Weakness in the gluteus maximus, tightness in the psoas muscle, or hip joint dysfunction with or without capsuloligamentous shortening can all contribute to decreased hip extension. As a consequence, the lumbar spine compensates and extends the hip via erector spinae contraction. This places strain on the lumbar spine and can be visualized during gait observation as hyperlordosis and muscle contraction. Tight hip flexors will cause a diminished toe-off, and a hypertonic quadratus lumborum will hike up the iliac crest on that side.

Question for Thought

What is the significance of decreased hip extension during gait?

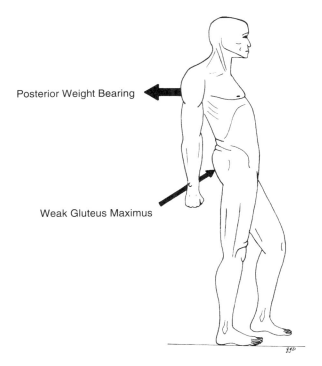

Posterior Weight Bearing

Weak Gluteus Maximus

Figure 5–5 Gluteus Maximus Gait

Observation of the direction in which the patellae point during gait can yield clues as to femoral version. The angle of version or torsion is the angle the femoral neck makes with the frontal plane as the femur is "twisted" on itself during development. This is evidenced by the fact that a femur bone resting on a level surface with the condyles lying flat will have the femoral head and neck angled off the surface slightly. Normally, the femoral neck is anteverted 12 degrees anterior to the transverse axis of the femoral condyles. Confusion often results when describing knee or patellar facing in relation to anteversion or retroversion. A better understanding can be gained if one holds constant the neutral orientation of the femoral neck and acetabulum. One then takes note of the effect that femoral version changes have on the orientation of the femoral condyles and patella (Figure 5–6). For instance, in femoral anteversion, the angle of version is increased as the femur is "twisted" more on itself. This causes more of the femoral head to be uncovered in the acetabulum; therefore, to have

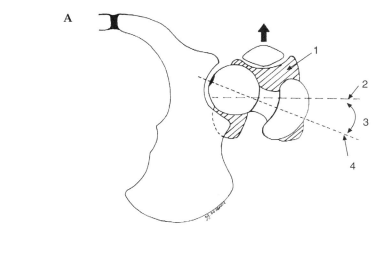

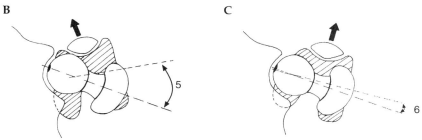

Figure 5–6 Knee and patellar orientation with anteversion and retroversion. **(A)** Normal: **(1)** femoral condyles, **(2)** transverse axis of femoral condyles, **(3)** angle of version, **(4)** axis of femoral neck and head. **(B)** Anteversion: **(5)** increased femoral version angle. **(C)** Retroversion: **(6)** decreased angle.

optimal weight bearing at the hip joint, the femur needs to be medially rotated during gait. Consequently, the individual stands or walks with the patella facing more medially, exhibiting a toe-in gait. A genu valgus posture is usually seen with anteversion.

In retroversion, the angle of version is smaller, the femoral condyles rotate externally, and the patient walks with a toe-out gait.[2] In retroverted hip joints, the added external rotation seen during gait can create muscle-shortening problems in the external hip rotators, especially in people who engage in prolonged gait activities, ie, running, unaccustomed walking. Genu varus is often associated with a retroverted hip joint.

Overall hip range of motion is normal in both anteversion and retroversion, but internal rotation is increased in the former, and external rotation is increased in the latter. This may create an imbalance of muscle length-strength parameters about the hip and pelvis and lower extremity. Femoral version provides us with a good example of the locomotor system's functional interdependence, in which biomechanical changes occurring at one area will cause changes elsewhere. For example, femoral anteversion is associated with an increased Q-angle at the knee (genu valgus deformity). This is further associated with a tight iliotibial band and pronated foot.[8] Additionally, sacroiliac joint dysfunction and a shortened Achilles' heel cord are commonly seen with a tight iliotibial band.[9]

Tight, shortened iliotibial bands are also commonly found in older adults who tend to be sedentary and manifest chronic hip and sacroiliac joint problems. It is important to identify short, tight iliotibial bands early on because these structures become relatively resistant to treatment if they are allowed to become chronically shortened. In identifying femoral version, one can educate patients on dysfunctional tendencies, ie, shortened iliotibial bands and the abovementioned problems associated with them, and teach them specific exercises to avoid difficulties. Granted, not much can be done for the actual femoral version abnormality, yet awareness of and attention to the clinical problems that may arise is important.

Posture

An individual's posture should be assessed to ascertain clues that yield information pertaining to his or her problem. However, as stated before, asymmetry is quite common in the human musculoskeletal system, and inferences drawn from postural distortions, especially those of a subtle nature, should be made with caution. This is meant not to downplay the importance of the postural attitude but to temper the clinical mind with discernment.

Posture should be assessed from all sides to visualize how the patient is oriented to gravity in relation to all planes. A plumb line can be used for reference. As one views from the posterior, the plumb line should ideally bisect the body in equal halves, and the head, shoulders, and pelvis should be level (Figure 5–7A). The feet should be equidistant and point slightly outward. The height of the iliac crests and posterior superior iliac spines (PSISs) can be ascertained by palpating each of them simultaneously. If an unlevel pelvis is present, a leg-length discrepancy may exist, and the rela-

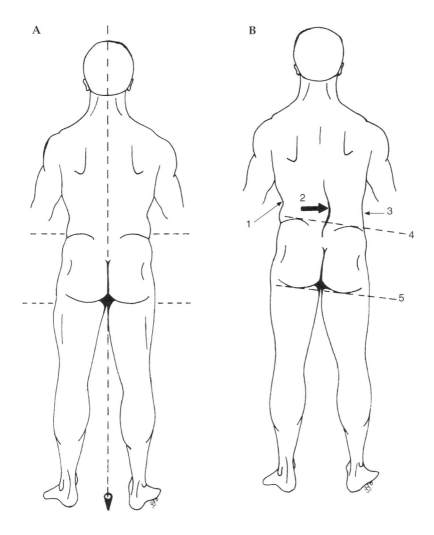

Figure 5–7 (A) Normal postural alignment. **(B)** Postural deviations seen with leg-length inequality: **(1)** indented waist, **(2)** lumbar scoliosis, **(3)** shallow curve at waist, **(4)** pelvic obliquity, **(5)** lower gluteal fold on side of short leg.

tive heights of the greater trochanter, fibular head or tibial tubercle, and lateral malleolus can be assessed to determine where the deficiency lies. This is not an accurate assessment by any means but simply serves as a clinical benchmark. For instance, pelvic torsion at the sacroiliac joints, where one ilium is counterrotated in relation to the other, can create an asymmetry in iliac crest heights without a leg-length insufficiency.[10] Asymmetric femoral neck angulation is not uncommon and can create uneven greater trochanter heights.[11]

The waist can appear indented more and the hip can seem to bulge more on the long-leg side of a patient with leg-length insufficiency[12] (Figure 5–7B). The arm on the side of leg-length insufficiency will appear to hang further away from the body in comparison to the arm on the long-leg side. Any lumbar scoliosis due to an oblique pelvis may be associated with increased skinfolds at the waist on the side of the scoliotic concavity.[12]

The contour of the spine should be observed for curves and distortions. The fullness of the erector spinae bulge can be compared for tone or spasm. The horizontal gluteal folds marking the inferior aspect of the gluteus maximus muscles should be level and symmetric bilaterally (Figure 5–8A). The fold will be lower on the side of a short leg or a sagging, atonic gluteus maximus, commonly found in chronic sacroiliac joint and hip lesions.[13] However, if the gluteus maximus is smaller from atrophy, the fold will appear shorter, level with the opposite side, or even higher, since the muscle belly does not sag as much due to shrinkage. In addition, the upper and outer quadrant of the gluteus maximus will appear flat if decreased tone is present.

Shortening and tightness of the adductors are apparent from observation of the medial contour of the thigh (Figure 5–8B). A faint letter "S" can be seen because the proximal short adductors (pectineus) seem bulkier in the proximal third of the thigh due to shortness and tightness, often seen in pubic symphysis and hip joint problems. The area at the junction of the long and short adductors appears deepened, and further distally, a small hollow from atrophy can be observed above the medial aspect of the knee.

As mentioned in Chapter 4, the layer syndrome[13,14] can commonly be observed from behind as one notices regions of hypertonic muscle groups alternating with adjacent regions of weak muscle groups. For example, in order from the feet upward, the hamstring muscles are usually tight, alternating with weak, atrophied gluteus maximus and lumbosacral erector spinae muscles. Next, the thoracolumbar erector spinae are found to be prominent and tight, alternating with hypoactive and weak interscapular and lower scapular fixator muscles. The upper trapezius muscles, levator scapulae, and cervical erector spinae are then seen to be tight at the top of the spine.

Viewed from the lateral, a plumb line should transect the auditory meatus, shoulder, thorax, lumbar vertebrae, and points slightly posterior to

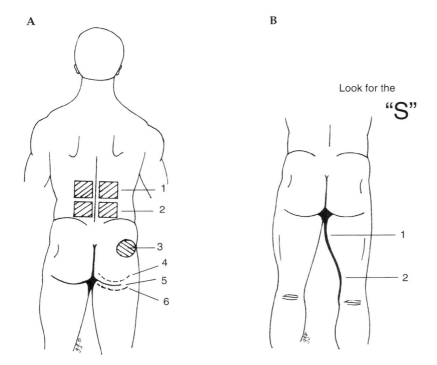

Figure 5–8 (A) Observations on posterior postural examination. Symmetry should be noted between the **(1)** thoracolumbar erector spinae and **(2)** lumbosacral erector spinae, **(3)** flattened area, **(4)** level of atrophic gluteus maximus, **(5)** shortened gluteal fold, **(6)** level of sagging, atonic gluteus maximus. **(B)** Hip adductor observations: **(1)** bulge due to short adductors, **(2)** atrophy of long adductors.

the hip joint axis and slightly anterior to the knee joint axis and the lateral malleolus (Figure 5–9). Posture as viewed from the lateral will yield information as to anterior or posterior pelvic tilting. More commonly one will observe an anterior pelvic tilt from two features that together constitute the pelvic crossed syndrome[13,14]: (1) weak gluteus maximus and shortened, tight iliopsoas muscles; and (2) weak abdominals and shortened and tight low back extensors. If the imbalance involves primarily the former, the lumbar lordosis will be increased and short, being confined to the lumbar spine only (Figure 5–10A). Slight flexion at the hip may be apparent. If it involves primarily the latter, the lordosis will be more shallow but longer, with the thoracic kyphosis starting higher up in the upper thoracic, forcing a forward head and neck position (Figure 5–10B).

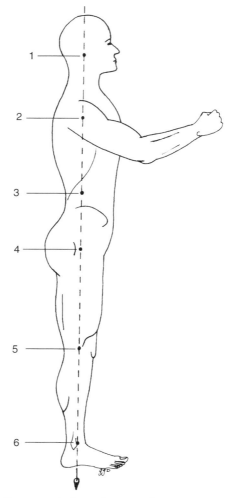

Figure 5–9 Normal alignment in lateral postural examination: **(1)** auditory meatus, **(2)** shoulder joint, **(3)** lumbar vertebrae, **(4)** slightly posterior to hip joint axis, **(5)** slightly anterior to knee joint axis, **(6)** slightly anterior to malleolus.

Tight and shortened hamstrings are often associated with a flat lordosis and posterior tilt of the pelvis, and the knees are commonly hyperextended (Figure 5–10C). If they are hypertonic in reaction to a weak gluteus maximus, the muscle belly will bulge and appear fatter. Flatness of the posterior thigh contour denotes weakness. The tensor fascia lata often cre-

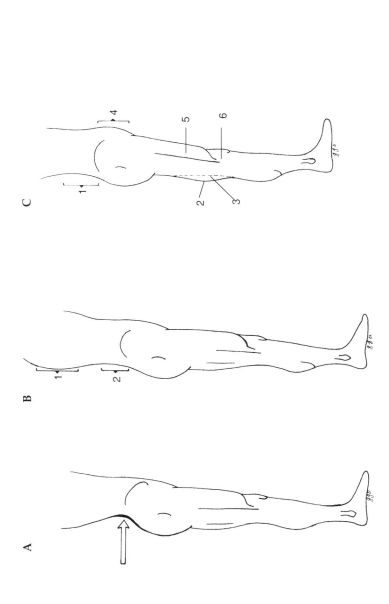

Figure 5-10 Postural observations from the lateral perspective. **(A)** Short lordosis. **(B) (1)** Shallow lordosis, **(2)** long thoracic kyphosis. **(C) (1)** Shallow lordosis, **(2)** hypertonic hamstrings, **(3)** atrophied hamstrings, **(4)** bulging lower abdominal muscles, **(5)** iliotibial band groove, **(6)** knee hyperextension.

ates a flattened contour in the upper anterolateral contour of the thigh due to shortening and tightness. Its pull through the iliotibial band creates a groove in the lateral aspect of the thigh.[13]

Seen from the anterior, the abdominals should appear symmetric when one compares the upper and lower quadrants and the two sides. Weak lower abdominal muscles commonly protrude, especially after multiple pregnancies. Tight obliques manifest themselves with a deep groove that is visible just lateral to the rectus abdominus muscle (Figure 5–11). The relative heights of the anterior superior iliac spines (ASISs) can be assessed and compared to the crest and PSIS heights observed earlier. If all three landmarks are lower on one side, leg-length insufficiency should be suspected.

Trunk Range of Motion

Gross trunk range-of-motion testing is not accurate in localizing joint signs, but it can be used as a quick general screening tool. Certain observations made during the various movements may yield valuable information.

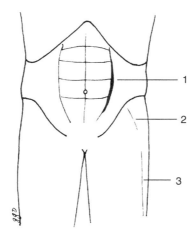

Figure 5–11 Anterior view of abdomen: **(1)** groove lateral to rectus abdominis muscle, **(2)** tensor fascia lata groove, **(3)** iliotibial band groove.

Flexion

Forward flexion should be performed smoothly, with the lumbar lordosis seen to reverse or at least flatten. Short and tight erector spinae muscles or lumbar joint dysfunction can create a persistence of the lordosis. In full flexion, the erector spinae muscles should fully relax, except for the iliocostalis thoracis, allowing the spine to rest on its ligamentous support.[15] In sacroiliac joint dysfunction, a pulling sensation is usually experienced and is localized to the lower back and affected sacroiliac joint. With some coaxing, the patient is able to flex further. However, in disc lesions, flexion is very difficult, and leg pain can become a predominant feature, usually increasing with progressive flexion.

During the forward-flexion maneuver, both PSISs can be palpated and observed for Piedallu's sign (Figure 5-12). If in full-trunk flexion one of the PSISs travels further than the other, a positive Piedallu's sign is present. Often while the patient is in the standing position, one PSIS is observed to be lower, yet during flexion it moves cephalad to emerge higher than the other PSIS. This is called the *overtake phenomenon*. That one of the PSISs travels further than the other is thought to be due to sacroiliac joint restriction. As the spine bends forward, the sacrum follows. If restriction in one of the sacroiliac joints is present, the ilium, and thus the PSIS, will follow and travel further cephalad than its fellow PSIS. This is not an exact test but serves as a quick screen. Often after manipulative reduction of a sacroiliac joint restriction, this test is seen to normalize.

While the patient is in the forward-bent position, the examiner can percuss the PSISs and spinous processes with the ulnar aspect of his or her fist to jolt the articular structures (Figure 5–13). The patient with joint dysfunction will experience a sharp pain that is short lasting. Pathology should be suspected when the pain elicited from percussion lingers, is severe, and causes the patient to cringe.

The return to the upright position can yield very important clinical clues. It should be done smoothly, starting with hip extension and followed by erector spinae contraction and spinal extension to neutral. At full flexion, a relaxation response in the erector spinae muscles should occur, causing the spine to hang by its ligaments. With joint dysfunction of the posterior facet joints, segmental reflex muscle guarding blocks this relaxation response. Upon the patient's arising from full-trunk flexion when the erector spinae should still be relaxed, the facilitated erector spinae muscles immediately contract and extend the facet lesion prematurely.[16] This causes a jab of pain and is called the *reversal sign*. Most back conditions can cause a tentative recovery to the neutral position, but a

A

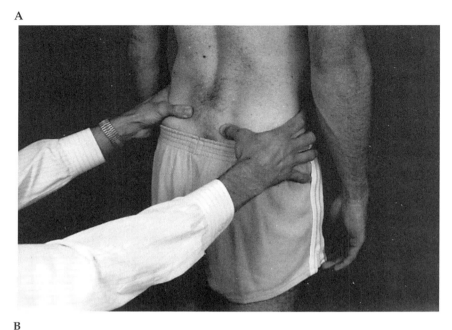

B

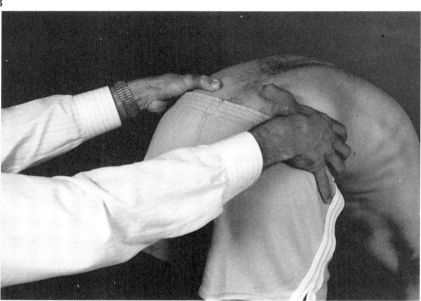

Figure 5–12 Piedallu's sign. **(A)** Note that right posterior iliac spine is lower. **(B)** Note that right posterior iliac spine "overtakes" left side with trunk flexion.

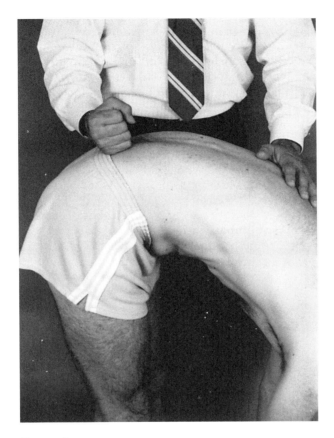

Figure 5–13 Percussion

slow, tortuous return should lead one to suspect pathology and not joint dysfunction.[17]

Extension

Trunk extension may be uncomfortable in sacroiliac joint lesions but is usually more so in lumbar facet joint dysfunction. Localizing combined extension, lateral flexion, and rotation (quadrant testing) to individual lumbar facet levels will help localize lumbar joint signs. This is similar to testing the whole lumbar spine with Kemp's test, but the combined movements are localized to the individual lumbar segments with the examiner's thumb.

Lateral Flexion

During lateral flexion of the trunk, the spine is seen to arc in a smooth curve with the erector spinae muscles on the convex side contracting eccentrically (Figures 5–14A and 5–15B). The pelvis should sway opposite to the side of lateral bending, and the PSISs should remain level.[18,19] Disruption of these events can be seen in hip and sacroiliac joint dysfunction, with the contralateral pelvic sway occurring minimally or missing altogether. A hypertonic quadratus lumborum muscle can limit lumbar side bending. This is evidenced by the lumbar spine's angling sharply at the thoracolumbar junction as the whole lumbar spine is "fixed" in place by the hypertonic quadratus lumborum (Figures 5–14B and 5–15A).

The PSIS opposite to the side of bending can usually be seen to rise up in relation to the other when dysfunction is present. Concentric contraction of the erector spinae group on the ipsilateral side of bending may signify disharmony of muscle function. Spasm or adaptive shortening of the hip abductors and/or adductors can also prevent normal pelvic motion in the frontal plane. Length and strength assessments of these muscles are indicated when inappropriate lateral pelvic sway is observed.

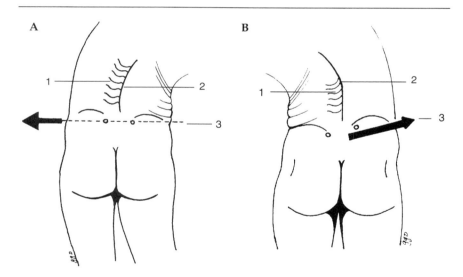

Figure 5–14 **(A)** Normal trunk lateral bending: **(1)** bulge of contracting muscle, **(2)** smooth lumbar spine curve, **(3)** lateral sway of pelvis while posterior superior iliac spines remain level. **(B)** Abnormal lateral bending: **(1)** contraction of muscles in concavity, **(2)** fixed lumbar spine, with angulation occurring at thoracolumbar region, **(3)** reduced lateral pelvic sway and elevation of posterior superior iliac spine.

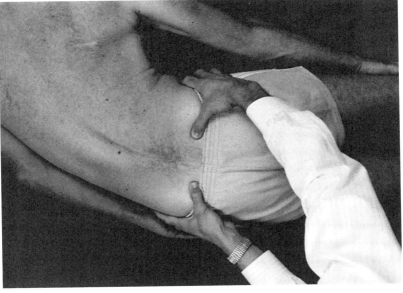

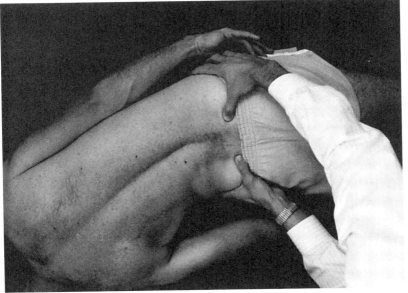

Figure 5–15 (A) Note angulation at thoracolumbar spine and rising up of right posterior superior iliac spine under examiner's right thumb. The left erector spinae muscle group is contracting; **(B)** Normal right lateral bending.

Sacroiliac Palpation: Gillet's Test

The following procedures are designed to accentuate normal gait parameters to assess sacroiliac joint function. The patient is asked to raise the knee as high as possible, and movement of the following landmarks is monitored with palpation: the PSISs, posterior inferior iliac spines (PIISs), sacral tubercle, and sacral apex (Figure 5–16). Because of its peculiar morphology, the sacroiliac joint has upper and lower aspects to it that seem to function separately. As a consequence, Gillet and Liekens[20] and Faye[21] advocate examining both parts by monitoring motion at the PSIS (upper aspect) and PIIS (lower aspect) in relation to the sacral tubercle and apex respectively. Essentially four areas are assessed: the upper and lower aspects of the sacroiliac joint on both the left and right sides. The following is a description of the examination of the right sacroiliac joint.

The examiner sits behind the standing patient and places his or her right thumb on the right PSIS and left thumb on the sacral tubercle to assess movement at the upper aspect of the right sacroiliac joint. A firm skin contact is necessary so that the examiner is not fooled by skin movement. The patient is asked to raise his or her right knee as high as he or she can, and the examiner monitors the movement of the right PSIS in relation to the sacral tubercle (Figure 5–17A). The patient's knee is usually raised bent.

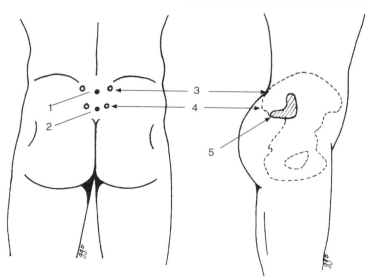

Figure 5–16 Sacroiliac joint palpation points: **(1)** S-2 tubercle, **(2)** sacral apex, **(3)** posterior superior iliac spine, **(4)** posterior inferior iliac spine, **(5)** sacroiliac joint.

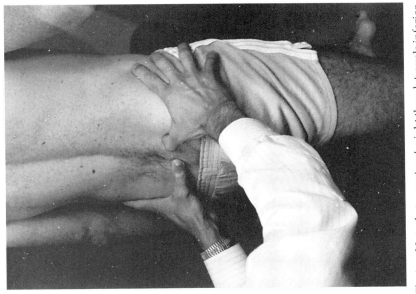

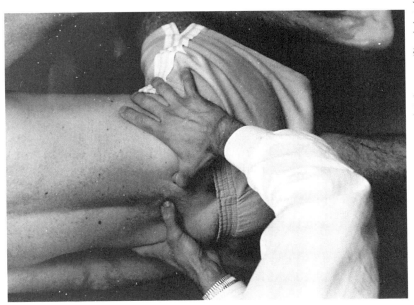

Figure 5–17 Palpation of upper aspect of right sacroiliac joint. **(A)** Flexion. Note that examiner's right thumb travels inferior. **(B)** Extension. Note that examiner's left thumb travels inferior.

However, Gillet and Liekens[20] and Schafer and Faye[22] mention that raising the straight leg physiologically blocks or restricts the pubic symphysis, forcing more movement to occur in the ipsilateral sacroiliac joint. This is thought to make more evident any joint restriction in that sacroiliac joint.

As the right knee is raised high, the right PSIS should be palpated to move inferior in relation to the sacral tubercle as the ilium goes through a posterior rotation through the sacroiliac joint. Faye[21] refers to this movement as *sacroiliac joint flexion,* and since we are monitoring at the level of the PSIS, it is termed *flexion of the upper aspect of the right sacroiliac joint.* The movement is perceived as a slight shifting or gliding motion of the PSIS relative to the sacral tubercle. Technically, the PSIS should move posteriorly and inferiorly, yet its inferior movement is more definite and can be as much as ½ in. No movement relative to the sacral tubercle denotes joint fixation or restriction. Initially during this maneuver, the entire pelvis en masse moves slightly around the contralateral femoral head, giving the illusion that the PSIS is moving. However, PSIS movement should be assessed relative to the sacral tubercle so as to monitor sacroiliac joint function.

Hypermobility may manifest itself with a clicking noise and increased motion during this maneuver. However, the clicking can also be coming from the femoroacetabular joint or iliotibial band, as in the "snapping-hip syndrome"[23]. This can usually be felt with the small finger of the palpating hand as it wraps laterally around the hip.

Maintaining the same anatomical contacts as above, the examiner then asks the patient to raise the left leg. In this instance, the sacral tubercle is now monitored in relation to the PSIS on the weight-bearing side, and it should be observed to move in a posterior and inferior direction (Figure 5–17B). This movement is called *extension at the upper aspect of the right sacroiliac joint.* This maneuver is mechanically similar to standing in a lunge-forward position with the right leg extended backward (Figure 5–18). However, for the sake of convenience, the patient is asked to raise the left leg instead, while relative sacroiliac joint extension is palpated for on the right side.

To monitor flexion motion of the lower aspect of the right sacroiliac joint, the examiner's right thumb is moved to the right PIIS, about 1½ in lower than the PSIS contact. The left thumb is moved to the sacral apex or the subcutaneous aspect of the sacrum just medial to the right thumb, thus straddling the lower aspect of the right sacroiliac joint. Again, the patient is asked to raise the right leg, and the right thumb contact is monitored in relation to that of the left (Figure 5–19A). What should be observed is a caudal and slightly lateral deviation of the thumb contacting the PIIS. An

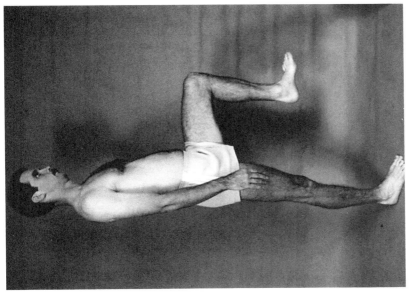

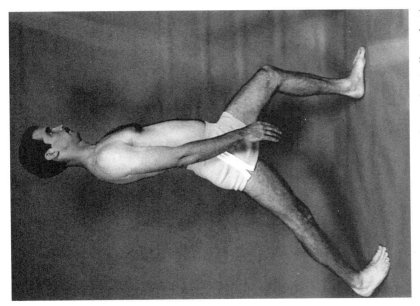

Figure 5–18 (A) This position is similar mechanically to that in Figures 5–18B and 5–17B. **(B)** Raising the left leg actually puts the right hip into relative extension.

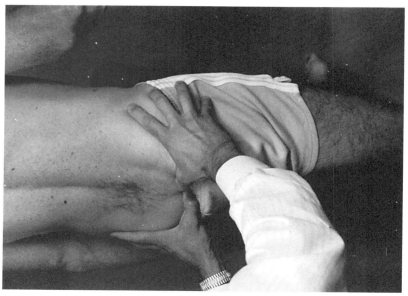

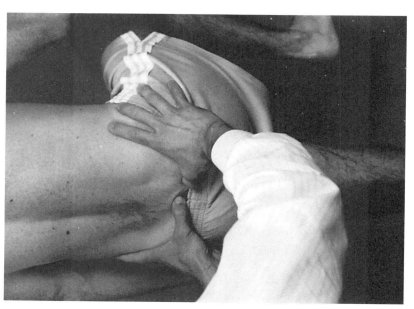

Figure 5–19 Palpation of lower aspect of right sacroiliac joint. **(A)** Flexion. **(B)** Extension.

alternative contact would be to palpate the ischial tuberosity with the right thumb while maintaining the sacral apex contact.

To assess extension of the sacroiliac joint's lower aspect, the examiner's palpatory contacts remain the same as above for the "lower" joint, but the patient is asked to raise the left leg (Figure 5–19B). The sacral contact is now monitored in relation to the iliac contact. The sacral apex should be observed to move inferiorly in relation to the PIIS contact.

In all the above maneuvers, the palpating thumbs, being astride the sacroiliac joint while contacting different osseous structures, should move independently if motion is free. If no movement is detected or if both thumbs move together as a unit, joint fixation can be suspected. Basically, flexion and extension movements should be palpated for at each of the following four locations: the upper and lower aspects of each sacroiliac joint. If all four locations are not assessed, joint problems are readily missed. Sacroiliac joint fixations often occur in multiples and especially in a diagonal fashion. For instance, restriction of the upper aspect of a sacroiliac joint is often associated with fixation in the lower aspect of the opposite side joint. Therefore, finding joint restriction in the upper poles should alert one to assess the lower poles as well. If one assesses only the upper aspects, important joint restrictions will be missed in the lower aspects. Similarly, if only flexion fixations are checked for, an important extension fixation will be missed if present.

During the knee-raising test, patients will often make compensatory movements in reaction to restricted sacroiliac or hip joint motion. When they raise a leg, the weight-bearing leg will bend slightly at the knee and extend at the hip to gain an increase in motion (Figure 5–20A). In addition, they will stick the buttock out laterally to aid in raising the knee higher (Figure 5–20B). Chronically stiffened sacroiliac joints can demonstrate a lack of motion at all palpation points. In such instances, ankylosis must be ruled out with radiographs before manipulation is undertaken.

In general, flexion movements are monitored with iliac contacts (PSIS, PIIS, or ischial tuberosity), and extension movements are monitored with sacral contacts (tubercle or apex). When the patient lifts the knee, the examiner's ipsilateral thumb should move with the appropriate contact. For example, as the patient's right leg is lifted, the examiner's right thumb should move with the palpated contact. If the examiner is monitoring the right sacroiliac joint, then the right PSIS or PIIS should be observed to move, depending on whether the upper or lower aspect of the sacroiliac joint respectively is being monitored. For an extension restriction, if the patient's left knee is raised while the examiner still monitors the right sacroiliac joint, the examiner's left thumb on the sacrum should move. Lack of

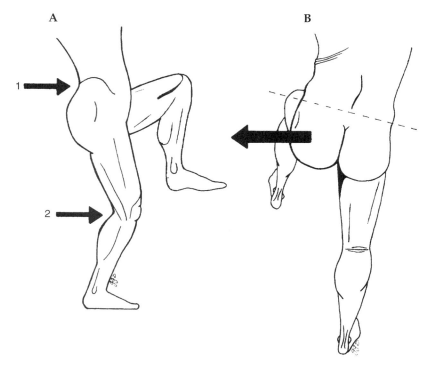

Figure 5–20 Compensation for stiff hip and sacroiliac joints in knee-raising test. **(A) (1)** Lumbar and hip extension; **(2)** knee flexion. **(B)** Patient sticks buttock out laterally.

movement indicates joint fixation. The type of fixation found determines the manipulative technique used, as is discussed in Chapter 7.

SITTING

Small Hemipelvis

An often-overlooked anomaly is a small hemipelvis (SHP) such that the height of the pelvis on one side is smaller than the other. About 20% to 30% of patients examined demonstrated an SHP.[24] Inglemark and Lindstrom[25] noted a significant association between leg length inequality and hemipelvis size. Commonly, an SHP is associated with an ipsilateral leg-length inequality, short upper extremity, and smaller face.[26] Therefore, finding one asymmetry on examination may lead to the observation of the others. A small hemipelvis will tend to manifest itself symptomatically during prolonged sitting postures, as compared to leg-length inequality, in which the effects are seen during standing.

While the patient is seated, the pelvic posture and attitude should be observed for obliquity, indicating pelvic torsion between the ilia at the sacroiliac joints or a small hemipelvis. Travell and Simons[12] explain the proper procedure used to assess a small hemipelvis. A clinical trial of placing a "butt lift" under the lower side can be done to level the pelvis and ascertain any corrective effects occurring in the spine and trunk above.

In an examination for an SHP, the patient must be seated on a firm surface, and the feet should be raised high enough to fit two fingers between the plinth and the patient's distal thigh[12] (Figure 5–21). Relative height assessments are then made of the anterior and posterior superior iliac spines and iliac crests. An SHP probably exists if all landmarks palpate lower on one side. Lumbar scoliotic deviation and shoulder height differences may be observed in the sitting position with SHP, as they are in the standing position with leg-length inequality. To correct this asymmetry, a "butt lift"[12] is used to level the pelvis while the patient is in the sitting position (Figure 5–22). This can be an important asymmetry to correct in someone who sits extensively.

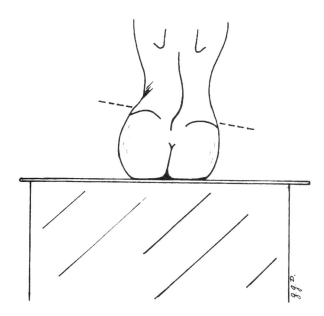

Figure 5–21 Right Small Hemipelvis

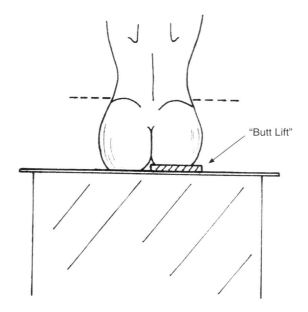

Figure 5–22 Correction of Small Hemipelvis with a "Butt Lift"

PSIS Measurement

The distance between the paired PSISs can be measured to compare with the measurement taken prone (Figure 5–23). A cloth tape measure will suffice. One should make sure to take a measurement from the same aspect of each PSIS. According to Mennell,[9,17] this distance should increase by ¼ to ¾ in when the patient goes from the sitting to the prone position. He says that its absence signifies sacroiliac joint disease and can be an early sign of ankylosing spondylitis. In addition, this movement is often decreased in older patients or in those who sit for prolonged periods of time and exhibit restricted sacroiliac joint motion in most of the four palpation points during the standing knee-raising test.

Lumbosacral Joint Versus Sacroiliac Joint

Sitting trunk rotation can yield important information differentiating lumbar facet from sacroiliac joint dysfunctions.[9] As the patient sits upright with hands interlocked behind the head, the examiner passively rotates the trunk by gently pulling on the ipsilateral arm and pushing on the con-

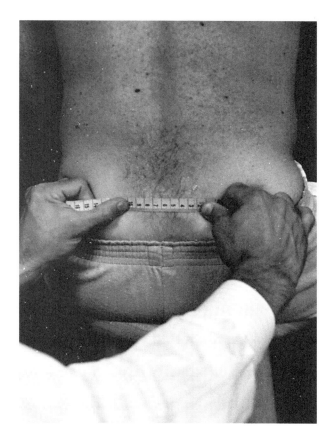

Figure 5–23 Sitting Measurement of Posterior Superior Iliac Spine Distance

tralateral scapula (Figure 5–24). A painful response can be elicited by the torsional stress placed on the ipsilateral (side to which the patient is rotated) lumbosacral and sacroiliac joints.

To differentiate lumbosacral from sacroiliac joint involvement, the patient is asked to slump backward onto the examiner (Figure 5–25). Pain in this position commonly is due to lumbosacral dysfunction, since this position stresses the lumbosacral region. If this maneuver is not painful, the patient is then rotated to the left while in this slumped position until the right ischial tuberosity (not the buttock itself) leaves the table (Figure 5–26). By twisting the sacrum between the ilia, this maneuver places a back-

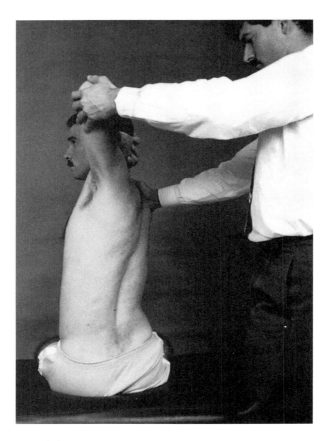

Figure 5–24 Trunk Rotation

ward torsion in the left sacroiliac joint and an anterior torsional stress in the right sacroiliac joint. Pain provoked on the left side indicates backward torsion dysfunction of the left sacroiliac joint. If the examiner now places his or her hand on the right ASIS and presses downward toward the table while maintaining the trunk in the torqued position, the backward torsional strain in the left joint will be relieved, and any elicited pain will be lessened.[9,17] The procedure is then repeated on the other side (Figure 5–27).

On the other hand, when the trunk is rotated to the left while the patient is in this slumped position, the patient can experience pain on the right side as the right sacroiliac joint is stressed in anterior torsion. As the right ASIS is pressed toward the table, the torsional stress is relieved, and any provoked pain due to a right anterior torsion dysfunction is diminished.

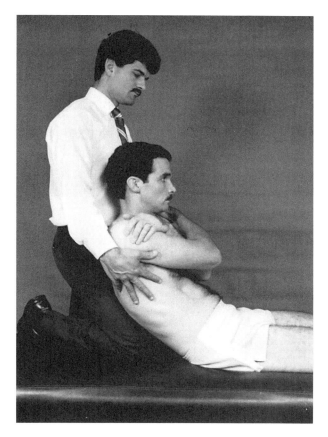

Figure 5–25 Backward-Lying or Slump Test

As an aside, this testing of sacroiliac torsional stress has been found to be useful as a therapeutic maneuver, especially in pregnant women exhibiting sacroiliac joint disorders. It is used mostly as a strong stretching mobilization. Also, this test does not differentiate involvement in the upper versus lower poles of the sacroiliac joint.

Piriformis Strength

When the hips are flexed to 90 degrees, the piriformis acts as a horizontal hip abductor. Therefore, one can test the strength of this muscle in the seated position by resisting the separation of the patient's knees (see Chapter 9, Figure 9–10). Weakness and pain are common with piriformis

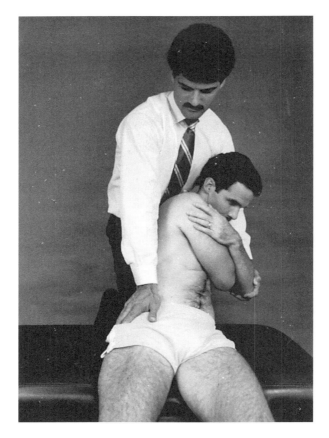

Figure 5–26 Backward torsion applied to left sacroiliac joint. Note pressure on the right anterior superior iliac spine to relieve torsional stress.

trigger points. Piriformis trigger points are often seen in association with sacroiliac and hip joint disorders.

SUPINE

Trunk Curl-Up

The patient is supine with knees bent, feet flat on the table, and arms across the chest or outstretched. The clinician monitors hip flexor recruitment by cradling the patient's heels and feeling if they lift during the test (Figure 5–28). The patient is instructed to do a posterior pelvic tilt and curl up until the scapulae come off the table. Ten repetitions are performed,

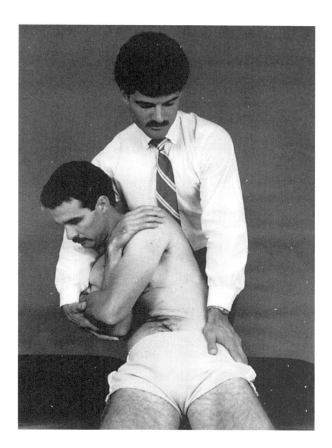

Figure 5–27 Backward Torsion Applied to Right Sacroiliac Joint

and the last one is held for 30 seconds. Any lifting of the feet, signifying hip flexor recruitment, extreme trunk shaking, or inability to maintain a posterior pelvic tilt indicates a positive test for weak abdominal muscles.[27]

A positive test for weakness or inhibition is usually due to tight erector spinae and/or psoas muscles that are reciprocally inhibiting the abdominal muscles. These would need to be assessed along with lumbar spinal joint mobility.

Pubic Symphysis

Pubic symphysis joint problems are not a common occurrence when compared to sacroiliac joint problems, but when they do exist, attention

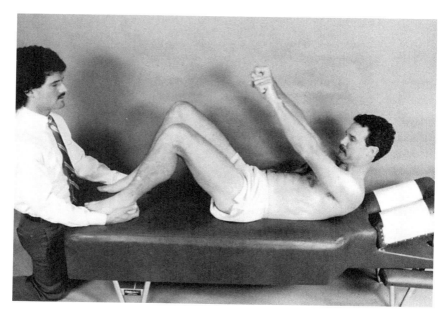

Figure 5–28 Trunk curl-up test. Note that patient is resting heels on clinician's hands.

should be given to them. The diagnosis of pubic symphysis joint dysfunction is generally presumptive and is based on three clinical criteria (Figure 5–29):

1. asymmetry of pubic tubercle relationship
2. tension in inguinal ligament/short hip adductors
3. tenderness at pubic tubercles and at inguinal ligament and hip adductor origins

Sagittal-plane rotation at the sacroiliac joint (positive- or negative-theta x-axis rotation of the ilia) appears limited in the presence of PS fixation,[20,28] and the standing knee-bending test then shows restriction of motion.

Tenderness and tautness are palpated for along the course of the inguinal ligament, especially at its origin and insertion. Typically, it will be tender to palpation in sacroiliac joint and pubic symphysis joint dysfunctions. Palpation of the symphysis pubis is accomplished by moving caudally from the midline lower abdomen until the joint is reached. The heel of the hand is

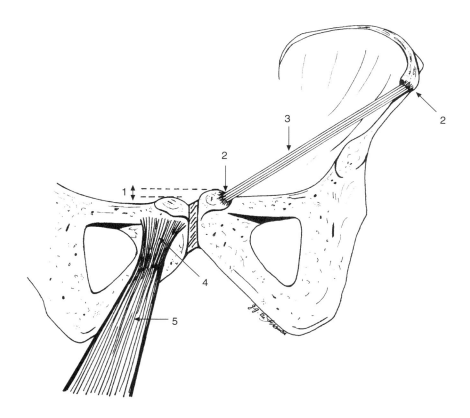

Figure 5–29 Clinical signs of pubic symphysis joint problem: **(1)** pubic tubercle asymmetry, **(2)** painful origin and insertion of inguinal ligament, **(3)** tension in inguinal ligament, **(4)** painful origin of adductor muscle, **(5)** tension in adductor muscle.

used, with the fingers pointing cephalad. The examiner is standing on level, with the pelvis facing cephalad. The examiner should exercise sensitivity and modesty when palpating this area. If it is deemed appropriate, the examiner can place the patient's hand and fingers under the examiner's until the pubic symphysis is reached. Next, using the index fingers, the

examiner compares the relative position and tenderness of each pubic tubercle. Pain and tension are present if this joint is in dysfunction. Sacroiliac
joint problems often coexist with pubic symphysis problems.[29,30]

Indirect joint provocation tests can be used. This entails flexing one
thigh on the chest while extending the other thigh off the table. This places
an extreme physiologic countertorque on the PS. A similar maneuver, incidentally, is performed to mobilize this joint, as discussed in Chapter 6.

While the patient is supine, the pelvis can be observed for asymmetry in
the anteroposterior dimension. The pelvis may seem to be slanting toward
one side, as there may be a small hemipelvis. These patients may have a
history of lower back, pelvic, or hip discomfort while lying supine due to
their asymmetry. An appropriately placed pillow can be an effective rem-
edy for them.

Sacroiliac Joint Distraction, Iliopsoas Palpation

The ASISs can be gently pressed apart simultaneously to gap the anterior aspect of the sacroiliac joints (Figure 5–30). The iliacus can be palpated
just medial and deep to the ASIS (Figure 5–31). Tenderness here is com-

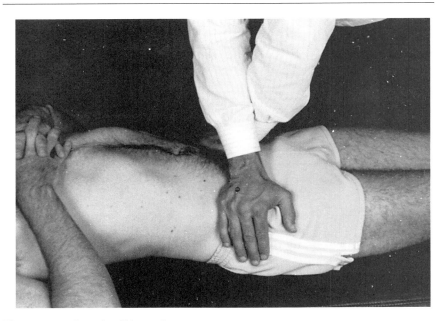

Figure 5–30 Anterior Distraction

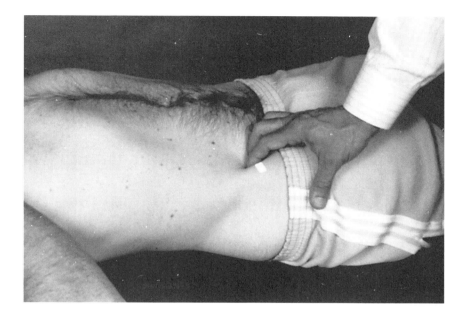

Figure 5–31 Iliacus Palpation (Marker Is on ASIS)

mon in hip and sacroiliac joint problems. Trigger points in the iliopsoas will also cause pain here. To palpate the psoas muscle directly, refer to Chapter 1. A short, tight psoas will palpate as taut and tender. Care must be used in this maneuver so as not to injure nearby viscera.

Straight-Leg–Raising Test

A straight-leg raise (SLR) should be performed to assess nerve tension and hamstring length (Figure 5–32). The knee should be held in extension, with neutral ankle position and neutral hip position with respect to rotation, abduction, and adduction. Hamstring tightness is noted in addition to any elicited pain. The SLR test is often touted as pathognomonic for nerve irritation when positive. However, just as "no man is an island," certainly no individual tissue is isolated from the rest of the musculoskeletal system. Tests designed to provoke a specific structure invariably affect adjacent structures. Muscles are connected to tendons, which are connected to bone, which when moved affect joints and their associated restraining tissues, including nerves and blood vessels.

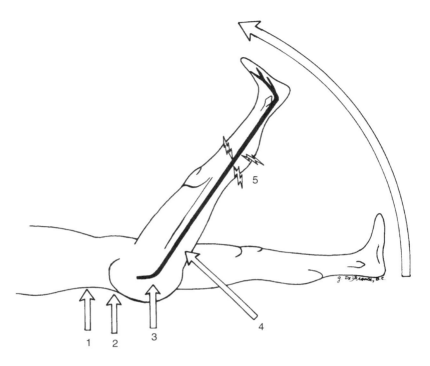

Figure 5–32 Structures moved or stressed during straight-leg–raising test: **(1)** lumbar facet joint, **(2)** sacroiliac joint, **(3)** hip joint, **(4)** hamstring muscles, **(5)** sciatic nerve.

Besides sciatic nerve tension, the SLR also affects the following structures: hamstring muscles, sacroiliac joint, hip joint, and even lumbar facet joints. Nerve irritation can be suspected if the SLR test is strongly positive[31–33] or if the well-leg–raising test is positive.[34] A sacroiliac joint problem can yield a positive SLR test but is usually seen at higher angles of elevation, usually above 45 degrees. The patient will experience pain in the joint, buttock, and/or proximal thigh as the ipsilateral sacroiliac joint is stressed in posterior rotation. The opposite leg should rise to normal range without difficulty, and the double-leg–raising test, which stresses the lumbosacral region by tilting both ilia simultaneously, should be negative. Shortened, tight hamstrings are commonly found in chronic sacroiliac conditions. They also aid in perpetuating joint dysfunction in the hip and pelvic joints. Some patients are "naturally" stiff and exhibit tight hamstrings. Of more clinical significance is asymmetry in hamstring length.

Hip Flexor Length

The examiner should assess passive hip flexion in each hip joint while observing for tissue contracture in the contralateral hip (Figure 5–33). This is best achieved by having the patient place one leg just off the edge of the examination table, with one flexed knee held against the chest. The other leg should hang off the table so that the thigh is horizontal and the leg dangles vertically.[35] The lumbar lordosis should be lost, and pressure is applied to increase thigh flexion onto the trunk. This is accomplished by the clinician's pushing the patient's foot on the side of the flexed knee with his or her thorax (see Chapter 9, Figure 9–16). Short hip flexors on the side with the leg off the table cause slight or even marked flexion of the thigh above the horizontal. If the rectus femoris is short and tight, the knee joint will extend so that the lower leg no longer hangs vertically but more diagonally. A tight iliotibial band and tensor fascia lata manifest as a deeper groove in the lateral aspect of the thigh and lateral migration of the patella.[35] In addition, the thigh may abduct slightly. A tight sartorius will cause flexion at the knee joint and slight external rotation of the thigh. Tight adductors are indicated by slight adduction of the thigh. Hip joint problems will manifest as groin pain on the side of thigh flexion. In a painful and/or restricted osteoarthritic hip joint, the thigh will be seen not to flex directly onto the chest but to deviate laterally from the line of the shoulder. Tight hip flexors are often associated with weak, inhibited gluteus maximus muscles. This should be assessed with the prone hip extension movement pattern (see below).

Gaenslen's Test

Gaenslen's test is a classic test for sacroiliac joint problems, since it imparts a strong extension force through the sacroiliac joint as well as the hip joint (Figure 5–34). When performed in the side posture, it is termed the *Gaenslen-Lewin* test and can be used to differentiate lumbosacral from sacroiliac joint problems, as described by Mennell.[17]

A Gaenslen's test can be performed on the supine patient to stress the sacroiliac joint by extending one thigh off the table and flexing the other thigh upon the chest. A strong stretch is also applied to the iliopsoas on the extended side, which may be uncomfortable to the patient. This is one of

A

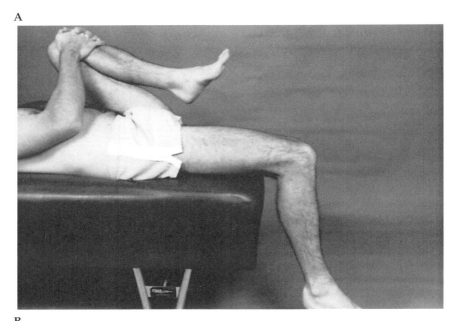

B

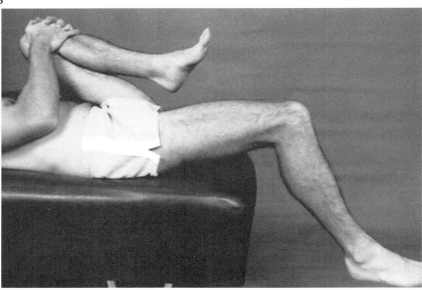

Figure 5–33 Hip flexor length test. **(A)** Normal finding. Note that thigh is resting flat on table and leg is hanging vertically off table. **(B)** Abnormal test. Note that thigh is off table, leg is slightly extended at knee.

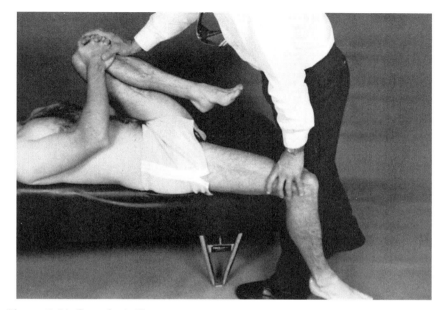

Figure 5–34 Gaenslen's Test

three provocative tests that can help localize a problematic sacroiliac joint. The other two are the Patrick-Fabere and Yeoman's tests.

Patrick-Fabere

The classic test for hip problems is the Patrick-Fabere test, in which the hip is flexed, abducted, externally rotated, and extended (Figure 5–35). Yet this test also effectively stresses the sacroiliac joint and is often positive in sacroiliac joint lesions. However, it is very common to find sacroiliac joint and hip joint problems existing concurrently.

A Patrick-Fabere test is performed by placing the ankle on the contralateral knee and forming a "sign-of-four" with the ipsilateral thigh and leg. Downward pressure is applied on the knee to stress the hip and sacroiliac joints while the contralateral ASIS is stabilized on the table. Pain in the groin can come from both hip and sacroiliac joint problems. Localized sacroiliac joint pain felt posteriorly incriminates that joint more.

Hip Adductor Length

By placing the sole of the patient's foot against the medial side of the opposite knee, and pressing the knee toward the table, one can assess the

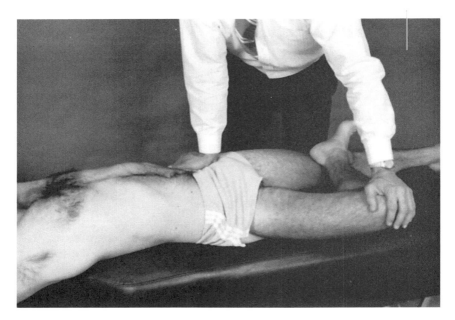

Figure 5–35 Patrick-Fabere Test

tension in the small adductors (Figure 5–36).[26] Another way of testing adductor length is to abduct the straight leg until tension is met and compare it with the other side (Figure 5–37). Then, if the long adductors are relaxed by flexing the knee (Figure 5–38), and if further abduction is possible, the long abductors are short and tight. If hip abduction in the plane of the table is limited when the knee is held in both the straight and slightly bent positions, the short adductors are tight.[35]

Hip Rotation/Posterior Shear/Hip Flexion-Adduction

With the hip joint held in 90 degrees of flexion, medial and lateral rotation can be examined by leveraging movement through the flexed lower extremity (Figure 5–39). Sacroiliac joint pain is often reproduced with external hip rotation in this position. Attention is paid to the end-feel and range of motion at the hip joint. Normally, a painless, leathery stop should be experienced. A more functional assessment of hip rotation is made in the prone position.

A posterior shear accessory movement can be applied to both the hip and the sacroiliac joints by pressing the femur into the table with the hip at

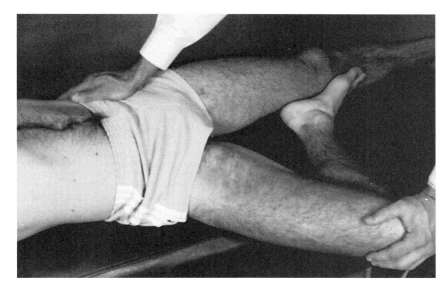

Figure 5–36 Length testing of short adductors. Note that foot is placed medial to knee.

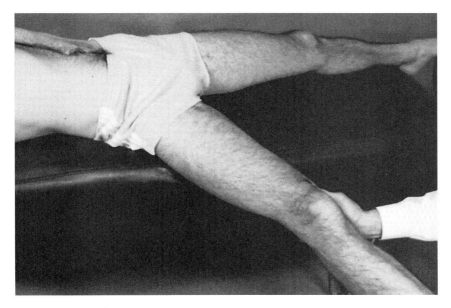

Figure 5–37 Length Testing of Long Adductors

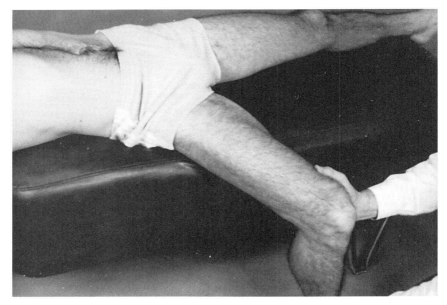

Figure 5–38 Knee Flexion Used To Relax Long Adductors

90 degrees of flexion (Figure 5–40). The examiner's other hand can simultaneously palpate the greater trochanter or sacroiliac joint sulcus to assess
motion. Slight adduction will tend to gap the sacroiliac joint posteriorly.
Small shifting movements can be felt, and pain provocation is looked for.

Maximal adduction while at 90 degrees of hip flexion stresses several
structures and is not a good localizing test (Figure 5–41A). Lewit[36] states
that this mostly stresses the iliolumbar ligament, as the posterior aspect of
the ilium is abducted from the sacrum and spine. By standing opposite the
side to be examined, the examiner grasps the flexed knee and pulls the
thigh into adduction, thus gapping the ilium from the sacrum and L-5.
Pressure is then applied along the long axis of the femur. This is similar to
the above posterior shear test except that much more adduction is used.
Restriction of hip adduction and pain provocation are noted.

To influence the sacroiliac ligaments, the thigh is flexed more onto the
trunk and adducted (Figure 5–41B). Pressure is also directed along the axis
of the femur. With the hip flexed to 90 degrees and strongly adducted,
pain experienced in the groin may be referred from the iliolumbar ligament or hip joint. Pain experienced in the buttock, posterior thigh, or lateral thigh with the hip flexed more than 90 degrees is usually from the

A

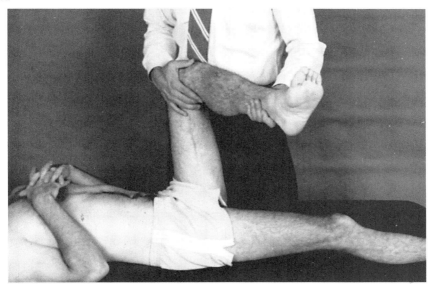

B

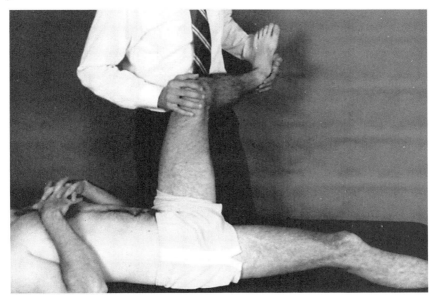

Figure 5–39 Hip rotation. **(A)** External. **(B)** Internal.

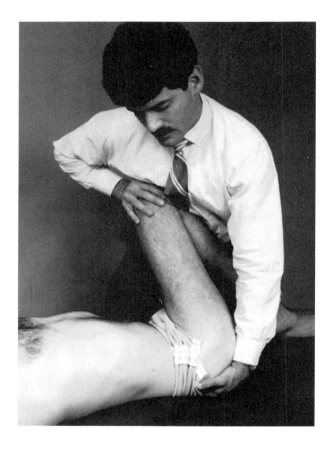

Figure 5–40 Anteroposterior shear of hip and sacroiliac joints. Note slight hip adduction.

---

sacroiliac ligaments.[36] Groin pain more often limits adduction in these tests and is more commonly due to hip joint problems.

Hip Joint Accessory Movements

If hip joint dysfunction is suspected, accessory or joint play movements should be explored in the supine position for posterior and lateral glides as well as long-axis extension with the hip in neutral, and inferior glide with the hip at 90 degrees flexion (Figures 5–42A through 5–42F).

A

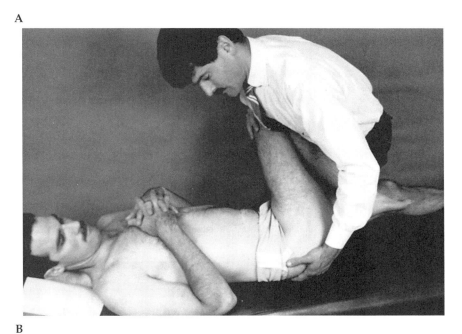

B

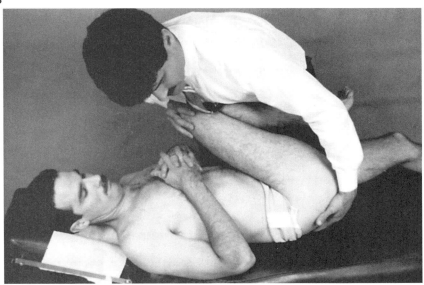

Figure 5–41 Hip flexion/adduction provocative test. **(A)** Note strong adduction at 90 degrees of flexion. **(B)** Note adduction with maximal flexion.

A

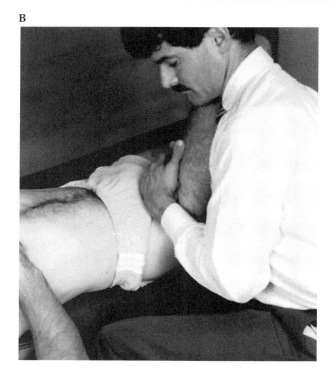

B

continues

Figure 5–42 Hip joint accessory movements. **(A)** Posterior glide. **(B)** Lateral glide. **(C)** and **(D)** Long-axis extension. **(E)** Inferior glide at 90 degrees flexion. **(F)** Same as **(E)** but with leg over shoulder.

Figure 5–42 continued

C

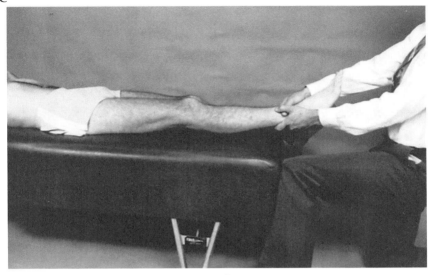

D

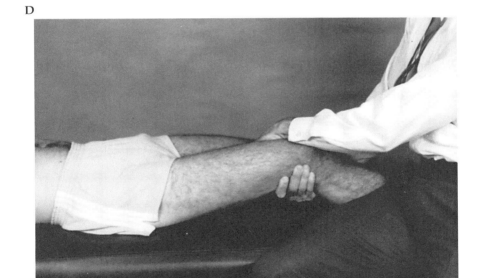

continues

Figure 5–42 continued

E

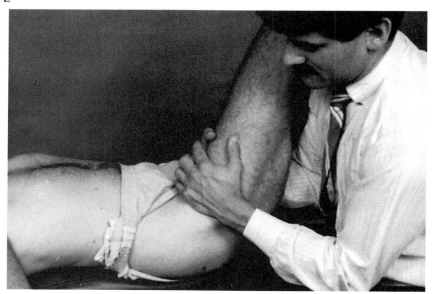

F

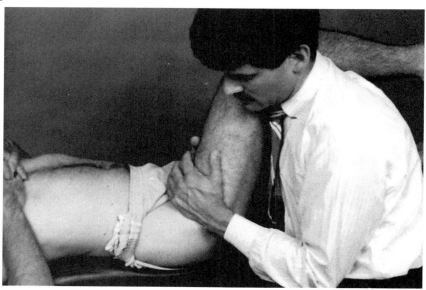

Double-Leg Raise and Lumbosacral Tilt

Two tests in the supine position can be used to incriminate lumbosacral versus sacroiliac joint dysfunction. A double-leg–raising test is performed to tilt the pelvis as a whole on the lumbar spine, thus stressing the lumbosacral joint (Figure 5–43). If lumbosacral joint dysfunction exists, the angle of leg raise will be less than that occurring in the single-leg–raising test with sacroiliac joint dysfunction.

Another maneuver stressing the lumbosacral joint in lateral flexion is performed next.[9,17] To perform this test, the supine patient's hips and knees are flexed to 90 degrees simultaneously while the examiner cradles both lower legs (Figure 5–44). With cradling of the lower legs, the pelvis is

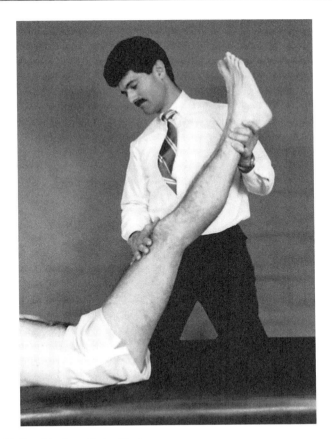

Figure 5–43 Double-Leg–Raise Test

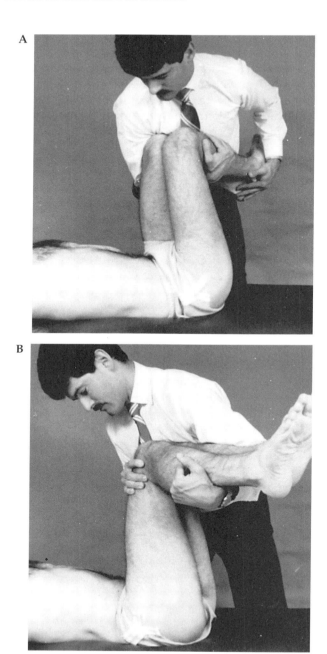

Figure 5–44 Lumbosacral tilt test. **(A)** To the left compresses left lumbosacral facet joint, distracts right joint. **(B)** To the right.

tilted to both the left and the right to gap and compress the lumbosacral joints alternately. Lumbosacral joint dysfunction is manifested by pain and restricted motion.

SIDE-LYING

Hip Abduction Movement Pattern

In the side-lying position, the patient is instructed to abduct the straight leg in the coronal plane. Simultaneous contraction of the tensor fascia lata and gluteus medius is looked for. Palpation of these muscles should be done only if visual observation is difficult, and even so, very light palpation must be used to reduce the chance of facilitating unwanted contractions. If the gluteus medius is inhibited and contracts poorly, the patient will have a tendency to roll the pelvis posteriorly in an attempt to recruit tensor fascia lata contraction. Flexion at the hip will be observed. External rotation signifies piriformis recruitment, and hip hiking signifies contraction of the quadratus lumborum. The leg can also be prepositioned in abduction without any hip flexion, and the patient is asked to hold the leg for 5 seconds. Limb shaking, leg deviations, and the pelvic movements described above are looked for and denote a positive finding for a poor hip abduction movement pattern.

If this test demonstrates poor hip abduction capabilities, the following should be looked for and treated: weak and inhibited gluteus medius, overactive hip adductors, overactive tensor fascia lata, overactive quadratus lumborum, and overactive piriformis. Sacroiliac, hip, thoracolumbar, and/or upper lumbar joint dysfunctions should be looked for, as they often accompany this poor movement pattern.

Quadratus Lumborum Trigger Point

One of the first things to test for in the side-lying position is the most overlooked muscle involved in myofascial pain syndromes of the lower back: the quadratus lumborum muscle (Figure 5–45). It can mimic lumbosacral, sacroiliac, and hip problems.[37] The patient lies on his or her side with the involved side up and the upper arm raised over the head and holding onto the top of the table; a roll cushion is placed under the waist, and the upper leg allowed to rest on the table behind the lower leg. Standing behind the patient, the examiner presses just lateral and deep to the erector spinae group, probing the length of the quadratus lumborum muscle from the inferior aspect of the 12th rib toward the iliac crest. A muscle harboring a trigger point will palpate firmly at its edge, eliciting

A

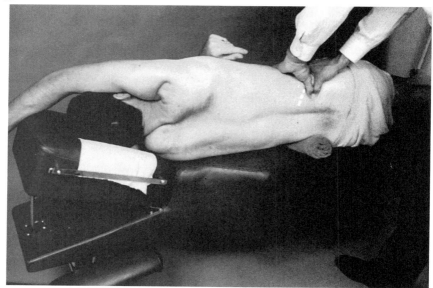

B

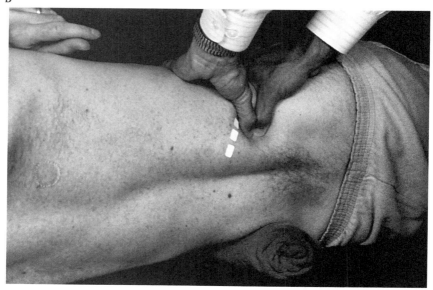

Figure 5–45 (A, B) Quadratus lumborum muscle trigger point examination. Twelfth rib is marked.

marked tenderness. Referred pain from the trigger points in the quadratus lumborum can travel to the ipsilateral sacroiliac joint, hip joint region, buttocks, and even groin. Trigger points in the quadratus lumborum are commonly found in association with sacroiliac and thoracolumbar joint dysfunctions and should be looked for routinely.[37]

Gluteal, Tensor Fascia Lata, and Piriformis Trigger Points

While the patient is in the side-lying position, other muscles just as important as the quadratus lumborum to examine are the gluteus minimus, gluteus medius, tensor fascia lata, and piriformis muscles. Trigger points in these muscles, including the quadratus lumborum, are regularly associated with sacroiliac joint dysfunction; however, gluteus minimus involvement is seen more frequently.[26] To find these trigger points, the triangular area between the greater trochanter and a line tracing the iliac crest is systematically palpated (Figure 5–46). Attention is given to the pain referral

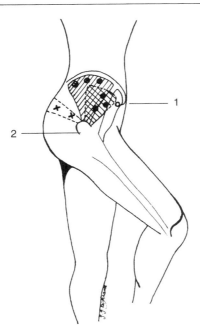

Figure 5–46 Hip trigger points (TPs): **(1)** anterior superior iliac spine, **(2)** greater trochanter. Open circle is tensor facia lata TP; anterior set of solid circles are gluteus minimus TPs; superior set of solid circles are gluteus medius TPs; X's are piriformis TPs.

characteristic for each of these muscles. With the patient's uppermost leg flexed at the hip and knee and resting in front of the lowermost leg, the gluteus maximus is relaxed so that the examiner can palpate these muscles. A line drawn from the PIIS to the top of the greater trochanter roughly outlines the superior border of the piriformis muscle.[26] Palpation of this muscle will be painful if trigger points are present. The piriformis trigger points refer pain to the buttock and posterior thigh, mimicking a radicular pattern.

Deep palpation is necessary for the gluteus minimus, since it lies deep to the gluteus medius and gluteus maximus in parts. Individual bands of muscle are difficult to identify, but point tenderness is easily elicited.[26] The more accessible anterior fibers are palpated anterior and posterior to the tensor fascia lata muscle.[26] The gluteus minimus trigger points refer pain down the posterior or lateral aspect of the thigh and lower leg, also mimicking a radicular problem.

The gluteus medius trigger points are commonly located just below the border of the iliac crest. Pain referred from gluteus medius trigger points centers on the lumbosacral and sacroiliac regions and buttock, mimicking lumbar, sacroiliac joint, and hip joint problems.

Tensor fascia lata trigger points are palpated just inferior and lateral to the ASIS. This muscle has a tendency to refer pain to the hip joint region and down the anterolateral aspect of the thigh as far as the knee.[26]

Hip abductor length can be tested in the same position in which one tests the quadratus lumborum muscle. The only difference is that the examiner lowers the patient's uppermost leg off the back of the examining table (Figure 5–47). Restricted adduction, seen as a lack of descent of the leg behind the table, indicates shortened hip abductors or hip joint dysfunction.

Hip abductor strength can be assessed in the side-lying position by having the patient hold the straight leg abducted against gravity. Pressure is applied by the examiner to the lateral aspect of the distal thigh. Adductor strength can be assessed by having the patient lift the bottom leg off the table against gravity while the examiner supports and holds the uppermost leg and thigh. The examiner then exerts pressure to the lower leg's distal medial thigh toward the table, and the patient is asked to resist.

Iliotibial Band

To test the resiliency of the iliotibial band, an Ober's test can be performed by holding the ankle of the uppermost leg while the patient is in a side-lying position, flexing the knee to approximately 90 degrees, extend-

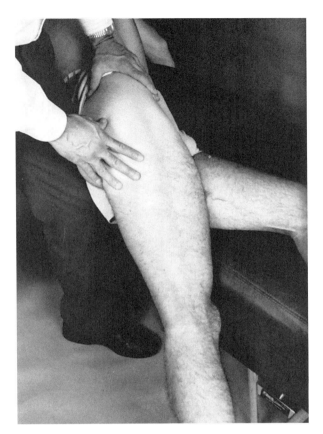

Figure 5–47 Hip Abductor Muscle-Length Test

ing the hip slightly, and allowing the knee to dangle from the iliotibial band toward the table (Figure 5–48). A shortened and tight band will not allow the knee to descend. Skin rolling over tight iliotibial bands is resistant and painful. The iliotibial bands feel coarse to the examiner and "bruised" to the patient. Tight iliotibial bands are commonly seen in chronic hip and sacroiliac joint problems.

Horizontal-Plane Gapping and Provocation of the Sacroiliac Joint

While the patient is still in the side-lying position, provocative or joint-stressing tests can be performed in the horizontal plane at the sacroiliac

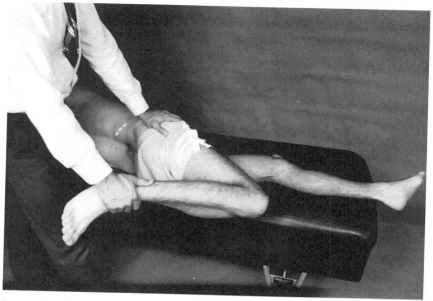

Figure 5–48 Ober's Test

joints. If the examiner places the fleshy part of his or her forearm over the anterior half of the iliac crest and presses toward the table, slightly anteriorly and slightly cephalad, a gapping of the sacroiliac joint can be imparted while the opposite hand palpates for it (Figure 5–49). Next, the examiner can compress the joint by placing the forearm on the posterior half of the iliac crest while pressing toward the table. The goal of these two procedures is to sense resiliency of the pelvic ring and to provoke the patient's presenting symptoms.

Sagittal-plane shearing of the sacroiliac joint can be accomplished by the examiner's standing behind the patient, facing slightly cephalad (Figure 5–50). The hand closest to the patient reaches anteriorly to cup the ASIS comfortably, while the other hand palpates the sacroiliac sulcus posteriorly. By leaning well over the patient so that the examiner's sternum comes in close proximity to the patient's uppermost hip, the examiner is in a strong position to impart an anterior-to-posterior shear on the ASIS of the iliac crest. The examiner's palpating hand can then discern shifting movements of the sacroiliac joint, as well as provoke any pain response from the patient. Obviously, the abovementioned procedures are then repeated on the opposite side.

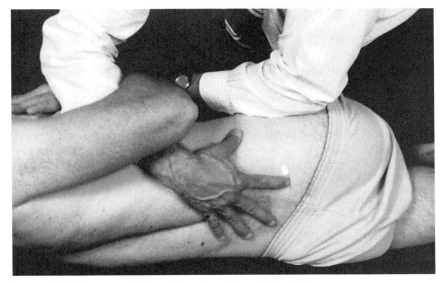

Figure 5–49 Horizontal-Plane Gapping of Sacroiliac Joint

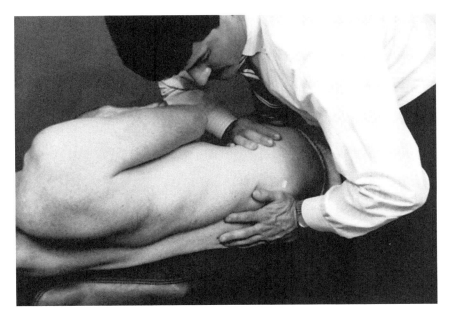

Figure 5–50 Sagittal-Plane Shearing of Sacroiliac Joint

Sacroiliac Joint Play in Torsion

With the patient in side-lying position, the examiner stands behind the patient and grasps the innominate by cupping the cephalad hand in front of the ASIS and pressing the caudad hand on the ischial tuberosity (Figure 5–51A). The ASIS is pulled as the ischial tuberosity is pushed in order to joint-play the innominate in posterior torsion. Restriction and pain provocation are looked for.

To test joint play in anterior torsion, the cephalad hand contacts the PSIS while the caudad hand cups the pelvis anterior to the acetabulum. To torque the innominate anteriorly, the PSIS is pushed while the acetabulum is pulled (Figure 5–51B).

PRONE

Measurement of PSIS Distance

Once the patient is prone, measurement of the distance between the two PSISs is performed again (Figure 5–52) and compared with that measured during the sitting examination. One should observe an increase in the distance by about ¼ to ½ in. Absence of this increase signifies ankylosis or chronic joint dysfunction.

Hip Extension Movement Pattern

To test the hip extension movement pattern, the patient is asked to raise the straight leg into hip extension (Figure 5–53). The activation sequence to look for is hamstring and gluteus maximus first, contralateral erector spinae second, and ipsilateral erector spinae last. Again, palpation should be done only if muscle contraction visualization is difficult, but it should be very light so as not to facilitate unwanted muscle contractions with tactile stimulation. The clinician should look for the following: reduced hip joint mobility; weak, inhibited gluteus maximus; overactive erector or hamstring muscles; or a shortened psoas muscle. Sacroiliac and thoracolumbar joint dysfunctions should also be searched for. What is commonly seen is an overactive erector spinae contraction occurring first, before the gluteus maximus contraction. Sometimes this occurs well up into the thoracolumbar area. It signifies a poor movement pattern, with hip extension being leveraged in the spine.

Heel-to-Buttock Test

The length of the quadriceps muscle group can be assessed while flexing the knee and trying to touch the heel to the buttock (Figure 5–54). This

A

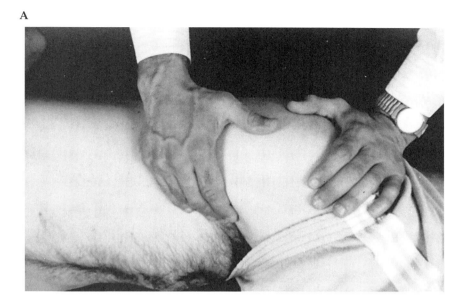

B

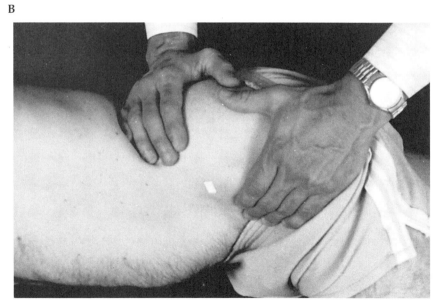

Figure 5–51 Joint play of sacroiliac joint. **(A)** Posterior torsion. **(B)** Anterior torsion.

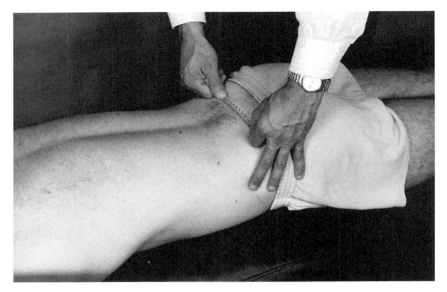

Figure 5–52 Prone Measurement of Posterior Superior Iliac Spine Distance

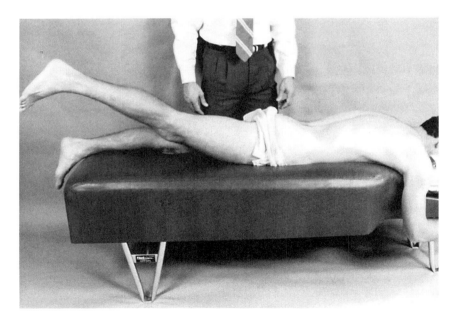

Figure 5–53 Hip Extension Movement Pattern

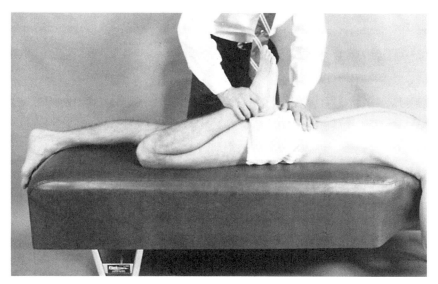

Figure 5–54 Heel-to-Buttock Test

maneuver additionally imparts an anterior torsion to the sacroiliac joint by virtue of the rectus femoris muscle attachments to the anterior aspect of the pelvis. Pain may be provoked in a symptomatic sacroiliac joint as a consequence. However, this test also extends the lumbar facet joints slightly, stresses the knee in flexion, and stretches the femoral nerve. Therefore, this test is not too localizing, and the findings should be interpreted in light of other findings uncovered during the examination. Lack of conditioning, long-standing hip and sacroiliac joint dysfunction, and knee problems are associated with rectus femoris muscle shortening that can limit this test. As mentioned earlier, some patients are "naturally" tight and, in this case, will never be able to touch their heel to their buttock. Yet they should display symmetry between the sides. Limitation of this test due to muscle shortening indicates the need to stretch the anterior thigh muscles. Tightness of these muscles can tether pelvic and hip joint function and needs to be assessed.

Hip Rotation/Piriformis Length

Internal and external hip rotation can be better assessed in the prone position by flexing the knee to 90 degrees and pushing the lower leg laterally and medially to cause internal and external hip rotation respectively (Figure 5–55). In femoral anteversion, the gross range of motion will be

A

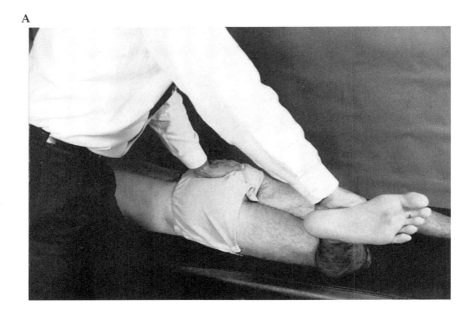

B

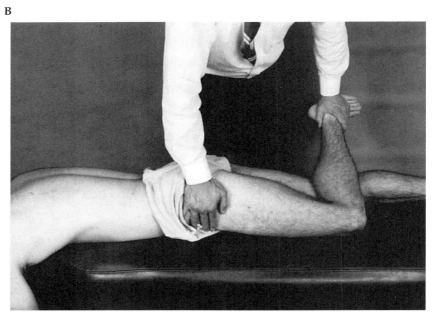

Figure 5–55 Hip rotation. **(A)** Internal. **(B)** External.

normal, but the percentage of internal rotation will be more than that of external rotation. The reverse is true in retroversion. The examiner assesses the range of motion of which the hip joint is capable and checks for end-feel. Sacroiliac joint pain can be provoked especially when the lower leg is pressed laterally.

Subtle sacroiliac joint gapping can be perceived by using a long-lever gapping technique, as shown in Figure 5–56. The examiner kneels next to the patient and uses his or her chest to stabilize the pelvis. The fingers of one hand palpate the sacroiliac sulcus nearest the examiner while the other hand presses the opposite leg laterally. Small shifting movements are palpated for. Localized reproduction of pain in the sacroiliac joint is found in dysfunction. This test can also be used to mobilize the joint.

The piriformis muscle is an important pelvic and hip joint structure often involved when sacroiliac or hip joint dysfunction is present. The length of the piriformis muscle is assessed by pressing the lower leg laterally, thus imparting a stretch to it. Care must be taken to be gentle. An overzealous application of this stretch can send the piriformis into spasm and create leg pain. By having the patient resist the examiner's lateral pressure on the lower leg, the strength of the piriformis can be checked.

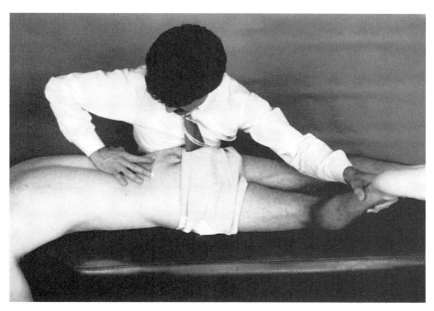

Figure 5–56 Long-Lever Sacroiliac Joint Gapping

Yeoman's/Gluteus Maximus Muscle Test/Hip Joint Play

Another classic provocative test for the sacroiliac joint is Yeoman's test, in which one imparts hip extension while stabilizing the pelvis to the table (Figure 5–57). This not only imparts an extension torque through the sacroiliac joint but also affects the hip joint and its anterior soft tissues, along with the lower lumbar facet joints (Figure 5–58).

As mentioned earlier, three provocative tests that reliably localize pain on testing to the problematic sacroiliac joint are the Patrick-Fabere, Gaenslen's, and Yeoman's. Mierau et al[38] found that two out of three of these tests were positive and localized pain to the affected sacroiliac joint in over 90% of the time. In very heavy or muscular patients, it is difficult to palpate the delicate movements of joint play. Thus, more information is gained by indirectly moving the joints through long-lever provocative testing, as above. For the average patient, especially if the problem is acute, the provocative tests will lateralize the problem to one joint or the other, and specific palpatory procedures can help further delineate the dysfunction.

One can test the gluteus maximus muscle in this position by pressing down on the distal posterior thigh while the knee is maintained in flexion

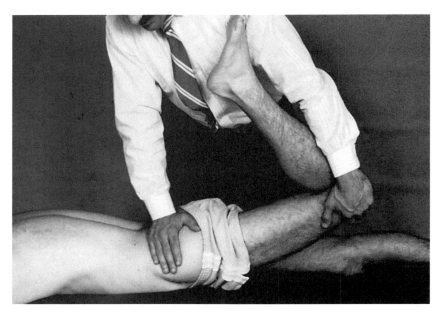

Figure 5–57 Yeoman's Test

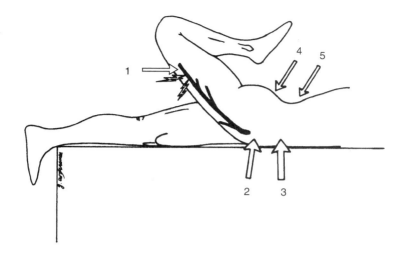

Figure 5–58 Structures moved or stressed during Yeoman's test: **(1)** femoral nerve, **(2)** hip joint, **(3)** psoas muscle, tendon, and bursa, **(4)** sacroiliac joint, **(5)** lumbar facet joints.

(Figure 5–59). The ability of the patient to hold the test position is first ascertained. In hip and sacroiliac problems, the gluteus maximus muscle is often weak and atonic. This becomes very evident to the patient in the above test.

To test passive hip joint extension directly, the hip is extended as in Yeoman's test above while the palpating hand presses on the greater trochanter to assess joint play (Figure 5–60A). Anterior glide can also be tested in the prone position, with the thigh resting on the table and the greater trochanter pressed toward the table (Figure 5–60B). The examiner looks for restricted motion and pain provocation.

Sacrotuberous Ligament

The examiner should palpate the sacrotuberous ligament for undue tension and pain by pressing into the height of the buttock between the ischial tuberosity and sacral apex (Figure 5–61). Normally, this ligament palpates as a firm, painless structure. Difficulty in locating the ligament can be overcome by palpating between the easily found sacral apex and ischial tuberosity. With practice, it becomes easier to locate the tough ligamentous structure. A difference in tension can usually be appreciated when

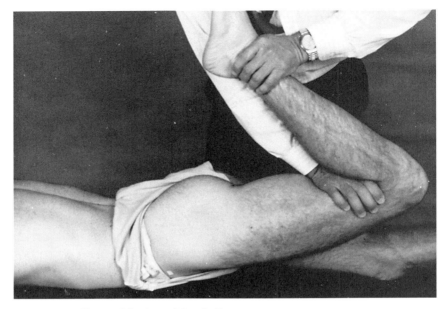

Figure 5–59 Gluteus Maximus Muscle Test

comparing sides. Deep pressure into the ligament may elicit a pain familiar to the patient that may otherwise elude conventional examination procedures. This ligament is commonly involved in traumatic falls to the buttock with attending sacroiliac and hip joint problems. If shortened and
painful, this ligament can create pelvic joint problems or allow them to
persist. Tightness and tenderness are indications for stretching and direct
pressure treatment, as described in Chapter 9. Pain from this structure can
be referred to the buttock region and down the posterior thigh (Figure
5–62). Resultant pelvic pain and pelvic organ dysfunction have been
known to occur due to somatovisceral reflex phenomena acting through
the S-2 to S-4 segments.[39]

Sacral Accessory Movements/Sacral Apex/Cranial Shear

Accurately directed pressures along the sacrum and sacroiliac regions
can yield important information concerning movement and pain provocation. While the patient is lying prone, the pelvis is supported by the two
ASISs and the pubic symphysis, forming a tripod. Applying pressure to
the sacral apex while at the same time palpating the sacroiliac sulci enables

A

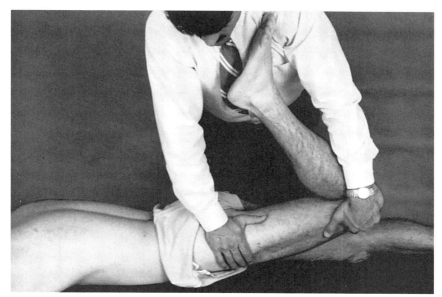

B

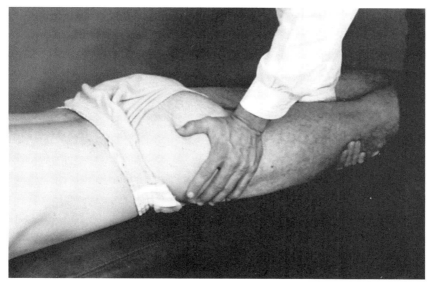

Figure 5–60 Hip joint play. **(A)** In extension. **(B)** In anterior glide.

A

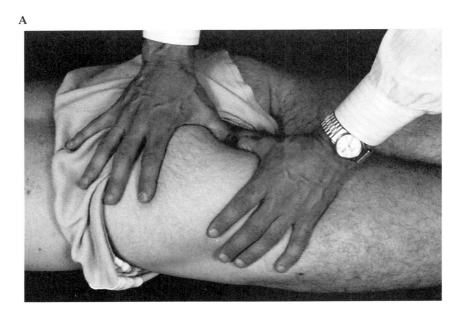

B

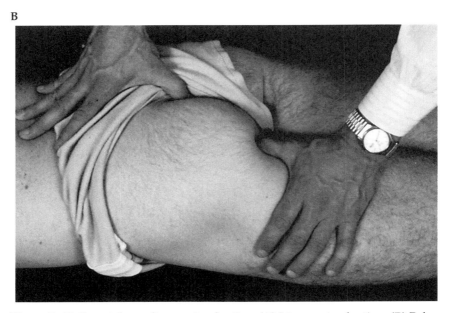

Figure 5–61 Sacrotuberus ligament palpation. **(A)** Ligament palpation. **(B)** Palpation of sacral apex and ischial tuberosity to locate extent of ligament.

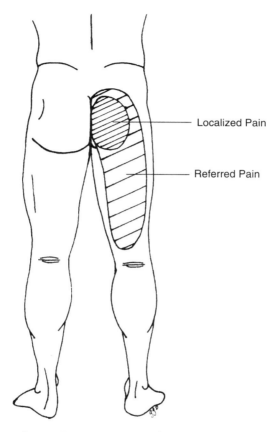

Localized Pain

Referred Pain

Figure 5–62 Sacrotuberous Ligament Pain Referral

one to feel a sense of suppleness and movement (Figure 5–63A). Pain that localizes to one of the sacroiliac joints upon pressing the apex of the sacrum in this position occurs often in acute sacroiliac joint lesions. However, effects can also be felt at the lumbosacral junction.

In another test to provoke sacroiliac joint pain, the examiner presses on the apex of the sacrum in a cranial direction[40] (Figure 5–63B). Pain provocation is looked for. A modification of this test would be to press concurrently in a caudal direction on the PSIS while pressing cranially on the sacral apex to effect a shear movement at the joint (Figure 5–63C). This may aid in lateralizing the pain to one side or the other.

Additionally, the examiner's thumb pad can be placed on the medial aspect of the PSIS and directed laterally to impart a localized gapping at

A

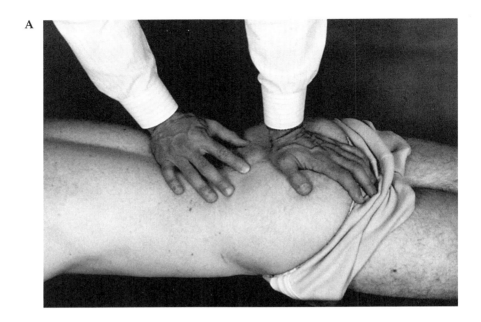

B

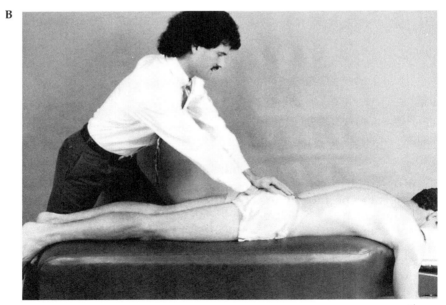

continues

Figure 5–63 **(A)** Sacral apex pressure. **(B)** Cranial shear. **(C)** Craniocaudal shear.

Figure 5–63 continued

C

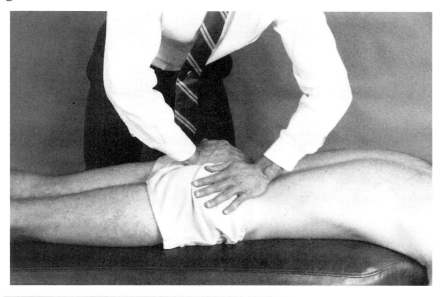

the joint (Figures 5–64A and 5–64B). The other hand can be placed over the thumb to reinforce the contact. Alternately, a double-thumb contact can be used against the medial aspect of the PSIS (Figure 5–64C). Although movement is very slight, pain provocation may be elicited. This maneuver may also elicit pain with an irritated iliolumbar ligament. In all these maneuvers, restriction and pain provocation are looked for. This information is then used to aid in mobilization and manipulation of the joint.

Sacro-Ilio Cross

Another provocative, as well as mobilization, technique is to contact simultaneously the PSIS and apex of the sacrum while imparting pressures in opposite directions (Figure 5–65). For instance, while facing perpendicular to the pelvis, the examiner places his or her cephalad hand on the sacral apex in the midline, using a pisiform contact. Crossing over with the caudal hand, the examiner places the other pisiform on the contralateral PSIS. Gentle oscillatory pressures are applied in opposite directions to sense resiliency and provoke pain. Findings are compared to those of the opposite side.

A

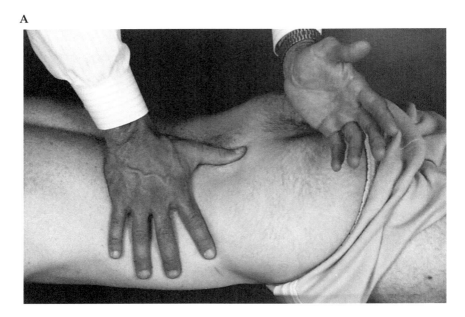

B

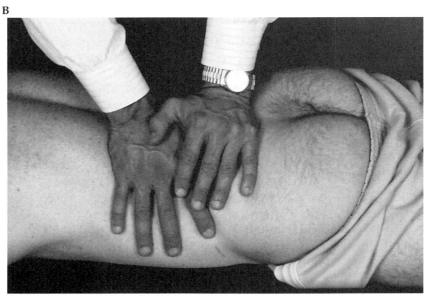

continues

Figure 5–64 Direct lateral gapping. **(A)** With thumb contact. **(B)** With reinforced contact. **(C)** With double-thumb contact.

Figure 5–64 continued

C

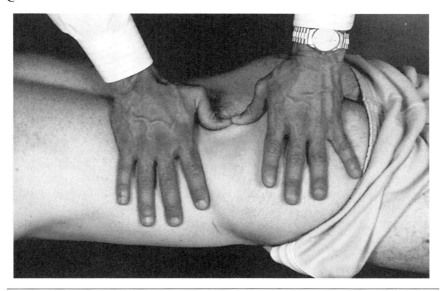

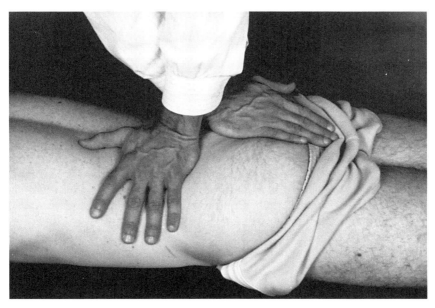

Figure 5–65 Sacro-Ilio Cross

Trunk Extension Differential Test

The trunk extension differential test can be used to take advantage of the fact that the erector spinae muscles generate substantial tension in and around the sacroiliac joints when they contract. The patient is asked to place the hands behind the back and raise the trunk off the table for a few seconds (Figure 5–66). Any change in the pain response in the sacroiliac region is noted. If there is pain on extending the trunk actively, the examiner has the patient repeat the procedure, but this time he or she stabilizes the painful side joint with firm pressure. If, upon active trunk extension, the pain response is diminished or absent with stabilization and the patient can accomplish the maneuver more easily, the pain is probably coming from the joint. However, if there is no change in the pain response with stabilization, yet active trunk extension is still more painful than lying prone, the erector spinae muscles are incriminated. If there is no change in the pain, whether the patient is prone, actively extended, or actively extended with stabilization, then inflammation or bone pathology should be suspected.

Static Palpation

Ligaments are never tender unless they are traumatized or unless the joint they support is dysfunctional.[17] Hence, the ligaments about the pelvic joints can be painful due to injury, dysfunction, or pain referral from some other site. The only area where the sacroiliac joint can be palpated directly is in its inferior aspect near the PIIS. The overlying tissues are often tender to palpation and can appear thickened in sacroiliac joint problems. The skin over each sacroiliac joint can be rolled while pain and tension are looked for. Chronic joint problems can yield sore, "bruised"-feeling ligaments for months and even years without the patient's being aware of the pain until it is palpated. As joint mobility and function are restored with treatment and exercise, this point tenderness abates.

In this author's personal experience, palpation of this area at one time revealed a pea-sized soft tissue abnormality, presumably in the ligamentous tissue, that created a very painful radiating sensation into the posterior buttock, thigh, and leg with tingling of the foot. Upon ischemic compression (sustained pressure) of the painful point and subsequent sacroiliac joint manipulation, the pea-sized structure was no longer palpable, and the radiating pain could no longer be elicited.

Coccyx

The coccyx is often painful in response to sacroiliac joint dysfunction, especially at the undersurface of its tip.[36] Tension and trigger points in the

A

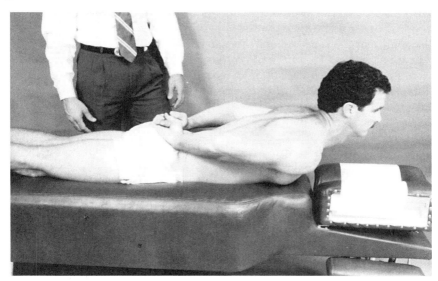

B

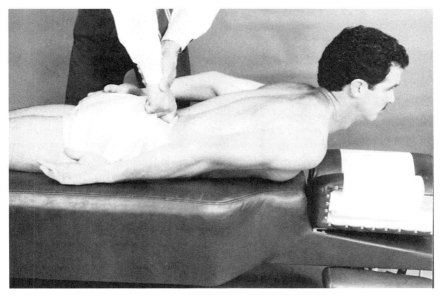

Figure 5–66 Trunk extension differential test. **(A)** Trunk extension without joint stabilization. **(B)** With joint stabilization.

levator ani and coccygeus muscles can also create coccydynia (coccyx pain).[26] Palpation of these structures is important, but thorough understanding of the anatomy is an essential prerequisite. Joint dysfunction and discopathy of the L-5 segment can also cause a painful coccyx.

In women, vaginal pain and dyspareunia can result from tension and trigger points in the bulbospongiosus and levator ani muscles. Travell and Simons[26] offer an excellent reference to the trigger point examination of this area.

The sacrococcygeal joint can be gently joint-played in various directions in an attempt to provoke the patient's presenting symptoms. An intrarectal examination rarely needs to be done for this. Externally, posterior to anterior and transverse pressures can be applied to the coccyx with the fingers. Refer to Chapter 6 for the discussion on mobilization of this joint.

Pelvic Floor

The pelvic floor can be a great source of pelvic pain. The levator ani, with its two main parts (pubococcygeus, iliococcygeus), is the most common source of referred perineal pain.[26] Lilius and Voltonen[41] mention that its pain can be referred to the sacrum, coccyx, rectum, and pelvic floor. Thiele[42] states that it can refer pain to the vagina, and Pace[43] includes the levator ani as a commonly overlooked source of low back pain. The coccygeus muscle is also known to refer pain to the perineum, coccyx, hip, or low back. The above two muscles make it difficult to sit if they harbor trigger points. In addition, defecation may be painful.

Digital rectal examination can greatly aid in finding as well as treating trigger points in the levator ani muscle.[26] The external anal sphincter should also be assessed for tone and pain. Once intrarectal, the examiner's finger can sweep across the expanse of the levator ani on either side of the midline. The coccygeus muscle can be identified by finding the coccyx and sacrococcygeal joint and moving laterally just anterior to the sacrospinous ligament. Tender and taut bands of muscle are searched for that reproduce the patient's symptoms. Thiele[42] discusses the various aspects of this examination.

RADIOGRAPHS

In addition to the standard lumbar radiographic series, consideration should be given to routinely using the anterior-to-posterior spot view with a 30-degree cephalad tube tilt (Figure 5–67). According to Yochum and

Rowe,[44] this is the best view for visualizing the sacroiliac joints. By opening the collimation laterally, the hip joints can be seen bilaterally. The view is taken with the patient either supine or standing and the tube tilted 30 degrees cephalad. The central ray is centered in the midline just below the level of the ASISs.

ERYTHROCYTE SEDIMENTATION RATE

With regard to laboratory testing, Borenstein and Wiesel state that "the most useful test in helping to differentiate medical from mechanical low back pain is the measurement of the erythrocyte sedimentation rate (ESR)."[45(p83)] The ESR essentially reflects the acute-phase response in reaction to tissue destruction. Systemically, the body responds to tissue injury with an increased level of plasma proteins made in the liver. Due to the

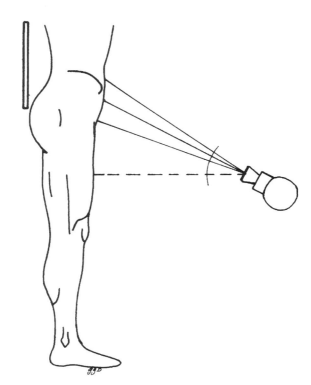

Figure 5–67 Radiographic Positioning

Table 5–1 Upper Limits for Erythrocyte Sedimentation Rates[32]

	Men	Women
Under 50 years old	15 mm/h	25 mm/h
Over 50 years old	20 mm/h	30 mm/h

increased level of these plasma proteins, the red blood cells tend to aggregate more, causing an increased rate of sedimentation in an upright tube. This rate of sedimentation is measured in 1 hour. Generally, the ESR is elevated in conditions of inflammation. These would include rheumatic disease, acute infections, tissue necrosis, malignant disease, and abdominal disease. As such, the ESR is a most practical and valuable screening test for the detection of medical pathology. Normal values vary depending on gender and age (see Table 5–1). Extremely high values (100 mm/hr and higher) most likely indicate malignancy.[46]

Chapter Review Questions

- What are the essential features of a manual functional examination?
- What effects do changes in femoral version have on gait appearance?
- Discuss the various postural findings that indicate joint and muscle dysfunctions common to the pelvic and hip areas.
- Relate palpation findings in Gillet's leg-raising test to manipulative technique setup.
- What three movement patterns should be examined for in the pelvic and hip areas?
- What are the clinical criteria for diagnosing pubic symphysis joint dysfunction?
- What provocative tests aid in diagnosing sacroiliac joint lesions?
- Explain the trunk extension differential test.

REFERENCES

1. Griner PF, Mayewsky RJ, Mushlin AL, et al. Selection and interpretation of diagnostic tests and procedures: principles and application. *Ann Intern Med.* 1981;94:553–563.
2. Hoppenfield S. *Physical Examination of the Extremities.* New York, NY: Appleton-Century-Crofts; 1976.

3. Ducroquet R, Ducroquet J, Ducroquet P. *Walking and Limping: A Study of Normal and Pathological Walking.* Philadelphia, Pa: JB Lippincott Co; 1968.

4. Robinson RO, Herzog W, Nigg BM. Use of force platform variables to quantify the effects of chiropractic manipulation on gait symmetry. *J Manipulative Physiol Ther.* 1987;10:172–176.

5. Herzog W, Nigg BM, Read LJ, Senior BPE. Quantifying the effects of spinal manipulations on gait using patients with low back pain. *J Manipulative Physiol Ther.* 1988;11:151–157.

6. Herzog W, Read LJ, Conway PJW, et al. Reliability of motion palpation procedures to detect sacroiliac joint fixations. *J Manipulative Physiol Ther.* 1989;12:86–92.

7. Ramamurti CP. *Orthopaedics in Primary Care.* Baltimore, Md: Williams & Wilkins; 1979.

8. Kessler RM, Hertling E. *Management of Common Musculoskeletal Disorders.* Philadelphia, Pa: Harper & Row; 1983.

9. Mennell JM. *Back Pain: Diagnosis and Treatment Using Manipulative Techniques.* Boston, Mass: Little, Brown & Co; 1960.

10. Bourdillion JF, Day EA. *Spinal Manipulation.* 4th ed. Norwalk, Conn: Appleton & Lange; 1987.

11. Hoskins ER. The development of posture and its importance: III short leg. *J Am Osteopath Assoc.* 1934;34:125–126.

12. Travell JG, Simons DG. *Myofascial Pain and Dysfunction: The Trigger Point Manual.* Vol 1. Baltimore, Md: Williams & Wilkins; 1983.

13. Jull GA, Janda V. Muscles and motor control in low back pain: assessment and management. In: Twomey LT, Taylor JR, eds. *Physical Therapy of the Low Back.* New York, NY: Churchill Livingstone; 1987:253–277.

14. Janda V, Schmid H. Muscles as a pathogenic factor in back pain. Proceedings of the 4th conference IFOMT. 1, 1980; Christchurch, New Zealand.

15. Peterson DH, Bergmann TF. The spine: anatomy, biomechanics, assessment, and adjustive techniques. In: Bergmann TF, Peterson DH, Lawrence DJ, eds. *Chiropractic Technique.* New York, NY: Churchill Livingstone; 1993;197–521.

16. Triano JJ, Schultz AB. Correlation of objective measure of trunk motion and muscle function with low-back disability ratings. *Spine.* 1987;12:561.

17. Mennell JM. *The Musculoskeletal System: Differential Diagnosis from Symptoms and Physical Signs.* Gaithersburg, Md: Aspen Publishers, Inc; 1992.

18. Faye LJ. *Motion Palpation of the Spine.* Huntington Beach, Calif: Motion Palpation Institute; 1981.

19. Gitelman R. A chiropractic approach to biomechanical disorders of the lumbar spine and pelvis. In: Haldeman S, ed. *Modern Developments in the Principles and Practice of Chiropractic.* New York, NY: Appleton-Century-Crofts; 1980:297–330.

20. Gillet H, Liekens M. *Belgian Chiropractic Research Notes.* Huntington Beach, Calif: Motion Palpation Institute; 1984.

21. Faye LJ. *Motion Palpation and Clinical Considerations of the Lumbar Spine and Pelvis.* Huntington Beach, Calif.: Motion Palpation Institute; 1986.

22. Schafer RC, Faye LJ. *Motion Palpation and Chiropractic Technic: Principles of Dynamic Chiropractic.* Huntington Beach, Calif: Motion Palpation Institute; 1989.

23. DeFranca GG. The snapping hip syndrome: a case study. *Chiro Sports Med.* 1988;2:8–11.

24. Lowman CL. The sitting position in relation to pelvic stress. *Physiother Rev.* 1941;21: 30–33.

25. Inglemark BE, Lindstrom J. Asymmetries of the lower extremities and pelvis and their relation to lumbar scoliosis. *Acta Morphol Neerl Scand.* 1963;5:221–234.

26. Travell JG, Simons DG. *Myofascial Pain and Dysfunction: The Trigger Point Manual.* Vol 2. Baltimore, Md: Williams & Wilkins; 1992.

27. Lewit K. *Manipulative Therapy in Rehabilitation of the Locomotor System.* 2nd ed. London: Butterworths; 1991.

28. Nichols PGR. Short-leg syndrome. *Br Med J.* 1960;1:1863–1865.

29. Harris NH, Murray RO. Lesions of the symphysis in athletes. *Br Med J.* 1974;4:211–214.

30. Laban MM, Meerschaert JR. Lumbosacral anterior pelvic pain associated with pubic symphysis instability. *Arch Phys Med Rehabil.* 1975;56:548.

31. Kirkaldy-Willis WH, Hill RJ. A more precise diagnosis for low-back pain. *Spine.* 1979;4:102–109.

32. Jonsson B, Stromqvist B. The straight leg raising test and the severity of symptoms in lumbar disc herniation. *Spine.* 1995;20:27.

33. Supik AF, Broom MJ. Sciatic tension signs and lumbar disc herniation. *Spine.* 1994;19:1066–1069.

34. Hudgins WR. The crossed straight-leg-raising test. *New Engl J Med.* 1977;297:1127.

35. Janda V. *Muscle Function Testing.* Boston, Mass: Butterworths; 1983.

36. Lewit K. *Manipulative Therapy in Rehabilitation of the Locomotor System.* Boston, Mass: Butterworths; 1985.

37. DeFranca GG, Levine LJ. The quadratus lumborum and low back pain. *J Manipulative Physiol Ther.* 1991;14:142–149.

38. Mireau D, Yong-Hing K, Wilkinson A, Sibley J, Von Baeyer C. Scintigraphic analysis of sacro-iliac pain. Poster presentation. In: Vleeming A, Mooney V, Snijders C, Dorman T, eds. Proceedings of the First Interdisciplinary World Congress on Low Back Pain and Its Relation to the Sacro-iliac Joint; November 5–6, 1992; San Diego, CA.

39. Midttun A, Bojsen-Moller F. The sacrotuberous ligament pain syndrome. In: Grieve GP, ed. *Modern Manual Therapy of the Vertebral Column.* New York, NY: Churchill Livingstone; 1986:815–818.

40. Laslett M, Williams W. The reliability of selected pain provocation tests for sacroiliac joint pathology. *Spine.* 1994;19:1243–1249.

41. Lilius HG, Voltonen EJ. The levator ani spasm syndrome: a clinical analysis of 31 cases. *Ann Chir Gynaecol.* 1973;62:93–97.

42. Thiele GH. Coccygodynia: cause and treatment. *Dis Colon Rectum.* 1963;6:422–436.

43. Pace JB. Commonly overlooked pain syndromes responsive to simple therapy. *Postgrad Med.* 1975;58:107–113.

44. Yochum TR, Rowe LJ. Radiographic positioning and normal anatomy. In: Pine JW, ed. *Essentials of Skeletal Radiology.* Vol 1. Baltimore, Md: Williams & Wilkins; 1987:1–93.

45. Borenstein DG, Wiesel SW. *Low Back Pain: Medical Diagnosis and Comprehensive Management.* Philadelphia, Pa: WB Saunders; 1989.

46. Zacharski LR, Kyle RA. Significance of extreme elevation of erythrocyte sedimentation rate. *JAMA.* 1967;202:262.

Chapter 6

Mobilization

```
┌─────────────────────────────────────────────────────────────┐
│                    Chapter Objectives                          │
│                                                                │
│  •  to discuss general considerations concerning mobilization  │
│  •  to discuss mobilization theory                             │
│  •  to describe facilitation or muscle energy techniques       │
│  •  to describe joint mobilization techniques of the sacroiliac, pubic │
│     symphysis, hip, and sacrococcygeal joints                  │
└─────────────────────────────────────────────────────────────┘
```

GENERAL CONSIDERATIONS

Joints function to move. That movement is governed by joint architecture, soft tissue restraint, muscular contraction, and neurologic control. The absence of that movement, found on examination, forms the basis for the application of manipulative techniques designed to restore motion. The outdated concept that manipulation restores a bone that is out of place should be abandoned. Manipulation and mobilization are accurately directed forces that should be aimed at increasing motion in already restricted joints. In this regard, we are concerned with restoring passive physiologic and/or accessory movements. Passive physiologic movements are those same movements performed passively that the patient can perform actively, eg, hip flexion, abduction. Passive accessory movements are those involuntary movements that occur when an operator imparts motion to the joint. For instance, a patient cannot voluntarily perform long-axis extension (joint distraction) of the hip joint. Neither can anterior or posterior glide or shear movements at the hip and sacroiliac joints be performed under a person's volitional control. Although small and involuntary, these accessory movements, also called *joint play movements*, are very important for normal, painless movements to occur.

What guides the practitioner in the use of manual techniques is the presence of "joint signs." These are pain, restriction of motion, and spasm. These joint signs, when present, help determine the type of mobilization that needs to be performed.

The use of manual methods to treat musculoskeletal ailments is an ancient form of therapy. The main goal is to impart movement to painful, restricted joints and muscles to enhance mobility and relieve pain. As in any field, terminology can be confusing. Manipulation and mobilization are actually considered specific types of passive movement therapy. The distinction between the two depends on parameters of amplitude and speed of movement, and the patient's ability to remain in control of the movement. This chapter discusses mobilization, and the following chapter discusses manipulation.

MOBILIZATION THEORY

Mobilization is a form of passive movement therapy that involves oscillatory movements of various amplitudes executed in certain parts of a joint's range of motion. The movement imparted is still under the control of the patient, should he or she decide to halt it. Mobilization also includes sustained stretches of variable vigor at the end range. The different amplitudes of mobilization are divided into four types or grades by Maitland[1] for ease of assessment and application (Figure 6–1). A fifth grade, grade V, is reserved to denote a manipulative thrust. The four grades of mobilization are as follows:

Grade I: a small-amplitude movement executed at the beginning of the joint's range

Grade II: a larger-amplitude movement occurring within the range but not extending to the limit or engaging any stiffness or spasm

Grade III: a large-amplitude movement that engages stiffness or spasm by extending to the limit of range

Grade IV: a small-amplitude movement at the limit of range that engages stiffness or spasm

Sometimes, after a grade V manipulation has been performed, grade IV oscillations are performed to stretch the joint's capsuloligamentous structures effectively. Although it is not part of Maitland's descriptions of mobilizations, I refer to this technique as a grade VI mobilization.

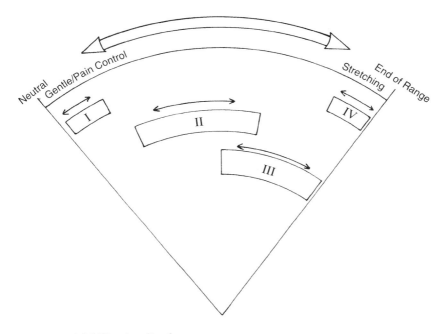

Figure 6–1 Mobilization Grades

Grades II, III, and IV can be applied either more or less vigorously and denoted with a plus (+) or minus (–) sign (II+, II–, III+, III–, etc.) respectively. The usual frequency of oscillations is two to three cycles per second for about 20 seconds, more slowly and gently for painful joints and more quickly and abruptly for chronically stiff joints.

The choice of the mobilization grade used depends upon the type of pain reaction and end-feel found during the examination of joint motion. Therefore, it is important to determine clinically whether the resistance to joint motion is from pain or spasm and whether it is from articular or peri-articular tissues. For example, muscle spasm exhibits a "twanglike" end-feel, and the muscle contraction may be visible. When reflex spasm is encountered during mobilization movements, the treatment movement should be a sustained stretch just at the point of onset of pain or spasm. The pain and spasm should subside in about 20 seconds, at which time the joint can be challenged slightly more.

Similarly, pain is a predominant feature in acute conditions, and painful joints, especially if irritable, demand respect. The speed and amplitudes of oscillations must be guided by the joint's pain response. Grade I and II oscillations are used mostly to reduce pain through mechanoreceptor stimulation. Gentle, slow oscillations can allow enough improvement to occur so that movements of greater amplitude can follow. A regular rhythm is implemented to "lull" the extremely painful joint into quiescence and allow the patient to relax with the movements. Just as a painful myofascial trigger point can be "deactivated" by sustained pressure (ischemic compression), a painful joint motion can be rendered less so with continued gentle oscillating movements. It is amazing how a series of gentle grade I or grade II mobilizations can effectively calm down a painful osteoarthritic hip joint.

The beginning and ending pressures of the oscillations should be equal in rate, and the changing from on-pressure to off-pressure should be almost imperceptible so that they seemingly blend with each other. Usually, in joints that are not as painful, the beginning pressure is quicker than the off-pressure. However, if joint pain is provoked more with the off-pressure, then it should be the faster component. This causes a kind of recoil or rebound mobilization. Take, for instance, a posterior-to-anterior oscillation on the lower pole of the sacroiliac joint that elicits pain upon its release. To mobilize better in this case, the on-pressure is made slower than the off-pressure in order to cause a rebounding mobilization from anterior to posterior. This is a very useful procedure in cases of painful coccydynia. Slow, gentle on-pressures followed by quick, almost abrupt, off-pressures will at first elicit a painful response. However, after 30 to 60 seconds of these "rebounding" oscillations are performed, the pain usually subsides.

Shortened capsuloligamentous tissues are characteristic of chronic conditions in which stiffness is more of a feature than pain. These joints can be handled more firmly without reprisal, especially near the end range of motion. Grade III and IV mobilizations are best used in this situation. These aid in stretching adaptively shortened or scarred capsuloligamentous structures. Maitland[1] describes a staccatolike oscillation combined with sustained stretching. Combining small grade IV amplitudes of oscillation near the end range with larger grade III amplitudes interposed works well. The larger amplitudes tend to abate any pain caused by the smaller end-range oscillations.

Where in the range the pain and/or spasm occurs is also important. Grades I and II are used mostly to reduce pain if its onset occurs early in the range, whereas grades III and IV are used to stretch stiffened tissues felt later in the range.[1]

Mobilization techniques can often be used as preparatory maneuvers performed prior to a grade V manipulation, especially in chronic conditions. This creates greater relaxation of the periarticular soft tissues as well as the patient.

FACILITATION TECHNIQUES

Facilitation techniques, also termed *muscle energy* or *muscle relaxation techniques, proprioceptive neuromuscular facilitation (PNF)*, and *postisometric relaxation (PR)*, are also used as a means of mobilizing joints by releasing tension in shortened or hypertonic muscles. These are covered in more detail in Chapter 9. However, in brief, relaxing and lengthening muscles by utilizing neuromuscular reflexes associated with muscle contraction has the effect of increasing mobility in the neighboring joints. Generally, the tight muscle is contracted isometrically for a few seconds in the direction opposite the restriction or tightness. Upon relaxation, stretching of the muscle is performed to lengthen it to a new length or "barrier." For example, to increase hip extension using a muscle energy technique, the psoas muscle can be stretched. The patient lies supine with the thigh and leg on the involved side off the table. The clinician then applies a gentle floorward stretch to the distal thigh until a resistance is met. The patient is then instructed to contract or press the thigh up against the clinician's resistance for 8 to 10 seconds (near maximum contraction if performing PNF, minimally for PR techniques), after which he or she is instructed to relax ("let go"). The thigh is then allowed to drop further floorward, thus increasing hip extension. The process is repeated again at the new muscle length achieved. The isometric contraction is associated with a reflex-mediated inhibition that occurs after the contraction and lasts for several seconds. This is taken advantage of, and the muscle is passively stretched for that period.

To utilize the reciprocal inhibitory effects of antagonistic muscle group contractions, the patient can be asked to press the thigh actively floorward after his or her 8- to 10-second contraction, rather than having the clinician passively press it. Respiration can be recruited to enhance facilitation and inhibition. The patient inhales a deep breath and holds it for a few seconds to enhance overall muscle facilitation during the muscle contraction. Upon exhaling, he or she is instructed to relax. In general, exhalation is associated with reflex neuromuscular inhibition, thus enhancing the relaxation of the muscle.

MOBILIZATION TECHNIQUES

The following section deals with various mobilization techniques for the sacroiliac, hip, and symphysis pubis joints. The techniques are arranged according to the patient's posture and explained with regard to their setup and actual performance. Contraindications to manual techniques are discussed in Chapter 7.

Sacroiliac Joint

Prone

Sacro-Ilio Cross. With the patient prone, the clinician stands perpendicular to the patient's pelvic region. The clinician's cephalad hand makes a pisiform contact in the midline on the sacral apex. The caudal hand is then crossed over the cephalad hand by making a pisiform contact on the opposite-side PSIS. The clinician positions himself or herself such that his or her sternum is over his or her contacts. By pressing downward in the direction of each forearm, he or she imparts a sagittal-plane shearing force to the sacroiliac joint by oscillating the sacrum in relation to the ilium (Figure 6–2). The mobilizing force actually comes from movement at the hips and trunk being transferred through the shoulders and arms. To lessen the strain on his or her back, the clinician can take a wide stance to lower the center of gravity. Repeated oscillations into a restricted joint create mobility that is perceived as increasing springiness or pliability at the joint. This also serves as an excellent premanipulative maneuver for the sacroiliac joint.

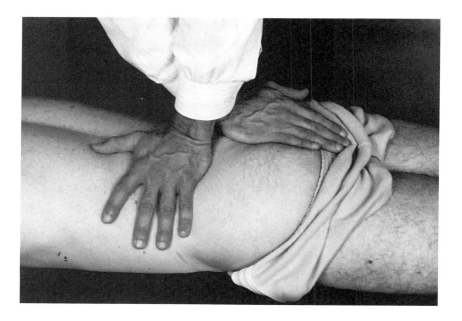

Figure 6–2 Sacro-Ilio Cross

Direct Gapping. The clinician again positions himself or herself perpendicular to the patient's pelvis. He or she then places the thumb pad just medial to the opposite PSIS (Figure 6-3A). The clinician's other hand covers his or her thumb with a pisiform contact (Figure 6–3B). A mobilizing force directed laterally against the medial aspect of the PSIS will impart a slight gapping movement in the horizontal plane at the sacroiliac joint on the side opposite to where the clinician is standing. The movements should not be so firm that the pelvis and trunk move unless a more vigorous mobilization is warranted. However, a gentle rocking motion can be imparted to the immediate pelvic vicinity. On smaller and slender individuals, the cephalad hand can maintain a stabilizing contact on the near-side PSIS and sacrum, with the fingers pointing caudad. Meanwhile, the caudad hand can impart gentle oscillations with the thumb against the medial aspect of the PSIS on the opposite side. A double-thumb contact can be used on larger patients (Figure 6–3C).

Prone Gapping, Long-Lever. A prone gapping technique of the sacroiliac joint can be performed with the clinician kneeling perpendicular to

A

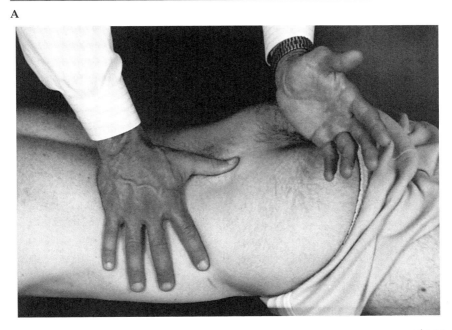

continues

Figure 6–3 Direct gapping technique. **(A)** Thumb contact. **(B)** Pisiform covering contact. **(C)** Double-thumb contact.

Figure 6–3 continued

B

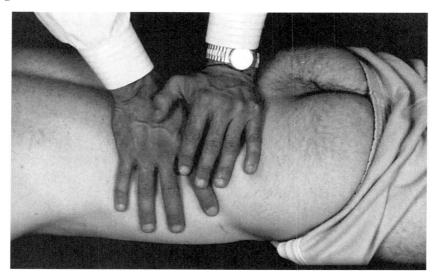

C

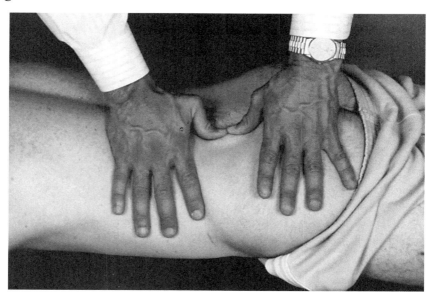

the patient's pelvis and stabilizing the ipsilateral ilium (right side) with the chest.[2] The patient's left knee is flexed to 90 degrees, and the clinician's caudad hand grasps the ankle and pushes it laterally to cause internal rotation of the left hip (Figure 6–4). Maximal internal rotation of the left hip, via a chain-reaction mechanism, will cause a gapping of both sacroiliac joints (Figure 6–5). This subtle movement can be monitored with the clinician's cephalad hand palpating the sacroiliac sulcus on the right or left side.

Extension Mobilization. This maneuver is similar to Yeoman's orthopedic test of hip extension (Figure 6–6). The clinician stands facing the patient just caudal to the level of the pelvis. The clinician extends the patient's contralateral thigh with his or her caudad hand by lifting it just proximal to the bent knee. To affect the upper aspect of the sacroiliac joint, the patient's PSIS is contacted with the clinician's cephalad pisiform or thenar eminence. Oscillations are performed as indicated. A variation of the above technique involves contacting the sacral apex instead of the PSIS (Figure 6–7). This affects the lower aspect of the sacroiliac joint.

Varied Sacral Pressures. With the patient prone, various directed pressures (accessory movements) are applied to the sacrum to cause joint mo-

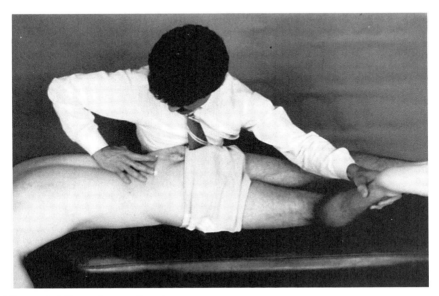

Figure 6–4 Long-Lever Gapping

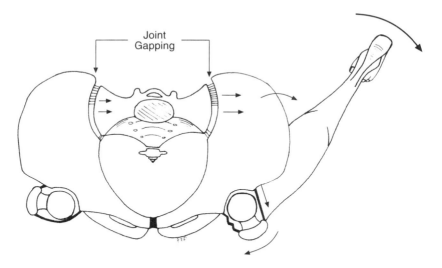

Figure 6–5 Mechanics of Long-Lever Gapping Technique

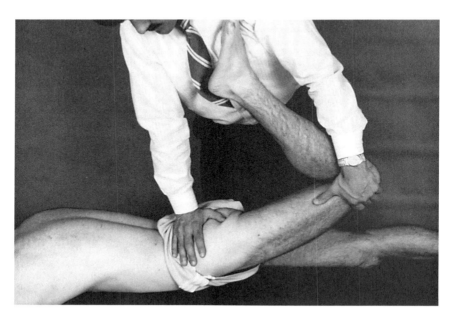

Figure 6–6 Extension mobilization for the upper aspect of the sacroiliac joint. Note posterior superior iliac spine contact.

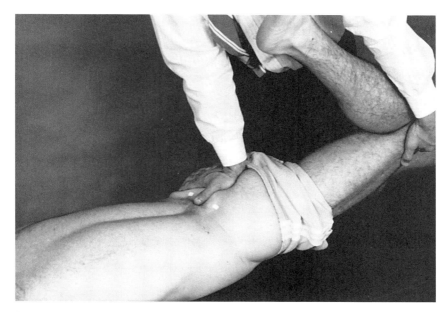

Figure 6–7 Extension mobilization for the lower aspect of the sacroiliac joint. Note sacral apex contact.

bilization movements that may possibly match the patient's signs and symptoms (Figure 6–8A). These pressures are applied in a posterior-to-anterior direction both centrally and to each side of the midline on both the upper and lower aspects of the sacrum. The sacrum can also be pressed in a cephalad direction from below while the iliac crest is pressed caudally (Figures 6-8B and 6–8C).

Side-Lying

Anterior Torsion. The patient lies on his or her right side with the left leg flexed slightly at the hip and knee so that the knee rests on the table in front of the right leg (Figure 6–9). The clinician can impart an anterior torsional mobilization to the left sacroiliac joint by standing behind the patient and contacting the patient's left PSIS with his or her right pisiform and the area over the left acetabular region with his or her left hand. The PSIS contact is pressed anteriorly while the acetabular contact is pulled posteriorly in an attempt to torque the ilium on the sacrum in an anterior direction. Gentle, rhythmic oscillations of varying amplitudes are then used, depending on pain and restriction.

A

B

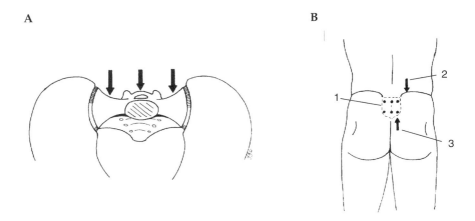

C

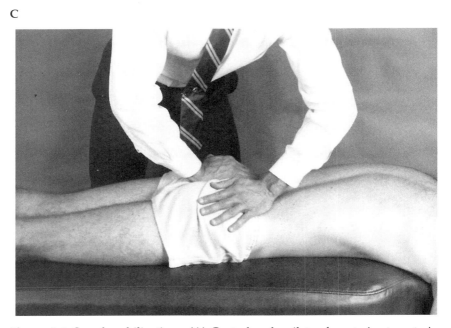

Figure 6–8 Sacral mobilizations. **(A)** Central and unilateral posterior-to-anterior pressures. **(B) (1)** Outline of sacrum and indicated spots for posterior-to-anterior mobilizations; **(2)** caudally directed mobilization on iliac crest; **(3)** cranially directed mobilization on sacral inferior-lateral angle. **(C)** Combination craniocaudal shear at SIJ.

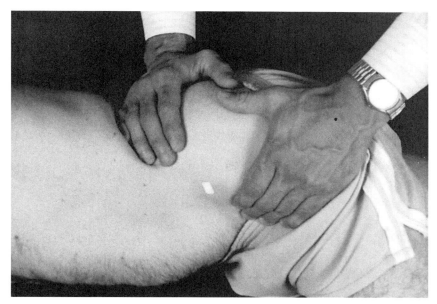

Figure 6–9 Anterior Torsion Mobilization

Posterior Torsion. The patient assumes the position described for the previous technique; however, the clinician reverses the contacts by cupping the right hand over the ASIS and placing the left hand on the ischial tuberosity (Figure 6–10). By pushing on the ischial tuberosity and pulling on the ASIS, the clinician can impart a posterior torsion to the sacroiliac joint.

The movements in the above two techniques are subtle, with the intent of mobilizing the uppermost sacroiliac joint. Therefore, the motion should be directed locally without rocking the entire pelvis.

General Flexion with Facilitation. In the side-lying position, the patient flexes the uppermost thigh as far as possible. The clinician stands in front of the patient, facing somewhat cephalad, and places the patient's uppermost knee against his or her thigh. The patient is asked to press his or her knee into the clinician's thigh for 8 to 10 seconds, thus contracting the hip extensor muscles. The patient is then asked to inhale deeply and relax on the exhale, being told to "let go." Upon sensing relaxation, the clinician increases the patient's hip flexion by pressing with his or her thigh in a headward direction. When a new resistance is met at a higher angle of flexion, the procedure is repeated. The patient can remain passive during the stretching phase or can assist the stretch with an active contraction of

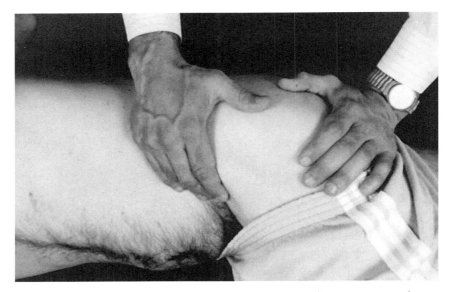

Figure 6–10 Posterior torsion mobilization. Note hand placement reversal compared to Figure 6–9.

the hip flexor muscles. The goal is to increase hip flexion to the point of stretching the hip and sacroiliac joints. This is a very effective technique to use during acute situations, as a premanipulative maneuver, or in working with chronic joint stiffness commonly seen in patients over 50 years old. Often the patient experiences decreased pain and tension in the hip and sacroiliac regions after this procedure is performed.

Sagittal Shear. The patient is placed in the side-lying posture with the clinician standing behind the patient at the level of the pelvis. The clinician places his or her left thenar eminence over the sacrum, and his or her right hand gently cups the patient's ASIS anteriorly. By stabilizing the sacrum posteriorly with his or her thenar eminence, the clinician attempts to impart a posterior shear of the ilium on the sacrum by gently pressing in an anterior-to-posterior direction through the ASIS (Figure 6–11). It must be emphasized that the ASIS contact should be comfortable. To ensure this, the ASIS is cupped in the palm of the clinician's hand. Alternatively, the clinician can stabilize the ASIS contact and press from posterior to anterior on the sacral base.

Lower-Joint Gapping Technique. The patient is in the same position as above, but the clinician stands in front of the patient facing the pelvis. By

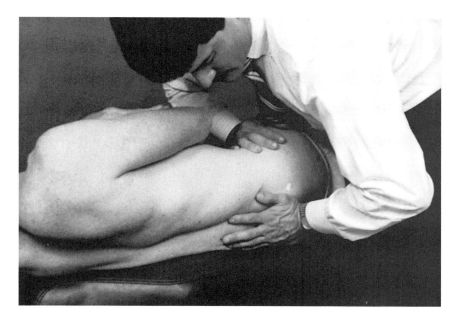

Figure 6–11 Sagittal-Plane Shear

getting into a low stance, he or she places his or her sternum over the patient's uppermost hip. The medial and most inferior aspect of the ischial tuberosity is contacted with the caudal hand's pisiform while the cephalad hand grasps the rim of the iliac crest. The elbow of the caudad hand is held below the level of the ischial tuberosity contact. Pressing toward the ceiling with the ischial contact and pressing floorward with the iliac contact stresses the ilium in such a way as to gap the lower aspect of the patient's right sacroiliac joint (Figure 6–12).

These last five side-lying techniques are excellent maneuvers to perform when the patient finds it difficult to lie supine or prone, as, for example, during pregnancy.

Supine

Backward Lying with Torsion. This maneuver is similar to the examination technique performed earlier. It can be used as an effective stretching mobilization for the sacroiliac joint. The patient slumps back against the clinician and torsion is applied to the trunk (Figure 6–13). The ASIS is pressed toward the table as the trunk rotation is accentuated. A slight lifting traction is applied to the trunk so that a tractionlike torsion is applied

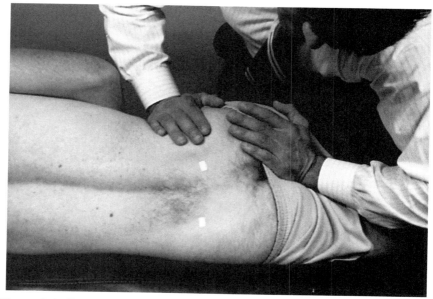

Figure 6–12 Lower-joint gapping technique. Note low lifting angle of ischial contact.

to the sacroiliac joint on the side of ASIS contact. This is particularly useful in pregnant women, especially during house calls or if they have difficulty reclining due to pain.

Anterior-to-Posterior Shear. The patient lies supine with the right thigh flexed to 90 degrees and slightly adducted. The clinician faces perpendicularly to the patient, standing on the patient's left side. The clinician grasps the patient's flexed knee with his or her right hand and pulls the thigh toward him or her so that the pelvis rotates up off the table slightly. He or she then contacts with the left hand the patient's right sacroiliac sulcus. Mobilizing oscillations are directed by the clinician's right arm down through the patient's flexed femur to create an anterior-to-posterior shear force of the ilium against the sacrum. The pelvis is rotated off the table only to the extent that the clinician's fingers of the left hand can gain access to the sacroiliac sulcus to monitor the mobilizing oscillations (Figure 6–14).

Pubic Symphysis

Pubic symphysis (PS) fixations are suspected when asymmetry of the pubic tubercles is observed[3,4] and when unilateral tension and tenderness are found in both the inguinal ligament and the short hip adductors (see Chapter 5, Figure 5–29). Sagittal-plane rotational movements at the sacroiliac joints appear to be hindered when PS fixations are present.[5] Motion palpation of the PS is difficult to perform, and overall assessment of its functions is generally by clinical suspicion. Restoration of motion can be accomplished by simple mobilizations and facilitation techniques. The mobilizations are more like stretches. High-velocity maneuvers are usually not necessary.

General Countertorque Technique. This and the following technique are applied to both sides to cause a general mobilization of the PS joint. The

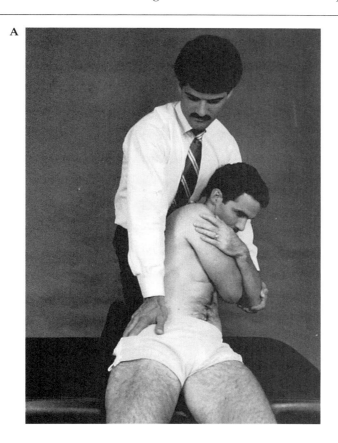

A

continues

Figure 6–13 (A, B) Backward lying with torsion. The ASIS is stabilized as the sacroiliac joint is tractioned and rotated on the side of contact.

Figure 6–13 continued

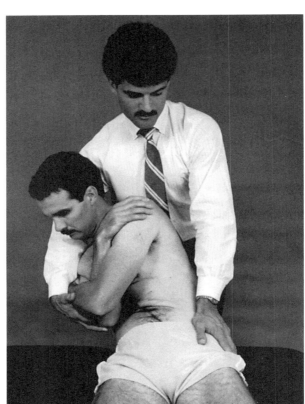

patient is supine, with the right thigh and leg near the edge of the table and the other thigh flexed up onto the chest or as far as possible. The patient can hold the left knee up to the chest with both hands, with the clinician supporting it for control. The other thigh is allowed to drop to the table surface or, if the patient is flexible enough, off the table. The clinician applies a firm stretch to the right distal femur while stabilizing the left thigh upon the patient's chest (Figure 6–15). This is held for 30 seconds, with small-grade IV oscillations being applied afterward for another 20 to 30 seconds. The procedure is then performed on the other side.

Countertorque with Facilitation. Since the above procedure stretches the psoas muscle on the right, a facilitation technique designed to stretch

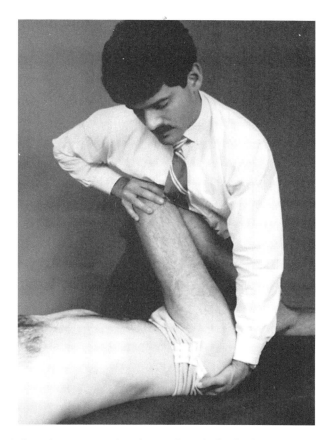

Figure 6–14 Anterior-to-posterior shear. Note slight thigh adduction.

this muscle will accomplish similar results. The patient is placed in the same position as above but this time is instructed to resist gently the downward pressure on the right distal femur ("hold" or "pull up gently against my hand") for 8 to 10 seconds (Figure 6–16). He or she then inhales deeply and, upon exhaling, is told to "relax" or "let go." Only when the clinician senses relaxation in the right hip flexors after the isometric contraction and exhalation (postisometric relaxation) does he or she encourage or coax more hip extension on the right. The hip is extended until resistance is met with, and the procedure is repeated again. This whole process is performed three to five times, depending on the tightness of the hip flexors, and repeated on the other side.

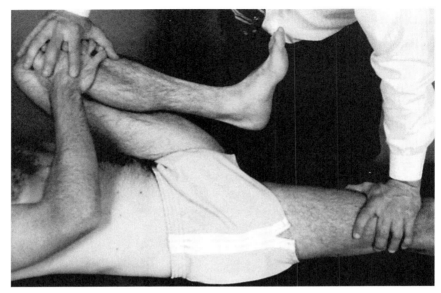

Figure 6–15 General Pubic Symphysis Countertorque

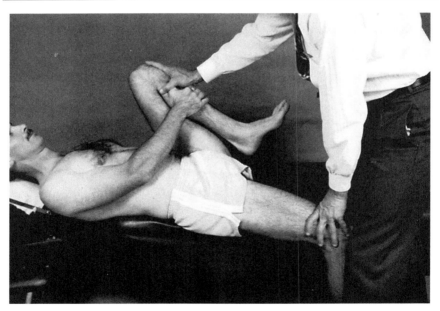

Figure 6–16 Countertorque Using Psoas Muscle Facilitation Stretch

Abduction Facilitation. This maneuver and the next two are considered general "shotgun" techniques to create mobility at the PS. The patient is supine with knees bent and feet flat on the table. The clinician holds the knees together to resist their active separation on the part of the patient (Figure 6–17). After several seconds of resisting strong abduction, the patient relaxes, and the pain and tension at the inguinal ligament and adductor insertions are reevaluated.

Adduction Facilitation. The patient is supine, with knees bent and feet resting flatly on the table. The clinician places his or her forearm lengthwise between the patient's knees to act as a block to movement. The patient is instructed to adduct the knees strongly (Figure 6–18). After several seconds of contraction, the patient relaxes, and the pain and tension are reassessed at the inguinal ligament and/or adductor tendon insertions.

Adduction Facilitation with Thrust. The patient is positioned as above, but with knees held together. The clinician holds the medial aspect of each knee with his or her hands and instructs the patient to adduct strongly. The clinician applies a high-velocity, low-amplitude impulse thrust in an

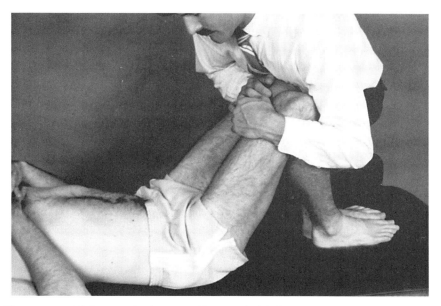

Figure 6–17 Abduction facilitation. Clinician holds knees together against patient resistance.

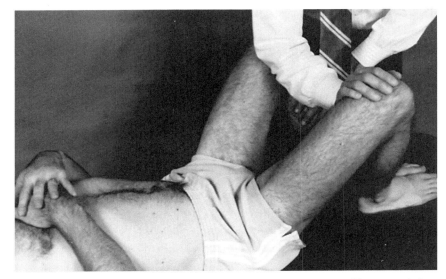

Figure 6–18 Adduction facilitation. Clinician resists adduction of knees with forearm.

---

attempt to separate the knees slightly (Figure 6–19). This maneuver attempts to cause a gapping at the PS.

Hip Joint

The hip joint is a large synovial joint capable of global motion. Mobilization is directed at increasing physiologic as well as joint play movements. In addition, the combined movement of flexion with adduction is probably the most important movement to test and treat. If this maneuver can be performed painlessly, then mobilization in flexion and adduction performed as separate movements is rarely needed.[6] The physiologic movements include flexion, extension, abduction, adduction, and medial and lateral rotation. The accessory movements include anterior, posterior, and lateral glides; long-axis extension; posterior shear at 90 degrees flexion; and caudal glide at 90 degrees flexion.

Mobilization Using Physiologic Movements

Combined Flexion/Adduction. Lewit[7] describes this maneuver in the treatment of what is termed "ligament pain."[8] Two positions are assessed

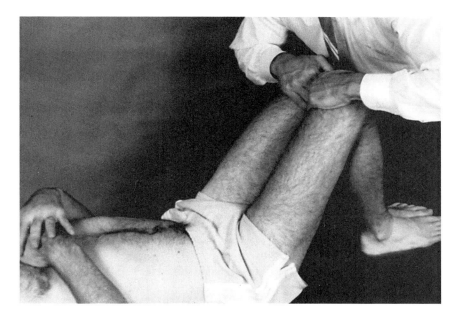

Figure 6–19 Adduction Facilitation with Impulse Thrust

and treated. The first is with the hip in 90 degrees of flexion, with strong adduction being applied (Figure 6–20A). This position stresses not only the hip joint but the iliolumbar ligament,[7] and pain may be experienced in the groin. The second entails flexing the hip maximally and then applying strong adduction (Figure 6–20B). This tends to affect the sacroiliac joint ligaments, and the patient usually feels discomfort in the buttock that can radiate into the posterior or posterolateral thigh. In both of these positions, longitudinal pressure is applied along the axis of the femur by pressing on the knee. If resistance is met, postisometric relaxation can be used to overcome it. This technique is usually uncomfortable when restriction is met, and care must be taken not to overwhelm the patient with discomfort, as this is quite easy to do.

To perform this maneuver, the patient is supine, and the clinician stands opposite to the side in question. The clinician reaches across and flexes the hip to 90 degrees or maximal flexion, depending on which position reproduces the patient's symptoms more. The thigh is then adducted strongly but carefully. While holding this combined flexion/adduction position, the clinician applies pressure back along the axis of the femur. The patient

A

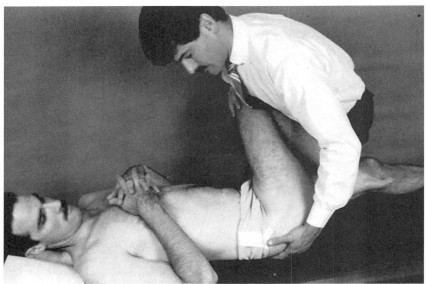

B

Figure 6–20 "Ligament pain" mobilization. **(A)** Hip flexion at 90 degrees. **(B)** Hip flexion maximal. Adduction is applied in both positions.

is then instructed to abduct the thigh to resist the clinician's pressure of adduction for 10 seconds and to relax. Further adduction is then coaxed, and the above process is repeated three to five times.

Maitland[6] describes a similar technique. The thigh is maintained in flexion/adduction as it is moved through an arc from 90 to 140 degrees of flexion (Figure 6–21A). An abnormal arc of motion is indicated by a painful restriction somewhere along its length. At such a point, thigh flexion can be advanced painlessly only if the thigh is abducted slightly. This is represented diagrammatically in Figure 6–21B as a small peak in the flexion/adduction arc traced by the knee. Mobilizations of various grades are applied at the point along the arc that is restricted and painful. Maitland[6] describes three methods to use when approaching the painful point in the arc during mobilization. The first is to adduct the thigh directly into the center of the painful point, wherever it lies on the arc. Grade IV mobilizations can be used to increase the range of adduction at this painful point.

The second method entails holding the thigh in the flexion/adduction position but starting below the level of the painful point in the arc. While maintaining this combined position, the clinician flexes and extends the thigh in such a way as to "rub" back and forth over the painful spot along the arc (Figure 6–21C). The amount of adduction pressure needs to be monitored to create as little pain as possible.

The third method is a combination of the first two and seems to be the most important.[6] It has two parts. The thigh is adducted toward and just below the painfully restricted part of the flexion/adduction arc and then extended (Figure 6–21D). From this new position, the movement is reversed by flexing the thigh just to the level of the painful point and then abducting it back to the starting position, nudging the painful point from the opposite direction. The second part of this mobilization is the mirror-image maneuver of the first part in that it moves toward and above the painful point in the arc as the thigh is flexed, rather than extended, upon meeting the painful restriction. This movement is then retraced by extending the thigh along the arc to the painful point and abducting it back to the starting position. This whole maneuver is repeated again, nudging the painful point first from below and then from above, observing for any change in signs and symptoms.

Abduction. A position similar to the Patrick-Fabere test can be utilized to mobilize hip abduction. The only difference is that the foot of the flexed and abducted leg is placed along the medial aspect of the opposite knee, resting on the table. The clinician then oscillates the hip joint into abduction by

A

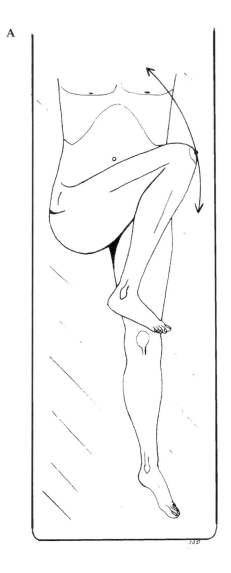

continues

Figure 6–21 Combined flexion/adduction. **(A)** Normal arc traced by knee. **(B)** Bump in arc signifies where knee has to be abducted slightly to bypass painful point. **(C)** Mobilization back and forth over painful point. **(D)** Mobilization above and below painful point alternately.

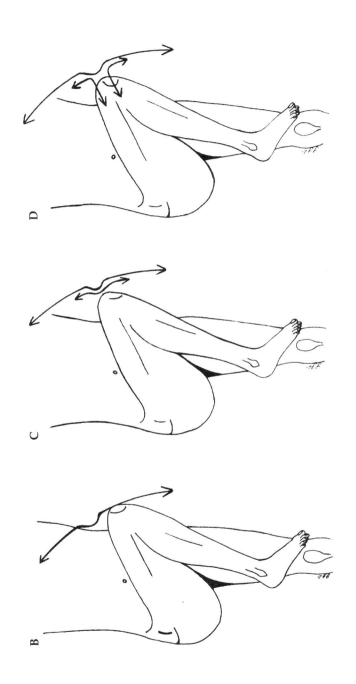

Figure 6-21 continued

pressing the knee toward the table. The opposite ASIS is supported firmly but comfortably (Figure 6–22). A facilitation technique can be performed using this same positioning. The patient presses the knee up against the clinician's hand for a count of 10 seconds. Upon relaxation, the clinician coaxes the knee closer to the table. This is repeated three to five times.

Medial and Lateral Rotation. Even though *rotation* here is meant to apply to the hip joint, in reality it describes the motion occurring around the femoral shaft. A roll-and-slide movement actually occurs at the femoral head in the acetabulum. In other words, the ball-like femoral head is not neatly spinning around an axis in the acetabular fossa. This is because the femoral head is offset from the femoral shaft's axis by the femoral neck.

Medial hip rotation is usually more commonly involved than lateral rotation, but assessment ultimately determines which motion or motions to treat. Three positions can be used to mobilize medial and lateral rotation, depending on the joint signs and symptoms.

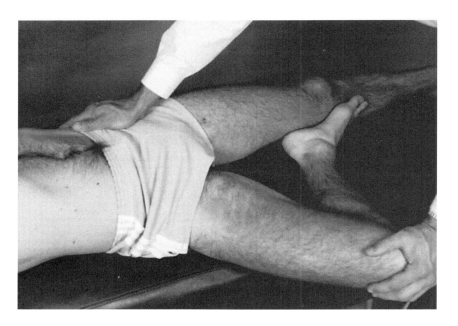

Figure 6–22 Hip Abduction Facilitation

In the first position, the patient is supine, with a pillow or roll placed under the distal thigh to relax the hip in a few degrees of flexion (Figure 6–23). The clinician grasps above and below the knee joint and gently rolls the knee medially from the neutral position, using the appropriate grade mobilization. This is a very important technique for treating painful hip joints when using grade I and II mobilizations.[6] Gentle rolling of the thigh medially relaxes the patient, affords effective pain relief, and prepares the joint for further mobilizations. The knee can also be rolled laterally if so indicated by joint signs and symptoms.

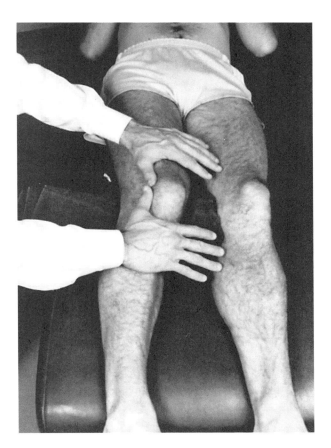

Figure 6–23 Medial hip rotation mobilization. Note towel rolled under knee.

A

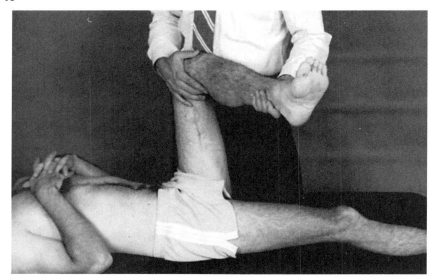

B

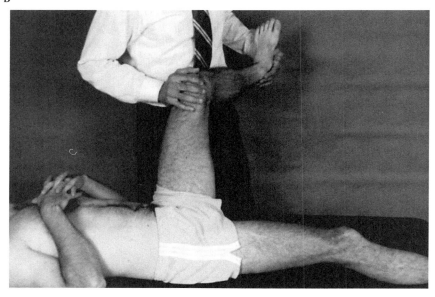

Figure 6–24 Hip rotation, supine at 90 degrees flexion. **(A)** Lateral. **(B)** Medial.

The second position to use for medial or lateral rotation is with the patient supine but with the hip and knee flexed to 90 degrees (Figure 6–24). The clinician supports the lower limb at the knee and ankle. By swinging the lower leg laterally around the axis of the vertically situated femur, he or she rotates the femur medially. The reverse movement is used for lateral femoral rotation. The appropriate mobilization grade is used, depending on joint signs and symptoms.

The third position involves placing the patient prone and bending the knee to 90 degrees (Figure 6–25). The clinician is on the same side and grasps the ankle with his or her caudal hand. His or her cephalad hand contacts and supports the patient's pelvis. By pressing the patient's lower leg laterally, he or she rotates the femur internally. To impart external femoral rotation, the leg is pressed medially. Laterally pressing the lower leg also stretches the piriformis muscle and gaps the sacroiliac joint.

Extension. The patient is placed prone. The clinician stands on either side of the patient and grasps the flexed knee with his or her caudal hand. His or her other hand contacts the greater trochanter while he or she lifts the thigh off the table to impart hip extension (Figure 6–26). This move is best for grade IV mobilizations. If extension is painful, lesser grades can be performed in the supine position by supporting the knee and heel so that the hip and knee are in slight flexion (Figure 6–27). Lowering the knee toward the table and lifting the heel away from the table allow the thigh to extend gently toward neutral. If the patient is large, gravity can be used as an assist by placing the patient supine, with the involved side close to the edge of the table. The thigh and leg are then lowered off the table with mobilizing oscillations.

Mobilization Using Accessory Movement

Long-Axis Extension in Neutral. In this technique we are actually referring to the axis of the femur. Due to the inclined angle of the femoral neck in relation to the femoral shaft, true long-axis distraction of the joint entails a more laterally directed mobilization. This technique can be performed in both supine and prone positions. Patients seem to relax more in the prone posture. In the supine position, the clinician grasps the lower leg just proximal to the ankle joint with both hands. The patient's leg is lifted very slightly and tractioned along the axis of the femur (Figure 6–28). The traction can be sustained and combined with muscle facilitation by having the patient resist the traction gently and inhaling deeply. Upon exhaling, the

A

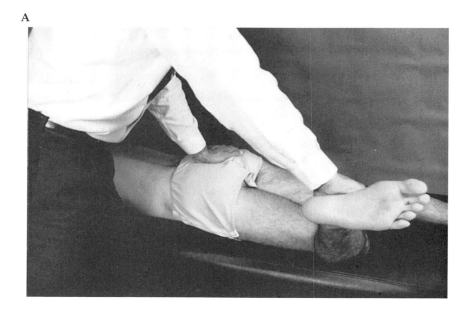

B

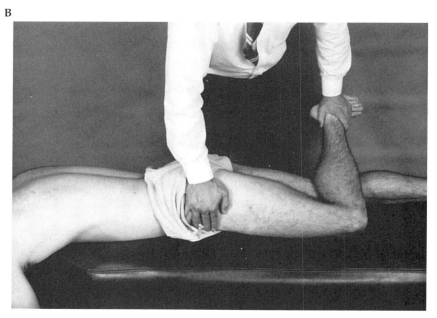

Figure 6–25 Hip rotation, prone. **(A)** Medial. **(B)** Lateral.

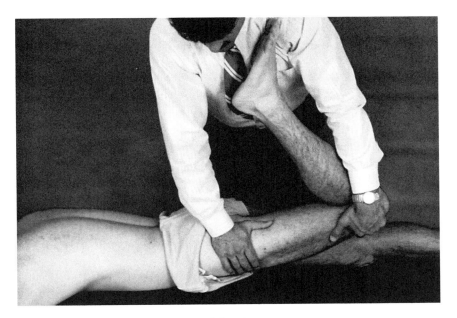

Figure 6–26 Hip Joint Extension Mobilization

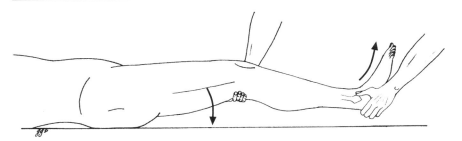

Figure 6–27 Supine Hip Extension Mobilization

patient is instructed to relax, and the traction is gently increased. The movements can also be oscillated according to joint signs and symptoms. This is an excellent technique to reduce joint irritability and pain if done gently with traction or lower-grade mobilizations.

Caudal Glide in Flexion. The patient's hip is flexed to 90 degrees and the knee is flexed fully, if this is tolerable. The clinician kneels next to the

A

B

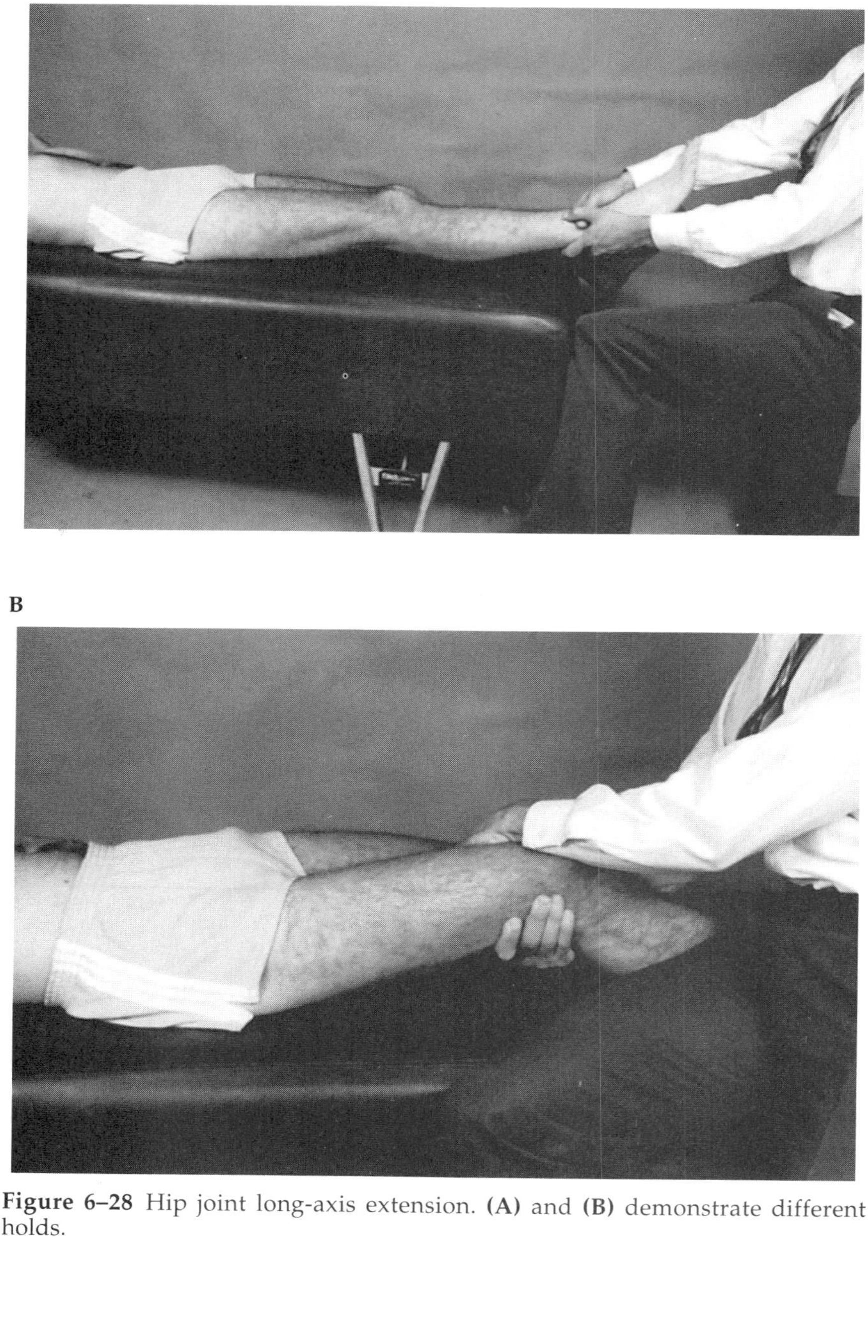

Figure 6–28 Hip joint long-axis extension. **(A)** and **(B)** demonstrate different holds.

patient's hip, facing cephalad, and wraps his or her hands around the most proximal aspect of the patient's thigh, encircling both the lower leg and thigh or just the thigh (Figure 6–29A). If knee flexion is limited, the lower leg can be placed over the clinician's near shoulder (Figure 6–29B). The patient's thigh and clinician's body should move as one during the mobilization. The movement entails pressing posteriorly (toward the table) and pulling caudally with the hands while the clinician's shoulder leverages the knee or distal femur slightly cephalad. The hands are almost performing a scooping motion.

Lateral Glide with Flexion. The patient's thigh is flexed to 90 degrees. The clinician is kneeling to the side of the patient, facing the hip joint. The clinician encircles the proximal thigh with both hands overlapped. The patient's thigh is hugged by the clinician's hands, shoulder, and chest while the clinician's trunk and the patient's thigh move as one unit. As in the above technique, a scooping action is performed by pressing posteriorly (floorward) and laterally (Figure 6–30). The above two techniques can also be used as thrust (grade V) techniques.

Posterior Glide. The clinician places his or her caudal hand under the patient's medial distal femur, supporting the thigh. His or her cephalad hand is placed over the most proximal aspect of the femur, on level with the greater trochanter. The patient's distal thigh is raised very slightly as the clinician's cephalad hand presses the greater trochanter toward the table (Figure 6–31).

Anterior Glide. Essentially, this is the reverse of the above technique. The hand positions are the same except the patient is prone (Figure 6–32). In these last two techniques, various degrees of abduction can be employed, depending on joint signs and symptoms.

Sacrococcygeal Joint

This joint is often the site of pain, either from local dysfunction or referred from the lumbosacral area. It is important to assess the coccyx by palpation for tenderness in relation to imparted movements. Care must be taken to distinguish pain from movement versus pain from palpation pressure.

Maitland[1] discusses the use of posterior-to-anterior, anterior-to-posterior, and transverse pressures applied to the coccyx externally. Contact on the coccyx is taken using the thumb pads, and mobilizing oscillations are directed in various directions. The thumbs must be placed deep enough to

A

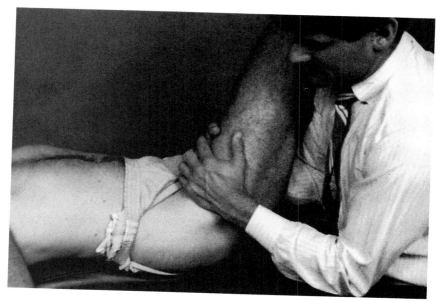

B

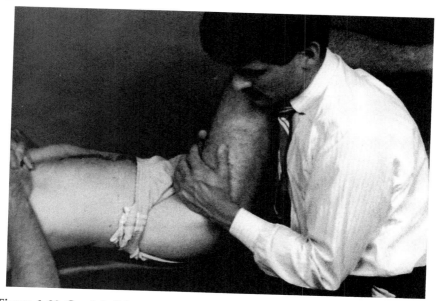

Figure 6–29 Caudal glide in flexion. **(A)** and **(B)** demonstrate different holds.

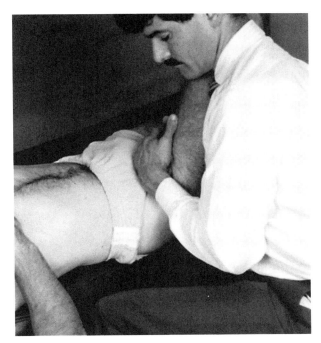

Figure 6–30 Lateral Glide with Flexion

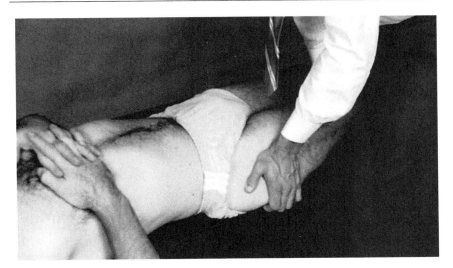

Figure 6–31 Posterior Glide

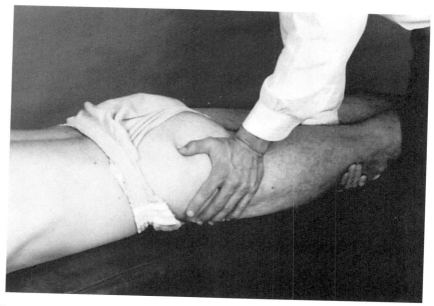

Figure 6–32 Anterior Glide

contact the coccyx, especially the lateral aspect when one is doing transverse mobilizations. Gentle movements are used and modulated according to joint signs and symptoms.

States[9] mentions a manipulative technique that can be adapted here for mobilization (Figure 6–33). The patient lies prone, and the clinician places his or her cephalad hand on the patient so that his or her thumb covers the coccyx and his or her fingers spread laterally over the iliac crest. The caudal hand covers the thumbnail with a pisiform contact, and the fingers wrap around the cephalad hand's wrist. Tissue slack is removed in a cephalad direction in such a way that the thumb slides onto the sacrococcygeal joint. Pressure is then applied in a cephalad and downward direction for mobilization. States[9] mentions using a thrust technique, but this should be performed with care.

Lewit[7] describes a muscle facilitation technique using the gluteus maximus muscle to aid in mobilizing the coccyx (Figure 6–34A). The concept entails contracting the gluteus maximus muscle to facilitate levator ani muscle contraction. The patient is prone, and the clinician stands at the level of the patient's knees, facing cephalad. The clinician's hands are crossed to contact each buttock at the level of the anus. The buttocks are

A

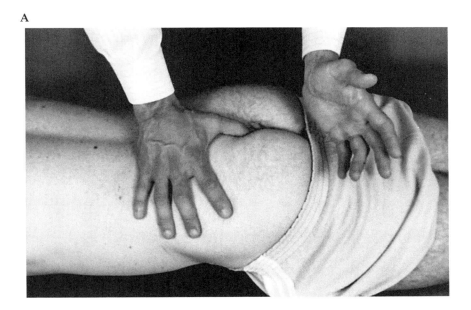

B

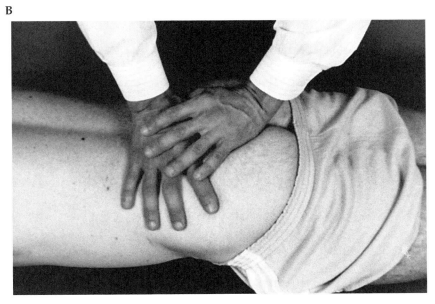

Figure 6–33 Sacrococcygeal mobilization. **(A)** Thumb contact reinforced by **(B)** pisiform contact.

A

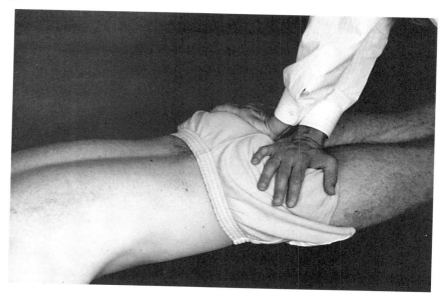

B

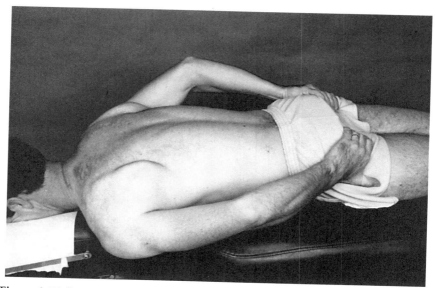

Figure 6–34 Postisometric relaxation of gluteus maximus muscle. **(A)** Clinician assisted. **(B)** Patient home exercise.

separated to tension by the clinician, and the patient is instructed to press the buttocks together for 10 seconds. The patient inhales and upon exhaling is told to relax and "let go." The buttocks are then stretched further apart by the clinician, and the procedure is repeated three to five times. Afterward, the coccyx should be less tender to palpation. Patients can be instructed in performing this on themselves for home use (Figure 6–34B).

Another effective technique has the patient lying on his or her side (Figure 6–35A). The clinician faces the patient from the front, leans over the pelvis, and contacts the medial aspect of the "down" side gluteus maximus muscle with his or her caudal hand. The contact can be made as close to the coccyx as possible with the thenar eminence or pisiform. Traction is made toward the table, and a soft tissue pull is generated via the gluteus maximus fibers affecting the coccyx. Either sustained traction or oscillations can be used, depending on which is better tolerated by the patient. The patient can also assist by gently contracting the gluteus maximus against resistance while he or she inhales. Upon exhaling, he or she is told to relax, and pressure is applied to traction the gluteus maximus when relaxation is sensed. The patient is asked to lie on the other side, and the procedure is repeated. However, instead of turning the patient over, one

A

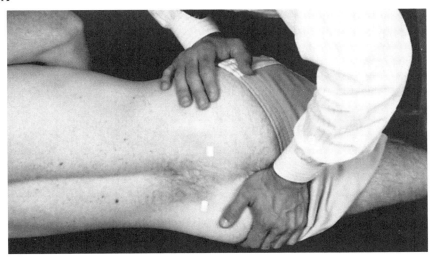

continues

Figure 6–35 Lateral traction on gluteus maximus muscle. **(A)** Downward traction. **(B)** Upward traction.

Figure 6–35 continued

B

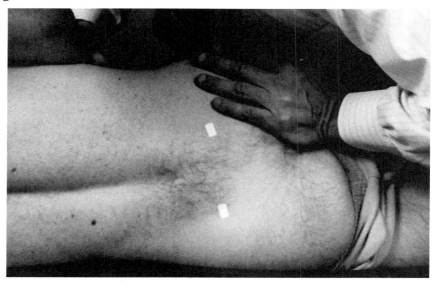

can simply contact the medial part of the gluteus maximus on the "up" side and traction upward (Figure 6–35B). Either a pisiform contact or finger contacts can be used to traction upward.

Although rarely indicated, if the above techniques fail to bring about relief, then the coccyx may need to be mobilized per rectum. A well-lubricated gloved finger is gently inserted into the rectum as per the protocol for performing a digital rectal examination. The coccyx is gently held between the intrarectal finger and the externally placed thumb. Gentle, mobilizing oscillations are attempted in flexion, extension, side tilt, and long-axis extension.

Chapter Review Questions

- What is the difference between mobilization and manipulation?
- What are passive physiologic movements?
- What are accessory joint movements?
- What are joint signs?

- What are the different grades of joint mobilization?
- How are painful, acute joint conditions mobilized differently from stiff, chronic ones?
- What is one of the most important movements to test for and treat in hip joint conditions?
- Discuss the various ways to mobilize the sacrococcygeal joint.

REFERENCES

1. Maitland GD. *Vertebral Manipulation.* 5th ed. Boston, Mass: Butterworths; 1986.
2. Grieve GP. *Common Vertebral Joint Problems.* New York, NY: Churchill Livingstone; 1981.
3. Bourdillion JF, Day EA. *Spinal Manipulation.* 4th ed. Norwalk, Conn: Appleton & Lange; 1987.
4. Greenman PE. *Principles of Manual Medicine.* Baltimore, Md: Williams & Wilkins; 1989.
5. Schafer RC, Faye LJ. *Motion Palpation and Chiropractic Technic: Principles of Dynamic Chiropractic.* Huntington Beach, Calif: Motion Palpation Institute; 1989.
6. Maitland GD. *Peripheral Manipulation.* 2nd ed. Boston, Mass: Butterworths; 1977.
7. Lewit K. *Manipulative Therapy in Rehabilitation of the Locomotor System.* Boston, Mass: Butterworths; 1985.
8. Hackett GS. *Joint Ligament Relaxation Treated by Fibro-osseous Proliferation.* Springfield, Ill: Charles C Thomas, Publisher; 1956.
9. States AZ. *Spinal and Pelvic Technics.* 2nd ed. Lombard, Ill: National College of Chiropractic; 1967.

Chapter 7

Manipulation

Chapter Objectives

- to describe what characterizes a manipulable lesion
- to describe what happens when a joint is manipulated
- to review grade VI mobilizations
- to discuss the audible click sound
- to discuss slack removal in joint manipulation
- to discuss contraindications to manual techniques
- to describe sacroiliac and hip joint manipulation techniques

Manipulation is actually a specific type of passive manual treatment. It is a skillful art that demands much training and experience of the practitioner who wishes to become proficient in its use. A weekend course in manual technique does not qualify someone to perform expert manipulations any more than singing in the shower prepares one for a concert tour. Manipulative therapy demands practice, experience, and ability.

Manipulation is performed to restore joint play at dysfunctional joints. It is thought to work by (1) releasing entrapped synovial folds or plica; (2) relaxing hypertonic muscles; and (3) disrupting articular or periarticular adhesions.[1] Fibrosis of the periarticular tissues can be a result of trauma and inflammation, immobilization, or degenerative joint disease.

Manipulation is defined as a high-velocity, low-amplitude thrust or impulse directed at restoring joint play. It is performed at the end of the usual passive range of motion, is usually associated with an audible "click," and, because of its speed, is not under the voluntary control of the patient. In relation to the four grades of mobilization, it is given the designation grade

V. It is similar to a grade IV mobilization in amplitude and position in the joint's range but differs in the velocity of delivery.[2]

A sixth (VI) grade of mobilization essentially is a small-amplitude mobilization (IV) applied after a grade V manipulation has removed the joint's physiologic elastic barrier (Figure 7–1). This is further explained later in this chapter.

Manipulative techniques can be short-lever or long-lever. Short-lever techniques entail taking direct contacts near the joints to be moved, ie, spinous and transverse processes, whereas long-lever techniques take advantage of leverage gained through trunk and limb movements. Long-lever techniques are performed in such a way as to localize a manipulative thrust to a particular region or joint. A classic long-lever technique involves placing the patient in a side-lying position, with the uppermost thigh flexed and adducted in relation to the trunk (Figure 7–2). The uppermost shoulder is stabilized or pressed posteriorly to create a moment of torque in the spine and pelvis. The use of the thigh as the long lever aids in leveraging tension into the spinal or pelvic joints. There are numerous refinements of the above description, depending on which joint and which type of movement restriction are treated.

WHAT CHARACTERIZES A MANIPULABLE LESION?

Various terms describe the manipulable lesion. Among these are *subluxation*, *joint dysfunction*, *somatic dysfunction*, *fixation*, *joint blockage*, and *segmental dyskinesia*. A variety of factors characterize a manipulable lesion. Since manipulation is a force that imparts mobility to restricted joints and tissues, the mobility characteristics of the lesion should be assessed. In this

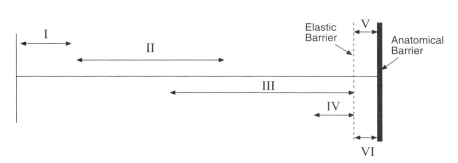

Figure 7–1 Mobilizaton grades. Note that grade VI is a mobilization performed after a grade V manipulation.

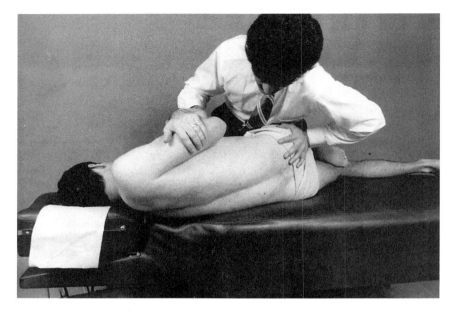

Figure 7–2 Classic Side-Lying Positioning for Sacroiliac Joint Manipulation

regard, decreased regional and intersegmental motion should be a characteristic of the manipulable lesion that is looked for. Included with this is a lack of joint play, termed *joint dysfunction*, which is a central feature of the manipulable lesion. Soft tissue changes such as thickening or atrophy of the periarticular tissues can be present (see Chapter 4, the section "Soft Tissue Changes"). Pain and localized skin hypersensitivity also characterize the manipulable lesion, as do muscle spasm, especially if localized, and muscle imbalances. A positive response to manipulative treatment is a logical but not too often thought of characteristic.

WHAT HAPPENS WHEN A JOINT IS MANIPULATED?

A joint's total range of motion is divided up into three zones of movement: active, passive, and paraphysiologic (Figure 7–3). An elastic barrier of resistance separates the joint's passive range of motion from the paraphysiologic space. The limit of anatomical integrity represents the ultimate barrier: that of the restraining soft tissues in the form of a joint capsule and ligaments. Manipulation entails moving a joint with a high-velocity, low-amplitude thrust that is outside the patient's control to

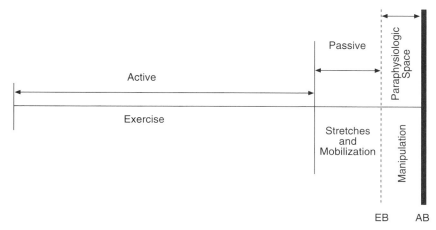

Figure 7–3 Range of motion. EB, elastic barrier of resistance; AB, anatomical barrier.

prevent it, yet accurate enough to enter the paraphysiologic space after all the "slack" is removed. "Slack" is the motion in the active and passive ranges that needs to be taken up prior to engaging the elastic barrier. It is the sudden movement beyond the elastic barrier of resistance that is usually associated with the "click" sound common to manipulation. However, further movement would impose upon the integrity of the joint's soft tissue and risk injury. Although quick, the distance traversed during a manipulation is very small, usually on the order of ⅛ in. Manipulation is usually associated with an audible click or pop due to a joint cavitation phenomenon.

Exercise works within the active range of motion, and mobilization affects more the passive range of motion; neither affects the paraphysiologic space. It is manipulation that affects the paraphysiologic space. Mennell[3] states that exercise, being a voluntary activity, cannot restore joint play, an involuntary joint motion. The same can be said for passive stretching techniques. In fact, Mennell[3] states that exercise will delay the recovery of a dysfunctional joint if the joint play is not restored first. Exercising a dysfunctional joint too soon in treatment can cause painful exacerbations and reflex muscle reactions. Exercise therapy is most important, even mandatory, especially in locomotor disturbances. However, it should be used only when joint play has been restored. To exercise without restoring joint play would be like loosening a rusty hinge by repetitively swinging the door back and forth, regardless of the squeaking and grinding. Although movement is attained, and noisily so, it occurs at the expense of the hinge's structural integrity. It would make much more sense to oil the hinge first and then work it in with movement—movement that would be easier, quieter, and more in harmony with the hinge's structure. In the above analogy, the movement is exercise, the squeaking and grinding are pain, and the lubricating oil is the restoration of joint play.

Therefore, in the overall treatment of joint injuries, the active, passive, and joint play (paraphysiologic) ranges of motion must all be assessed. Often the active and passive ranges of motion are seen to increase after a manipulation. A common example is an improvement on the straight-leg–raising test following a sacroiliac joint or hip joint manipulation. This is due to tension in the hamstring muscles being relaxed in response to arthrokinetic reflex action. Joint mechanoreceptors are thought to be stimulated during manipulation, and this in turn creates reflexogenic muscle tone changes in the muscles that serve the joint.

In 1947, two anatomists from Great Britain, Roston and Haines,[4] researched joint dynamics occurring during a manipulative thrust. Using the metacarpal-phalangeal joint as their model, they observed under radiologic examination the joint's reaction to axial traction. The results were plotted, and a load separation curve was graphically displayed. Tension was plotted on the horizontal x-axis, and joint separation in millimeters was plotted on the vertical y-axis.

The load separation curve illustrated by Figure 7–4 demonstrates that as the joint "slack" is taken up, tension builds, and at the end of a joint's passive range of motion, a sudden gapping of the facet surfaces occurs with a coexistent audible joint click.

Unsworth et al[5] evaluated the synovial fluid and concluded that the crack sound was due to a cavitation phenomenon involving a bubble of carbon dioxide that forms and breaks (cavitates). A radiolucent intraarticular space is also produced after the manipulation. It takes 20 minutes for the gases to be absorbed and the joint to stabilize. During this time, an audible click will not be heard if a second manipulation is attempted. In the meantime, the joint is considered physiologically unstable due to its reduced coaptive force. Normally, the intra-articular pressure of synovial joints is subatmospheric and affords coaptive stability. For example, the femoroacetabular joint can be stripped of all its muscular, capsular, and ligamentous attachments, and the femoral head will still remain in the acetabular fossa. It is only upon drilling a hole through the acetabular floor from inside the pelvis that the femoral head easily falls out of the socket as the subatmospheric coaptive force is released. In this regard, Sandoz[6] states that it is good practice to rest the joint approximately 20 minutes

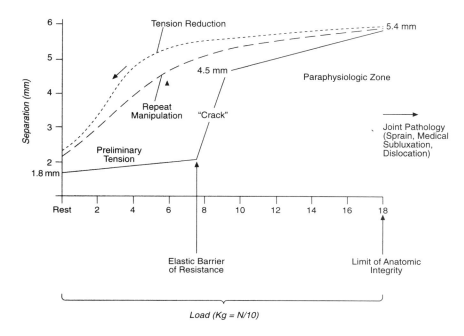

Figure 7–4 Load separation curve. An audible "crack" is heard at 8 kg of tension as the joint surfaces are separated and the paraphysiologic space is entered. Small dashed line denotes the release of tension. Note that the separation of surfaces does not return to original starting point. The middle curve indicates a second attempt at manipulation immediately after the first one. No crack sound is elicited. *Source:* Reprinted from *Chiropractic Technique* by T.F. Bergmann, D.H. Peterson and D.J. Lawrence, p. 289, with permission of Churchill Livingstone, © 1993.

post manipulation before regular activities are resumed, ie, to have the patient lie down during the joint's refractory period or limit his or her activity for that time.

Sandoz[6] summarizes that the following events occur at the moment of intrusion into the paraphysiologic space: (1) a sudden separation of the joint surfaces; (2) an audible cracking sound; and (3) appearance of a radiolucent space in the joint. Sandoz[6] also mentions that the active and passive ranges are increased temporarily after a manipulation as the paraphysiologic space is added to them. He comments that one must remain cautious when manipulating a joint during its refractory period due to the absence of the protective elastic barrier. The only barrier of resistance present in such a situation is the limit of anatomical integrity. Forceful manipulation can risk injury to the soft tissue–holding elements of the joint.

GRADE VI MOBILIZATION

The loss of the elastic barrier can be used to an advantage when one wants to mobilize (not manipulate!) these soft tissue restraints after a manipulation. Without the elastic barrier present, the capsuloligamentous tissues can be directly stretched. Although the term is not used in the existing literature, I refer to this as a *grade VI mobilization*. The grade V manipulation removes the elastic barrier, and a gentle, small-amplitude, mobilizing oscillation afterward can help stretch the articular soft tissues. Thus, a grade VI mobilization is analogous to a grade IV mobilization performed after a manipulation (V). This is particularly effective in chronically stiff hip joints, using a long-axis extension maneuver described later. Grade VI mobilizations using the sacro-ilio cross and anterior or posterior torsion techniques are also useful in chronic sacroiliac joint dysfunctions.

Aside from the mechanical aspects of a manipulation, it is recognized that important effects can be attained via neurophysiologic reflexogenic phenomena.[7-13] It is thought that stimulation of the joint receptors initiates an afferent barrage to the central nervous system, where neural connections result in efferent effects to other structures. Korr[8] discusses how the sympathetic nervous system is physiologically situated between the somatic and visceral systems, possibly allowing one to affect the other. He feels that chronic segmental facilitation of the sympathetic nervous system due to a somatic dysfunction (subluxation, fixation, somatic lesion) can create visceral consequences of disease. It is not unusual for the experienced manipulative practitioner to observe functional "organic" changes in response to restoring locomotor (somatic) function. Dysmenorrhea, dyspareunia, enuresis, and functional bowel disturbances have been known to improve after treatment for pelvic joint problems for which patients have presented.

Also noted are changes in the locomotor system at sites distant from the primary area treated, ie, midthoracic or cervical muscle spasm or range of motion improving after administration of a sacroiliac manipulation. These changes are mediated by the all-important nervous system. Manipulation should not be regarded as simply restoring motion in a restricted joint. Joint manipulation helps to reestablish the functional biomechanics of the locomotor system while simultaneously stimulating the nervous system via reflex phenomena.

By stimulating joint mechanoreceptors, joint manipulation supplies a means of input to the nervous system on a reflex basis. Theoretically, dysfunctional joints and soft tissues supply the nervous system with abnormal afferent input that can engage reflex mechanisms causing undesirable effects. Such consequences can be referred pain, muscle spasm, vasomotor changes, and even subtle visceral changes. Manipulating a dysfunctional joint can reduce its abnormal afferent input and subsequent reflexogenic effects and have far-reaching beneficial effects. Any input into the system causes a response, even if it is not observable on the exterior.

WHAT ABOUT THE AUDIBLE "CRACK"?

The significance of a joint's audible "crack" during a manipulation is debatable. Many manipulators feel that for optimal results it is necessary to gap the joint until it clicks. Others feel that it is not. In referencing Mierau et al, Gale[14] mentions that manipulation has been found to be superior to mobilization in increasing overall mobility. We need to keep separate the terms *mobilization* and *manipulation*. The former pertains to passive movements performed up to but not entering the paraphysiologic space. The latter entails entering the paraphysiologic space and is usually associated with an audible click. Similarly, Hadler et al[15] showed significantly better results with manipulation than with mobilization.

It is commonly observed that patients improve even when the manipulative technique is not associated with an audible crack. Certain patients have joints that just do not "crack," regardless of the force used, how often they are manipulated, or the expertise of the manipulator. Nevertheless, the joint's range of motion and patient's symptoms seem to improve more rapidly when the joint is cavitated. That is not to say that every joint manipulation performed on every patient should result in a "click," especially on the first attempt. Nor is it to say that an audible click should be the sole goal. However, somewhere along the patient's clinical course, if manipulation is indicated, the cavitation phenomenon is certainly welcomed.

The joint should be "caressed" and coaxed to move. If it clicks, so be it. If it does not, further coaxing can be attempted, but brute force should never be used, especially if only to fulfill the near-neurotic whim of hearing an audible click. Some manipulative practitioners have been accused of being too rough by performing too vigorous a manipulation in order to hear that infamous "pop." Unfortunately, some are too rough. Joints that are stiff and fixated actually invite correction. Thus, a practitioner weighing 160 lb who finds himself in a wrestling match with a joint weighing a few ounces should reevaluate how he approaches manipulation.

In chronically stiff joints, manipulation should be used carefully. Years of poor joint function, adaptive shortening of periarticular tissues, and fibrosis do not readily reward the practitioner with an audible click, at least not in the beginning. This is common in problems of the sacroiliac and hip joints, where some of the largest and most powerful ligaments in the body are found. Several visits over a few days using mobilization first and then manipulation may produce a joint cavitation.

Meal and Scott[16] mention how weather can affect the ability of a joint to make an audible crack. They observed that when a low-pressure weather system was present, the joints under study cracked more easily, with less tension and creating less noise.

Question for Thought

How is it that weather can affect joint conditions?

SLACK REMOVAL

Most of the work in manipulation involves taking all the slack out of the surrounding tissues while guarding neighboring joints that do not need to be manipulated. When a joint is taken to the end of its passive range of motion, right up to the elastic barrier, all slack is said to have been removed. This "preparation" of the joint is culminated by the grade V thrust itself, which is directed at the joint, not the entire patient. More specifically, it is directed at the joint restriction. The amount of force needed is minimal, but the speed of execution is rapid so as to overcome the inertia of the restriction. The move incorporates finesse and feel rather than force. The quick, short impulse allows safe entrance into the paraphysiologic zone.

The importance of removing all tissue slack and taking a joint to tension before manipulating it can be illustrated by a simple experiment (Figure 7–5). Suppose a bedroom door is slightly stuck in its doorjamb and we want to open it, but we want to do it in an unusual way. We tie a strong industrial rubber band to the door knob at one end and anchor the other end to a crank. Next, we crank up the tension in the rubber band just to the point where the door will fly open. The band is so tense that if we were just to flick it with our finger, the door would immediately fling open. Do you think it would matter from which direction we flicked the rubber band? Not really. As long as the rubber band was "preloaded" to the threshold tension needed to open the door, and as long as the direction of that tension was applied correctly, the door would fling open with minimal force

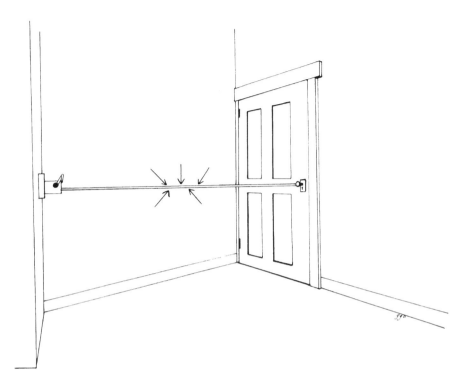

Figure 7–5 Door analogy and slack removal. Arrows indicate the various directions of applying finger flick.

in the direction we wanted. What the finger flick would actually be doing would be supplying us with just enough force to overcome the inertia holding the door closed.

The finger flick itself would not require tremendous effort, nor would the direction of its application to the rubber band be important. The only thing that would be important would be that it occurred, but in conjunction with the correct preload tension. Most of the effort in opening the door would be generated by the rubber band. So, too, is slack removal related to joint manipulation. This is especially true when joints surrounded by large, powerful muscles and ligaments are manipulated.

Most errors in manipulation arise from the inadequate removal of tissue slack. Unfortunately, many people apply too much of the effort to the actual impulse thrust. The amount of tissue tension generated during slack removal is inversely related to the amount of impulse thrust required. If

little slack is removed prior to a manipulation, one of two things will occur. Number one, the thrust will be dissipated in the extra slack that is still
present, and the joint's paraphysiologic space will not be reached. Number two, the extra slack needing to be taken up will most likely be incorporated with the impulse thrust. This creates a high-velocity, high-amplitude
thrust from the active and passive ranges of motion right up to and
through the elastic barrier, resulting in a painful manipulation. This as-
sault and battery must be avoided at all costs. Problems with manipulation arise when the overzealous or impatient practitioner takes the joint
through active, passive, and joint play ranges all in one quick movement.
The joint mechanoreceptors react too briskly to be "fooled," and reflex
muscle guarding is usually recruited, resulting in an unsatisfactory maneuver, to say the least.

Traction and slack removal should be performed slowly and gently,
with the practitioner being astute to any reaction from the joint, muscles,
or patient in general. Needless to say, an uncomfortable position is not
conducive to a relaxed patient. It is good practice to ask the patient if he or
she feels comfortable just before the impulse thrust is delivered. Be mind-
ful of the patient who may be too embarrassed to volunteer this information.

The goal is to generate just enough tissue tension around the joint via
slack removal so that a high-velocity, low-amplitude impulse is all that is
necessary to "open the door." The vulnerability of the patient should be
recognized and respected at all times, together with the realization that we
manipulate living, feeling human beings, not just restricted painful joints.

CONTRAINDICATIONS

Mobilization and manipulation are indicated when one determines that
a joint's accessory or joint play movements need to be restored. According
to Maitland,[2] hypermobile joints may need to be mobilized (not manipulated!) to reduce pain and increase their function, not to increase their
range of motion. In this regard, grade I and II mobilizations are used to
stimulate mechanoreceptor activity and reduce pain. Manipulation, on the
other hand, should not be used on hypermobile joints. Generally, mobilization and manipulation are used to increase joint motion. However, there
are instances when mobilization and manipulation techniques are contraindicated.[17] These can be grouped into absolute and relative contraindications and are listed in Exhibits 7–1 and 7–2.

There are usually no arguments over the absolute contraindications, but
the relative contraindications carry some disagreement among field prac-

Exhibit 7–1 Absolute Contraindications to Manipulation

- Malignancy
- Infections
- Fractures
- Bone disease
- Ruptured ligaments
- Acute inflammatory arthritis
- Large-disc prolapse with signs of cord compression
- Cauda equina syndrome

titioners, depending on their experience. Relative contraindications demand careful assessment if manual techniques are to be considered for treatment. What may be a relative contraindication to an inexperienced clinician may not be one at all to an experienced practitioner. Conditions such as osteoarthritis, osteoporosis, and pregnancy, although not contraindications, should be handled with care. Problems can be avoided as long as the movements are gentle and match the integrity of the joint structures treated. Small-amplitude thrusts or impulses mean just that— small ⅛-in depths of movement. Control and gentleness at this depth rarely cause difficulties. Obviously, any increase in pain just prior to the thrust demands reassessment before following through with a manipulation.

Women in the third trimester of pregnancy need to be handled judiciously. Vigorous rotation movements to the pelvis and low back should be strictly avoided. The imminent threat of miscarriage also precludes manipulation.

Osteoarthritis often responds well to gentle mobilizations and manipulations. Commonly seen are patients with osteoarthritis of the hip, complete with groin pain, hip flexor gait, and radiographic evidence of arthrosis. These patients have usually been told that they will have to learn

Exhibit 7–2 Relative Contraindications to Manipulation

- Bone demineralization
- Bilateral root signs
- Sciatica with straight-leg raising less than 30 degrees
- Hypermobility
- Bleeding disorders/anticoagulant therapy

to live with their arthritis and disability and are placed on anti-inflammatory medications. Some are even told they may require total hip replacement surgery. Yet despite their poor prognosis, some, if not many, respond very favorably to manual methods. In addition to joint mobilizations and gentle manipulations, soft tissue manipulations are very necessary and useful.

Obviously bony ankylosis needs to be ruled out in the case of sacroiliac joint manipulation, if for no other reason than the futility of trying to manipulate a fused joint. Plain radiographs are not sufficient enough at times to delineate sacroiliac joint ankylosis where computerized axial tomography is.

What about the patient who is apparently in pain too acute for the application of manual techniques? Barring pathology, this can treated as a relative contraindication depending on the clinician's expertise; however, common sense should prevail, and anti-inflammatory strategies, such as electrotherapy, cryotherapy, and medication, can be used. Grade I and II mobilizations can be very effective in reducing pain and spasm over a 2- to 3-day period. Just as much good can be accomplished by patiently coaxing rather than rushing the process. What may seem to be an attempt at a quick, miraculous maneuver to fix the acute pain more often proves to be untimely, painful, and counterproductive.

SACROILIAC JOINT MANIPULATIVE TECHNIQUES

Side-Lying

The more common sacroiliac joint manipulations are carried out in the side-lying position. The type of joint restriction found on palpation examination determines how to position the patient for manipulation. In the assessment of sacroiliac joint motion, the patient is asked to raise one knee at a time while several bony landmarks are monitored via palpation. Attention is paid to which leg is raised and which palpation landmark is observed to be restricted, ie, the posterior superior iliac spine, sacral tubercle, or sacral apex. A general rule of thumb used to position the patient properly for manipulation is to reproduce in side-lying position the standing examination position in which the movement restriction was found. The palpation landmark found restricted in its movement is contacted for the thrust.

Upper-Pole Flexion Fixation

Take, for instance, a case in which the upper aspect of the right sacroiliac joint is restricted in flexion. As the examiner palpates and observes for movement of the right posterior superior iliac spine (PSIS) in relation to the sacral tubercle, he or she will notice lack of movement when the patient raises the right knee (Figure 7–6A). The examiner may also notice compensatory motions made by the patient subconsciously, ie, sticking the buttocks out laterally and/or bending the weight-bearing knee. To manipulate this dysfunction, the clinician places the patient in a position that best duplicates that examining posture. In this case, the patient is placed on the left side with the right thigh flexed (Figure 7–6B). The right PSIS is contacted and thrust upon to create motion in the upper aspect of the right sacroiliac joint. Reassessment should demonstrate the right PSIS to move more inferiorly when the right knee is raised.

Someone using the static model of "bone out of place" for manipulation may be inclined to ask, "Why contact the PSIS from the posterior to manipulate it anteriorly? Did not the motion assessment find a lack of posterior and inferior movement of the PSIS? Don't you want it to move posteriorly and inferiorly instead?" First, we are not trying to reposition a bone that is out of place. We are trying to increase a joint's range of motion. By contacting the PSIS, we gain leverage allowing us to gap the joint enough to allow motion to occur. Second, the patient's positioning and slack removal determine the motion to be induced. In this case, we are not trying to reposition the ilium more anteriorly by taking a posterior contact on the PSIS, although it seems so. Instead, we are trying to impart motion to the joint with an impulse thrust, regardless of its static neutral posture. The thrust overcomes the restriction, and the patient's positioning and slack removal, strongly favoring flexion, allow the motion to occur.

Upper-Pole Extension Fixation

If the upper pole of the right sacroiliac joint is fixated in extension, the examiner will notice a diminished excursion of the sacral tubercle in relation to the right PSIS when the patient lifts the left knee (Figure 7–7A). To manipulate this restriction, the clinician contacts the sacral base just medial to the downside PSIS (Figure 7–7B). The standing examination position is reproduced by placing the patient in the right side-lying position with the left thigh flexed (Figure 7–7C). The clinician should be positioned well over the manipulation contact. Reassessment should reveal the sacral tubercle to move more inferiorly when the patient again raises the left leg.

Lower-Pole Flexion Fixation

To assess a lower-pole flexion fixation of the right sacroiliac joint, the right posterior inferior iliac spine (PIIS) and sacral apex are palpated simultaneously while the patient raises the right knee (Figure 7–8A). The

A

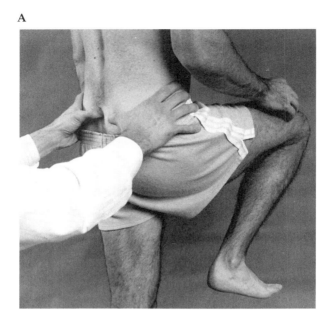

B

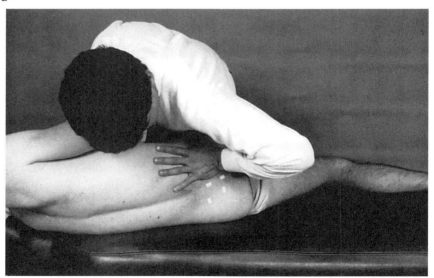

Figure 7–6 Right upper flexion fixation. **(A)** Palpation. **(B)** Manipulation.

A

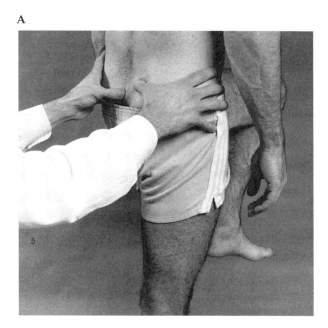

B

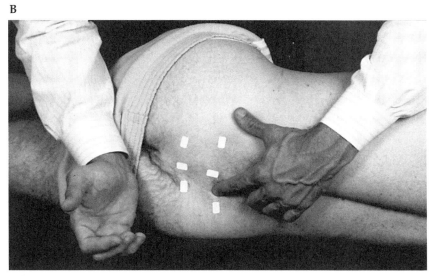

continues

Figure 7–7 Right upper extension fixation. **(A)** Palpation. **(B)** Point of contact. **(C)** Manipulation.

Figure 7–7 continued

C

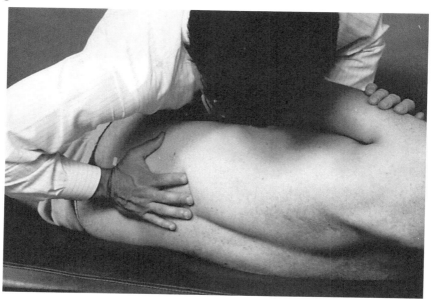

examiner should observe the PIIS to move inferiorly and slightly laterally in relation to the sacral apex contact. Lack of this motion indicates joint fixation. To manipulate this joint restriction, the clinician contacts the right PIIS or ischial tuberosity with the patient in a left side-lying position (Figure 7–8B). This essentially reproduces the standing palpation test in the side-lying position. Reassessment should show the right PIIS to move more inferiorly and laterally.

Lower-Pole Extension Fixation

A lower-pole extension fixation is assessed by simultaneously palpating the right PIIS and sacral apex while the patient raises the left knee (Figure 7–9A). The sacral apex should move inferiorly in relation to the PIIS contact. Lack of this motion denotes a loss of extension motion in the right lower pole. A pisiform contact is made on the downside of the sacral apex (Figure 7–9B). The patient is positioned in the right side-lying posture with the left thigh flexed (Figure 7–9C). Reevaluation should demonstrate increased inferior movement of the sacral apex when the patient lifts the left knee.

A

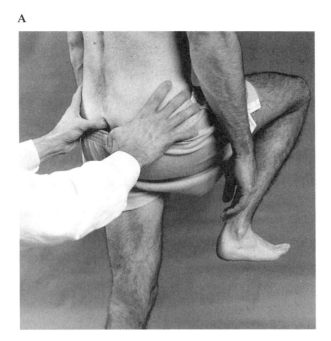

B

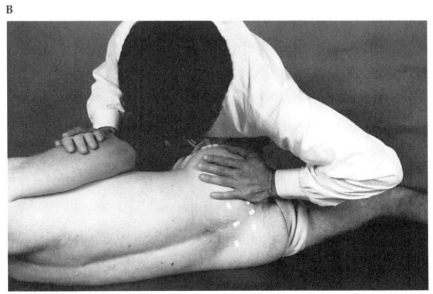

Figure 7–8 Right lower flexion fixation. **(A)** Palpation. **(B)** Manipulation.

A

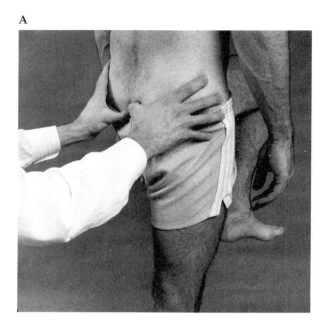

B

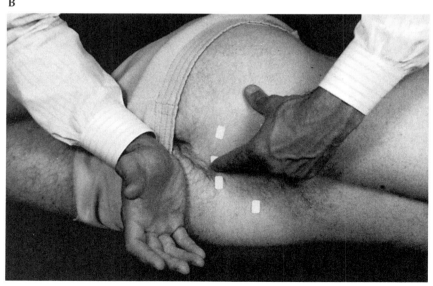

continues

Figure 7–9 Right lower extension fixation. **(A)** Palpation. **(B)** Point of contact. **(C)** Manipulation.

Figure 7–9 continued

C

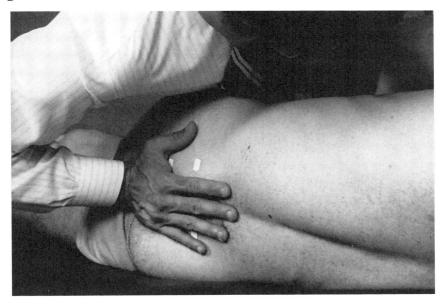

In all the above manipulations, the thigh is maximally flexed to "preload" the sacroiliac joint. The patient's arms are crossed in front of the chest. The clinician grasps the patient's forearms or uppermost deltoid with his or her cephalad hand and tractions headward. The impulse thrust is delivered only when every trace of "slack" is removed and the patient is relaxed. The joint must be taken to tension before manipulating. The pisiform aspect of the caudad hand makes the contact on the anatomical landmark that did not move during the motion assessment. In the case of large or flexible patients, the leg and thigh are placed in front of the clinician's knee to facilitate slack removal (Figure 7–10).

In a "body-drop" impulse, the clinician raises his or her torso a few inches and drops it suddenly to add inertia to the final impulse. The impulse itself is the final motion of the body drop and fine-tunes the amount of thrust delivered. The action is analogous to the workings of a bullwhip. The arm of the lion trainer and whip handle move through a large range of motion as they send the whip through its travel. The tip of the whip is accelerated at the last second through a much smaller range of motion as its direction of travel is reversed. The snapping sound is actually a mini–sonic boom as the tip of the whip is accelerated immensely.

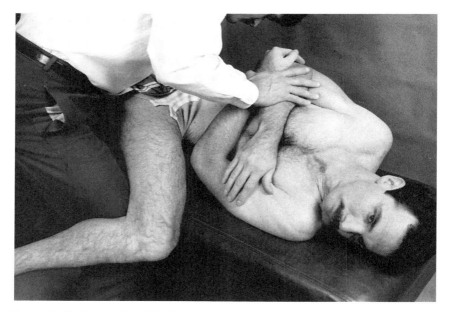

Figure 7–10 Alternative Side-Posture Position

Similarly, the manipulator's impulse is the fine-tuned terminal motion of the body drop.

A series of two to three thrusts graded in increasing intensity are delivered until the joint cavitates. The clinician is trying to coax the joint to move. The first thrust is light, followed by one of moderate intensity if a joint "release" was not experienced. If the joint still did not release, one last graded thrust of *slightly* more intensity can be tried. If a release is not felt or heard, the joint should be reevaluated for motion and not manipulated further. Often in such cases more motion is perceived on reassessment palpation as a result of the attempted manipulations' acting instead as firm mobilizations. This format is better than trying to release the joint with one big thrust. Generally, if all joint and soft tissue slack is removed, the joint manipulates very easily with minimal force. Sometimes the joint releases just from removal of all the slack.

Posttreatment soreness can be expected in some cases, and the patient should be informed of this. Painful flare-ups can occur, commonly in patients who exhibit signs of an unstable autonomic nervous system, stress, or an irritable joint in the vicinity of the manipulated joint. A flare-up may also occur if a few of the joint fixations present were not manipulated, being left unattended only to cause continued adverse reactions in the loco-motor system. For example, if one assesses only the upper poles of the sacroiliac joints for flexion fixations, important joint dysfunctions may be missed that may create flare-ups or slow clinical progress. For this reason, it is important to check both the upper and lower poles bilaterally for flex-ion and extension fixations. It is surprising how much pain and disability a single missed fixation can cause. Just manipulating a patient on one side and then the other without regard to careful assessment is asking for less than optimal results. At the least, provocative testing can be done to iden-tify the problematic side, followed by the knee-raising test to delineate fur-ther the fixations present on that side. Provocative testing entails maneu-vers that stress a joint to reproduce symptoms. The three best provocative tests used are the Patrick-Fabere, Gaenslen's, and Yeoman's tests. If two out of three of these tests are positive and localize the pain to the same joint, a high degree of confidence in lateralizing to the correct side of in-volvement is provided.

Prone

Upper-Pole Extension

A more direct way to impart extension in the sacroiliac joint is to place the patient prone and extend the thigh at the hip with the caudad hand (Figure 7–11). The PSIS on the fixated side is contacted with the cephalad hand and thrust upon. The thigh is lifted to tension, and the impulse is delivered when all joint slack is removed. The hip joint needs to be taken to its end range of extension. Leverage transmitted to the ilium via the anteriorly placed iliofemoral ligament (Y-ligament of Bigelow) imparts stress to the sacroiliac joint. Caution needs to be exercised because of the leverage generated by this technique and the possibility of affecting the lumbar facet joints.

Lower-Pole Extension

To affect the lower pole, the patient positioning is the same as in the previous technique, but the sacral apex is contacted with the pisiform of the manipulating hand (Figure 7–12). Thrusting, especially in these two techniques, is light and coaxing.

Supine

General Flexion

A general flexion manipulation can be used in the supine position. It is not specific to either the upper or lower aspects of the sacroiliac joint. This

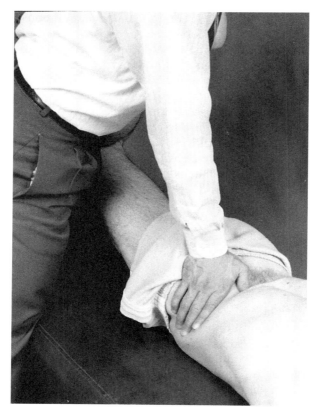

Figure 7–11 Extension Manipulation of Sacroiliac Joint's Upper Aspect

works well in patients who have difficulty assuming the prone or side-lying positions, ie, pregnant women. With the patient supine, the clinician stands on the involved side at the level of the pelvis, facing headward. The patient's thigh is flexed to 90 degrees and is slightly adducted with the caudad hand. The cephalad hand cups the anterior superior iliac spine and presses toward the table, taking up any slack. As the thigh is flexed to tension, a light body-drop impulse is delivered through both hands (Figure 7–13).

Caudal Glide

Quite frequently, patients present with a history of stepping into a hole unexpectedly and jamming the hip and back. A maneuver that is effective

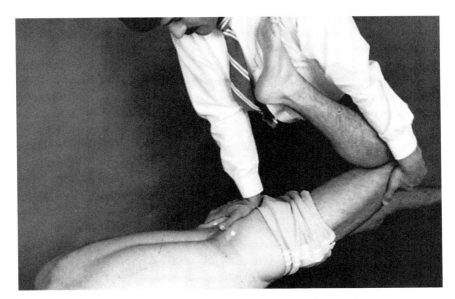

Figure 7–12 Extension Manipulation of Sacroiliac Joint's Lower Aspect

in this situation is a long-axis extension or distraction on the entire leg. To affect the sacroiliac joint, the straight leg is lifted off the table to 30 degrees and pulled with an impulse thrust (Figure 7–14).

In addition to these techniques, any of the maneuvers demonstrated in Chapter 6 for mobilization can be implemented for manipulation by using a grade V thrust. In all of these and the following techniques, manipulation is used when joint dysfunction or restricted motion is found during the examination.

HIP JOINT MANIPULATION

Side-Lying

Long-Axis Extension

The hip can be manipulated in long-axis extension by placing the patient in a side-lying position with the involved side up (Figure 7–15). It is used when long-axis extension in the hip joint is restricted. The uppermost thigh is flexed to 90 degrees at the hip, and the knee is flexed to allow the foot to rest behind the other knee. The flexed knee is adducted toward the floor. The clinician stabilizes the patient on the table with the cephalad

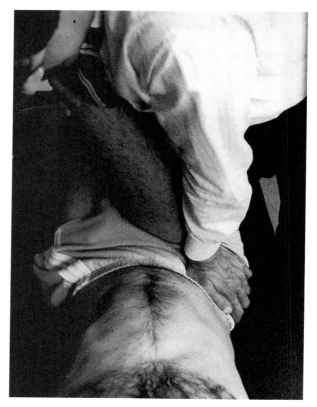

Figure 7–13 General Flexion Manipulation

hand. The clinician then places his or her knee and thigh against the patient's knee and thigh. The caudal arm is straight, and the greater trochanter is contacted with the heel of the hand. Slack is removed by tractioning the patient's thigh floorward with the clinician's knee and thigh. A body-drop impulse is made on the greater trochanter with the caudad hand to distract the femoral head from the acetabulum.

Prone

Extension

This maneuver is performed like the prone extension technique for the sacroiliac joint except that the greater trochanter is contacted by the ma-

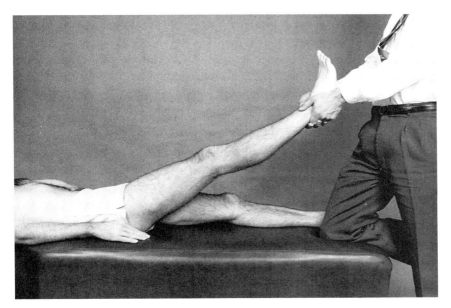

Figure 7–14 Caudal Glide Manipulation, Sacroiliac Joint

nipulating hand. All joint slack is removed by extending the hip to the end range, and an impulse thrust is delivered (Figure 7–16). This is not well tolerated in osteoarthritic hip joints and should be used carefully.

Lateral Rotation

With the patient prone and the clinician standing opposite to the side of involvement, the leg is flexed at the knee to 90 degrees. The lower leg is pulled toward the clinician with the caudad hand to impart lateral rotation at the hip joint. The cephalad hand contacts the opposite-side greater trochanter. With the hip held in extreme lateral rotation, a series of three to five impulse thrusts are made with the manipulating hand (Figure 7–17).

Long-Axis Extension

In this maneuver, the leg is grasped just proximal to the ankle. The clinician then tractions the leg in a long-axis direction to remove all slack and applies an impulse thrust, keeping the entire leg and thigh on the table (Figure 7–18). Patients are able to relax very well in this position.

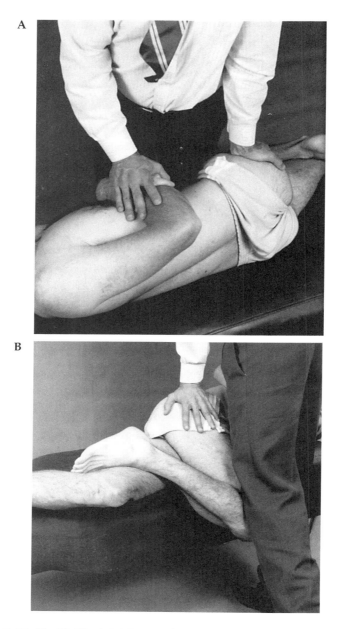

Figure 7–15 (A, B) Hip joint long-axis extension in side-lying posture. Note clinician's leg contact.

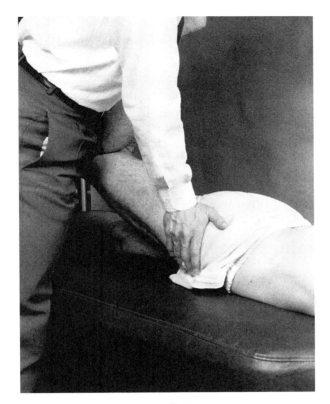

Figure 7–16 Hip Joint Extension Manipulation

Supine

Long-Axis Extension

This is the same maneuver as the previous prone technique except that it is performed in the supine position (see Chapter 5, Figure 5–42C). It differs from the sacroiliac caudal glide technique in that the leg and thigh remain on the table. An impulse tractional manipulation is applied. It must be emphasized that these techniques are to be performed gently and do not entail gross tugging. These are excellent techniques to follow up with grade VI mobilizations. That is, after the elastic barrier has been removed by a grade V manipulation, small-amplitude mobilizing oscillations are used to stretch the articular tissues further. This is very useful in treatment of chronic hip joint stiffness.

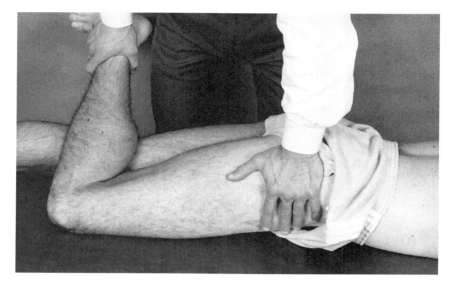

Figure 7–17 Hip Joint, Lateral Rotation Manipulation

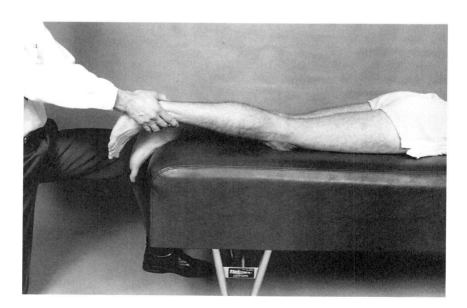

Figure 7–18 Hip Joint Long-Axis Extension

Caudal Glide at 90 Degrees Flexion

The patient is supine, with the thigh flexed to 90 degrees and the foot resting on the table. The clinician kneels beside the table on the same side and encircles the most proximal part of the thigh with both hands. If the patient's knee can fully flex so that the heel can touch the buttock, then the lower leg and thigh can both be encircled by the clinician. The clinician's shoulder is placed up against the mid- and distal thigh, and the hands, shoulder, and thigh move as one unit in a caudal direction to take up slack. At the point of restriction, an impulse thrust is given. The shoulder is pressed slightly headward as the hands scoop the proximal thigh floorward and caudally. This imparts a scooping movement to the technique (Figure 7–19A).

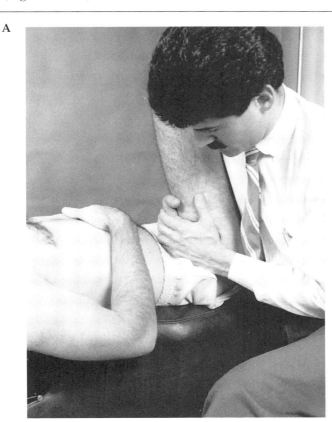

A

continues

Figure 7–19 (A) Hip joint caudal glide at 90 degrees flexion. **(B)** Lateral glide.

Figure 7–19 continued

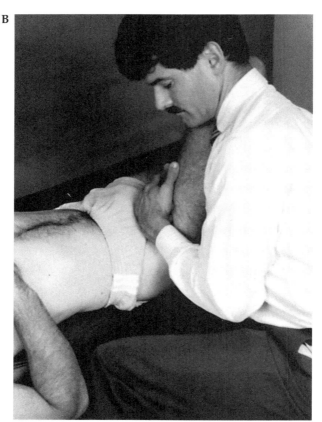

Lateral Glide at 90 Degrees

This technique is similar to the one above except that the direction of traction and impulse is lateral. To do this, the clinician faces perpendicular to the thigh and encircles its most proximal aspect. The shoulder is placed up against the middle and distal aspect of the lateral thigh, and the hands, shoulder, and thigh move as one unit laterally. The shoulder leverages slightly medially as the hands pull slightly floorward and laterally. This imparts a lateral scooping action to the maneuver (Figure 7–19B).

Posterior Shear at 90 Degrees

With the patient supine, the thigh is flexed to 90 degrees. The clinician places his or her leg nearest the patient on the table to afford a place on

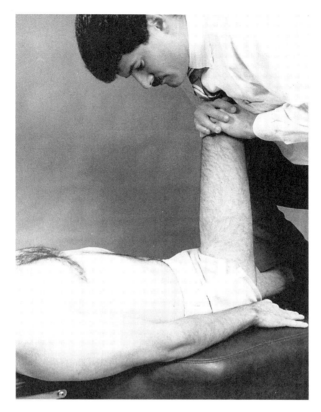

Figure 7–20 Hip Joint Posterior Shear at 90 Degrees Flexion

which the patient can rest his or her flexed lower leg. By leaning over the patient's bent knee, the clinician applies pressure down toward the table along the femoral shaft by resting his or her sternum on his or her hands, which are covering the patient's knee. After taking up all slack, he or she delivers a light body-drop impulse toward the table (Figure 7–20).

Chapter Review Questions

- What are the effects of joint manipulation?
- What are short- and long-lever manipulative techniques?
- What are the three zones of movement in a joint's range of motion?
- What are the two barriers to movement in a joint's range of motion?

- What causes the audible click heard during a manipulation, and what is its significance?
- What is the importance of "slack" removal during a manipulation?
- Name the contraindications to manipulation and mobilization.
- Describe a typical side-lying manipulative technique setup for sacroiliac joint dysfunctions.

REFERENCES

1. Shekelle PG. Spine update: spinal manipulation. *Spine.* 1994;19:858–861.
2. Maitland GD. *Vertebral Manipulation.* 5th ed. Boston, Mass: Butterworths; 1986.
3. Mennell JM. *Back Pain: Diagnosis and Treatment Using Manipulative Techniques.* Boston, Mass: Little, Brown & Co; 1960.
4. Roston JB, Haines RW. Cracking in the metacarpophalangeal joint. *J Anat.* 1947;81:165–173.
5. Unsworth A, Dowson D, Wright V. Cracking joints: a bioengineering study of cavitation in the metacarpophalangeal joint. *Ann Rheum Dis.* 1971;30:348–358.
6. Sandoz R. Some physical mechanisms and effects of spinal adjustments. *Ann Swiss Chiro Assoc.* 1976;6:91–141.
7. Palmer DD. *The Science, Art and Philosophy of Chiropractic.* Portland, Ore: Printing House Co; 1910.
8. Korr IM. Sustained sympathicotonia as a factor in disease. In Korr IM, ed. *The Neurobiologic Mechanisms in Manipulative Therapy.* New York, NY: Plenum Publishing Corp; 1978:229–268.
9. Lewit K. *Manipulative Therapy in Rehabilitation of the Locomotor System.* Boston, Mass: Butterworths; 1985.
10. Janse J. *Principles and Practice of Chiropractic: An Anthology.* Lombard, Ill: National College of Chiropractic; 1976
11. Sato A, Swenson RS. Sympathetic nervous system response to mechanical stress of the spinal column in rats. *J Manipulative Physiol Ther.* 1984;7:141–147.
12. Denslow JS, Korr IM, Krems AD. Qualitative studies of chronic facilitation in human motor neuron pools. *Am J Physiol.* 1947;105:229–238.
13. Kunert W. Functional disorders of internal organs due to vertebral lesions. *Ciba Found Symp.* 1965;13:85–96.
14. Gale PA. Joint mobilization. In Hammer WI, ed. *Functional Soft Tissue Examination by Manual Methods.* Gaithersburg, Md: Aspen Publishers, Inc; 1991: 194-214.
15. Hadler NM, Curtis P, Gillings DB, Stinnett S. A benefit of spinal manipulation as adjunctive therapy for acute low-back pain: a stratified controlled trial. *Spine.* 1987;12:703–706.
16. Meal GM, Scott RA. Analysis of the joint crack by simultaneous recording of sound and tension. *J Manipulative Physiol Ther.* 1986;9:183–195.
17. Haldeman S, Chapman-Smith D, Petersen D. *Guidelines for Chiropractic Quality Assurance and Practice Parameters.* Gaithersburg, Md: Aspen Publishers, Inc; 1993.

Chapter 8

Inflammation, the Soft Tissues, and General Treatment Considerations

Chapter Objectives

- to discuss inflammation and repair
- to discuss the effects of immobilization on the soft tissues
- to describe tissue structure and function of connective tissues, muscles, tendons, and ligaments
- to describe myotendinous junctions and insertional sites and muscle, tendon, and ligament injuries
- to discuss general clinical considerations for treatment by phase of healing

A common accompaniment to pelvic joint dysfunctions is problems of the associated soft tissues. The term *soft tissue* is general and vague but includes muscle, ligament, capsular, and fascial structures. Nerve and vascular components can also be included. However, a whole chapter can be written on each of the individual tissues involved, so for our purposes we contain our discussion to a brief review of connective tissue, muscle, tendon, and ligament.

It is foolish and naive to think that in treating locomotor disturbances, all one has to do is manipulate or mobilize a joint, especially since manual techniques mostly affect the soft tissues. Therefore, added attention must be paid to muscle and ligament problems. Joints affect their surrounding soft tissues and vice versa. Even the novice practitioner trained in manual methods recognizes local and often distant soft tissue changes in reaction to locomotor dysfunctions (see Chapter 4). These changes can be subtle or gross. Some subtle changes are periosteal pain points unknown to the patient unless examined for and painful, restricted skin rolling. Some gross changes are reflex muscle spasm secondary to joint inflammation and pain.

There is a saying that life is movement and movement is life. This is amply true of the locomotor system and its soft tissues, and especially true of hypovascular connective tissues like tendons and ligaments. Without a rich blood supply, they depend on movement to assist in diffusing nutrients throughout the extracellular compartment.

Immobility, on the other hand, creates the conditions in which degenerative processes can develop. Joints, muscles, and ligaments become "injured" just from being immobilized. If you totally immobilize a perfectly normal hip joint for several weeks, you will be hard pressed to move the joint without pain and dysfunction afterward. Histologically, fibrosis will be seen to infiltrate the framework of the tissues. Any trauma causing inflammation and repair will create scar formation and more fibrosis from the proliferation phase of inflammation. This is seen after immobilization from serious trauma.

But what about the person who becomes "physiologically immobilized"? Prolonged posturing, be it sitting, standing, or lying, coupled with a lack of physical movement, such as stretching and exercise, slowly robs the body of what it is designed for—speed, agility, and movement. Adaptive shortening and fibrosis occur as tissues seek to accommodate to the amount of activity applied. The tissues become less compliant and more physiologically immobile. More shortening and fibrosis occur, and the cycle continues. Acute and chronic soft tissue changes can be observed on examination (see Chapter 4).

INFLAMMATION AND REPAIR

After injury, a stereotypic inflammatory response occurs in the soft tissues that is designed to wall off, debride, and repair the damaged area. It was Cornelius Celsus, a first-century writer, who initially proclaimed the four clinical signs of acute inflammation: rubor, tumor, calor, and dolor. These changes of redness, swelling, heat, and pain are due to the stereotypic hemodynamic changes that are the hallmark of acute inflammation. Virchow later added the fifth clinical sign of *functio laesa*, or lost function. Inflammation can be acute or chronic. Acute inflammation is usually of short duration, typified by edema and exudation and a neutrophilic response. Chronic inflammation is of longer duration, associated with the proliferation of blood vessels and connective tissue and the presence of lymphocytes and macrophages. It can occur after unresolved acute inflammation or by itself from low-grade inflammation of long standing.

The acute inflammatory response usually lasts 1 to 3 days. Soon after, capillaries and fibroblasts proliferate, forming granulation tissue. This signals the start of repair. Small tissue defects heal rapidly with minimal scarring. However, large defects heal by secondary union. This is associated with increased granulation tissue formation and subsequent scarring. Wound contraction by contractile fibroblasts (myofibroblasts) occurs to repair the large defect. During the repair process, the wound is filled with granulation tissue, and more collagen is laid down, laying the groundwork for remodeling and maturation of the scar to occur. If the repair process takes a few days to a few weeks, the remodeling and maturation process may take many months to years, depending on the tissue involved and the extent of the injury. In the remodeling phase of healing, collagen fibers are oriented to the line of wound stress. In addition, a distinct increase in wound strength is observed.

Acute inflammation can either completely resolve, heal by scarring, abscess, or progress to chronic inflammation (Figure 8–1). Chronic inflammation occurs after an unresolved acute inflammation, repeated bouts of acute inflammations, or a low-grade inflammatory response unlike the traditional acute inflammatory process. It is characterized by its cellular response and proliferation of connective tissue and blood vessels. A low-grade chronic inflammation can persist for years, laying down more fibrotic tissue and creating more dysfunction.

Cantu and Grodin[1] discuss the differences between scarring and fibrosis. Both of these involve the production of connective tissue. However, whereas scarring is a local process occurring in the area of trauma, fibrosis affects the normal surrounding tissues and is more homogenous. It alters the actual structure of the connective tissue by inflammation that spreads via exudates to the surrounding nontraumatized tissues. Scarring limits mobility directly and by any secondary adhesions with neighboring tissues. Fibrosis, on the other hand, limits mobility because of its expansive effect on most of the surrounding tissue. An example would be capsulitis of the hip joint, in which the entire capsule is involved, not just specific areas of scarring. Fibrosis begins in response to an event noxious to the tissues. Factors triggering a fibrotic response include a neighboring inflammation, adaptive shortening due to poor posture or locomotor imbalance, joint dysfunction, and just immobilization itself.

Once the process starts, it can progress and create a self-perpetuating cycle. As the chronic low-grade inflammation continues and connective tissue is laid down, the fibrotic front advances, thickens, shrinks from myofibroblastic action, and restricts. Further dysfunction results, with continued irritation to the tissues. The cycle continues, and more fibrosis

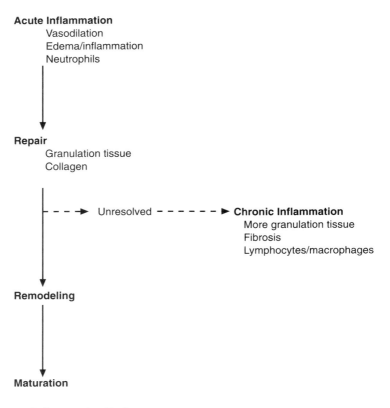

Acute Inflammation
  Vasodilation
  Edema/inflammation
  Neutrophils

Repair
  Granulation tissue
  Collagen

- - - ➤ Unresolved - - - - - - ➤ **Chronic Inflammation**
                                    More granulation tissue
                                    Fibrosis
                                    Lymphocytes/macrophages

Remodeling

Maturation

Figure 8–1 Inflammation Pathways

is produced. This continues until the inciting irritant is removed (Figure 8–2).

IMMOBILIZATION AND THE SOFT TISSUES

Immobilization creates fibrotic changes in the soft tissues affected.[2-4] Fatty fibrotic infiltrates can be grossly observed in capsular folds, creating adhesions. More infiltrate is deposited with longer immobilization times. Loss of ground substance occurs without significant loss in collagen fibers. This allows for the collagen interfiber distance to diminish and consequent cross-linking to occur. Without any directional stress applied to the tissues, new collagen is laid down in a disorganized, matted pattern. Tissue

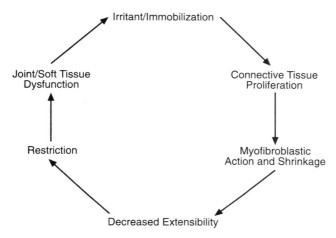

Figure 8–2 Effects of Immobilization

---

distensibility diminishes, creating more immobilization. Immobilization affects all the tissues of the musculoskeletal system. Joint capsules shrink[5] with irreversible changes seen after 8 weeks.[6] Ligaments fail at a lower threshold.[7] Muscle mass decreases, with a 20% loss of strength per week.[8] The maximal heart rate increases, and the $\dot{V}o_2$ max and plasma volume decrease.[9] The downside is that the effects from immobilization occur much more quickly than the beneficial effects gained from mobilization or exercise. Muscle force capacity is decreased 3% to 7% per day with immobilization, as compared to a gain of only 1% per day with activity.[10]

TISSUE STRUCTURE AND FUNCTION

Connective Tissue

Connective tissue is found throughout the body and is made up of cellular and extracellular components (Exhibit 8–1). It is arranged in dense regular, dense irregular, and loose irregular orientations (Exhibit 8–2). Clinically, we are concerned mostly with dense regular connective tissue, in the form of tendons and ligaments, and dense irregular connective tissue, such as joint capsules, aponeuroses, and periosteum. Fibroblasts and fibrocytes make up the cellular component. Fibroblasts produce mainly the fibers and ground substance found in connective tissues and later mature into the nonsecretory fibrocytes. In addition, cells of the reticuloen-

Exhibit 8–1 Connective Tissue Components

Cellular	Extracellular
• Fibroblasts	• Fibers: collagen, elastin, reticulin
• Fibrocytes	• Ground substance: water, proteoglycans
• Reticuloendothelial cells	

dothelial system are found in the connective tissues, especially during pathological conditions. Macrophages, mast cells, and plasma cells are among these. Macrophages function to phagocytize tissue debris, foreign material, and microorganisms, especially after injury. Mast cells release histamine and anticoagulants, and plasma cells produce antibodies for the body's immune response.

The extracellular part of connective tissue is made up of fibers surrounded by ground substance. The fiber types vary according to structure and function and are called collagen, elastin, and reticulin. Collagen is the main fiber type in connective tissue and is composed of four subtypes. Type I is the most ample form of collagen in the body and makes up a large part of the tissues affected by manipulation and mobilization, namely the joint capsules, ligaments, and tendons.[11] It affords tremendous tensile strength, especially if aligned in a dense pattern, as in tendons and ligaments. Elastin and reticulin are specialized fibers that recoil upon release of a deforming load. They are less able to withstand tensile forces and are limited in their distribution in the body when compared to collagen. For instance, elastin is found in the ligamentum flavum, the ligamentum nuchae, and the elastic walls of arteries. Reticulin is found mostly in the support framework of viscera and glands.

The ground substance secreted by fibroblasts forms the viscous matrix within which the cellular and fibrillar components of connective tissue are

Exhibit 8–2 Connective Tissue Types

Dense Regular	Dense Irregular	Loose Irregular
• Tendons	• Joint capsules	• Subcutaneous
• Ligaments	• Periosteum	• Mesentery
	• Aponeuroses	• Superficial fascia

embedded. It is made up of mostly water (70%) bounded by glycosami-noglycans, forming a gelatinous matrix. Hyaluronic acid and chondroitin sulfate are the two major types of glycosaminoglycans, with the former mostly binding water and the latter contributing to tissue cohesiveness.[1] This gel provides a medium through which diffusion of nutrients and wastes can occur. This is necessary because of the hypovascularity of connective tissue. It also provides elasticity, cohesiveness, and resistance to compression. By filling in the spaces between collagen fibers, the ground substance additionally maintains the appropriate collagen interfiber distance to prevent cross-linking and adhesion.[1]

Connective tissue functions to support, hold together, and provide a framework upon which tissues and organs are built. It also exhibits special deformation characteristics in response to various loads applied. It displays both viscous and elastic deformation properties whereby loads applied will result in nonrecoil and recoil actions respectively. In other words, its viscosity allows deformation to remain after a stretch, whereas its elasticity enables the tissue to recoil.

Muscle

Muscle tissue is specifically designed to generate tension. An individual muscle is composed of muscle cells, called *myofibers* or *muscle fibers*, that are grouped into bundles called *fasciculi*. Each myofiber contains the contractile proteins in the form of *myofibrils* (Figure 8–3). Muscle fibers occur in a variety of types, depending on functional and metabolic characteristics.[12] These are summarized in Exhibit 8–3. Connective tissue surrounds the fasciculi and muscle fibers and is called *perimysium* and *endomysium* respectively. The connective tissue wrappings on all three levels are actually confluent and allow passage for vascular, lymphatic, and neural elements. Muscle is very vascular tissue, and its perfusion is subject to activity-level changes. During activity, blood is directed through the capillary system. While the muscle is at rest, blood is diverted directly to venules.[13]

Anatomically, it is evident that muscle tissue and connective tissue are intimately related. The external fascial investments are continuous with the connecting tissue surrounding the individual muscle fibers, the endomysium. Therefore, treatments directed at muscle or myofascial structures cannot occur without affecting both simultaneously. Also, treatments directed at superficial fascial structures can affect muscles and fascia on deeper levels.

As discussed in Chapter 4, Janda[14] mentions how muscles of postural importance tend to shorten and become tight. In association with these are

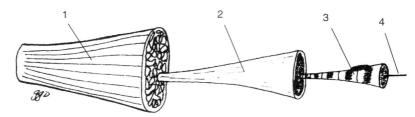

Figure 8–3 Muscle tissue: **(1)** muscle belly; **(2)** fascicle; **(3)** myofiber; **(4)** myofibril.

muscle groups that show a tendency to weaken. Length-strength assessment can supply us with this information, enabling stretching and mobilizing procedures to be used accordingly. Remedial exercises can be used on the weakened and inhibited muscles to reeducate them to proper function.

Muscles and Training

A muscle's response to training depends on the type of regimen used and the principles of overload, specificity, and reversibility.[15] Muscle fibers increase their capacity on a structural and physiologic basis to the extent that they are challenged by a specific training stimulus. As they adapt to the training demand imposed, the resultant changes plateau, and a new demand of higher intensity is needed for progress to continue. If the training stimulus is discontinued, the muscle becomes deconditioned, and the gains in structural and functional changes attained in training recede.

Low-intensity, high-repetition training induces muscle endurance if performed for 30 to 60 minutes on a regular basis. The intensity must be of sufficient magnitude to produce an overload, as must the duration of application. Endurance training increases the oxidative capacity of muscle and the percentage of high-oxidative muscle fibers.[16]

Exhibit 8–3 Striated Muscle Fiber Types

Fiber Type	Characteristics
Type I	Slow-twitch, fatigue resistant
Type IIA (fast red)	Fast-twitch oxidative, faster than Type I but less fatigue resistant
Type IIB (fast white)	Fast-twitch glycolytic, fast contraction, fatigues easily
Type IIC	Intermediate type, has characteristics of IIA and IIB
Type IIM (superfast)	Extremely fast contraction

High-intensity, low-repetition training creates muscle hypertrophy and increases in strength. Hypertrophy occurs via an increase in the muscle fiber's diameter. Due to the high loads imposed during this type of training, alternate-day routines are employed for adequate recovery to occur.

Injury Mechanisms

Clinically relevant injuries to muscle tissue are contraction or exercise induced, strain, contusion, and ischemia. Strenuous exercise and eccentric contractions are known to injure muscle fibers, resulting in postexercise soreness 1 to 3 days after the activity. Eccentric contraction generates more tension than isometric or concentric contractions and is associated with more myofibrillar damage and consequent postexercise soreness.[17] Intensive endurance exercises can injure muscle from metabolic buildup and ischemia.[18]

Strain injuries commonly occur after overstretching or a strong eccentric contraction. Injury usually occurs at the musculotendinous junction.[19] The precise reason for consistent failure to occur at the myotendinous junction is not clear but may be related to its structural makeup. Garrett and Tidball[19] discuss a study by Garrett et al in which electrically stimulated and nonstimulated rabbit muscles were subjected to tensile forces until failure and the effects were compared. The electrically stimulated muscles failed at the same length as the nonstimulated muscles but were able to sustain a higher force during stretching. Garrett and Tidball[19] comment that this is a significant finding demonstrating the ability of muscles to protect themselves and joints from injury. This study implies that muscles are better able to afford protection from injury and joint control if they can absorb more kinetic energy.[19]

Contusion injuries are caused by nonpenetrating blunt trauma. Inflammation occurs with hematoma formation. If severe enough, the hematoma can organize into osseous tissue, a condition called *myositis ossificans*. Interestingly, blunt injury responded faster in rat muscles that were mobilized than in those that were not.[20] Clinically, cross-fiber massage provides healing mobilization and works well after the acute phase in patients suffering from blunt trauma to muscle. As soreness and the muscle's ability to generate tension improve, postisometric relaxation and myofascial stretching aid greatly in recovery.

Increased pressure in compartments formed by tough fascial sheaths and bone can create nerve damage and decreased vascular perfusion, resulting in ischemic damage. Crush injuries, hemorrhage, or edema in a compartment can precipitate rapid pressure buildup with subsequent damage. Ischemia can develop at pressures lower than arterial pressure.[12]

This is potentially an emergency situation, with early recognition necessary since the amount and duration of pressure increase are proportional to the degree of injury.

Tendon

Tendons are the strongest soft tissue structures in the musculoskeletal system, owing to their high–collagen fiber composition and its dense parallel arrangement. Connective tissue organization in tendons is similar to that of muscle, with small bundles of fibers surrounded by an endotendineum, larger bundles by peritendineum, and the tendon itself invested in epitendineum. As in muscle, these layers of connective tissue are confluent and serve as passage for blood vessels. However, vascular injection studies have demonstrated avascular regions in tendon.[21]

Tendons are designed to withstand and transmit high tensile forces smoothly without any appreciable loss of energy, even though the Latin word for tendon is *tendere*, which means "to stretch." Observed longitudinally under light microscopy, the relaxed tendon demonstrates a regular wavy appearance, termed "crimping," that is a characteristic of the collagen fibers. Loads applied to tendons straighten out the crimping appearance (Figure 8–4A). Crimping apparently functions to dampen the shock from loads applied suddenly.

Most tendon injuries involve avulsion from bone or in-substance transection. Failure along the tendon's length is rare; disruption due to tensile forces more commonly occurs at the myotendinous junction.[19] Healing of tendon injuries has been shown to be greatly influenced by early intermittent passive mobilization[22] and continuous passive motion.[23] In one study, the mobilized tendons demonstrated greater strength than those of a control group in which mobilization was delayed.[22] The inflammatory stage in tendons lasts about 3 days, and full maturation of the injured area takes 2 to 3 months.

Ligament

Ligaments, like tendons, are cords or bands of dense regular connective tissue (Figure 8-4B). However, they display less uniformity to their parallel arrangement.[24] They also exhibit crimping, which is thought to add elasticity to ligament tissue.[25]

The word *ligament* is derived from the Latin word *ligare*, which means "to bind," and thus relates to their function of checking and stabilizing

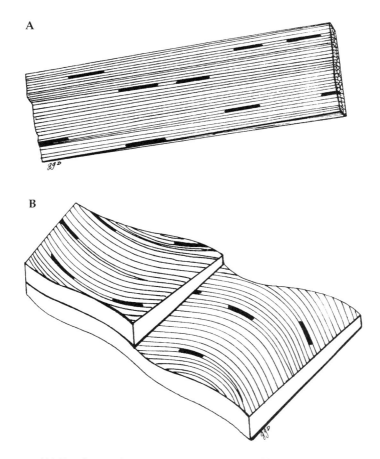

Figure 8–4 (A) Tendon without crimping pattern visible. **(B)** Ligament.

motion at joints. Attenuation of their function allows for excess joint motion and instability. Ligaments also play a neurosensory role.[26] Acting as sensory transducers, they supply the neuromuscular reflex system with afferent signals subserving proprioception. Ligaments are hypovascular, hypometabolic structures and consequently heal slowly when compared to other soft tissue structures. When strained maximally, they suffer stretch injury, partial tears, or full-substance tears. Ligaments are more prone to in-substance failure than to avulsion from bone.[26] Acute inflammation in ligaments lasts about 72 hours. Overlapping this are the repair and regeneration processes, lasting about 6 weeks. Maximal remodeling and maturation require up to 12 months or more.[27]

Ligament contraction has been observed to occur after injury.[27,28] Passive and active mechanisms have been postulated to signal ligament contraction. Ligaments held passively at a shorter length undergo collagen restructuring and cross-linking maintaining that length. Dahners[28] demonstrated active shortening mechanisms whereby actin, a contractile protein, contributed to the contraction of ligament. Interestingly, when normal stress-generated electrical potentials are simulated, this active ligament contraction is inhibited.[27] It seems that tissues normally emit stress-generated electrical potentials with mechanical loading and that a reduction of these potentials may signal the contraction process.

Myotendinous Junctions

A recent area of intense study in musculoskeletal tissues is the myotendinous junctions. Biomechanical studies have consistently shown that the interface between muscle and tendon is the weakest link in the contractile unit.[19] Tension developed in the muscle is transmitted to the tendon across the myotendinous junction, a highly specialized structure. Indirect injuries, or stretching and overcontraction injuries, tend to occur at the myotendinous junction more frequently than at other sites. The ends of the muscle fiber do not terminate as smooth conical insertions in the connective tissue matrix of the tendon. The membrane of the myofibril is invaginated, allowing greater surface area contact with the tendon collagen fibers (Figure 8–5). However, the terminal portions of the myofibril are less extensible and therefore more prone to tearing.[1]

Insertional Sites

Another area of weakness in the system is tendon, ligament, and capsular insertion sites to bone. A transitional zone of only 1 mm in width allows the change from collagen to bone to occur (Figure 8–6). Within this zone, a blend of different tissues occurs such that collagen progresses to fibrocartilage, calcified fibrocartilage, and finally bone.[29] These sites are also avascular, being dependent on tissue diffusion for nutrition. They often become painful in response to regional and even distant locomotor dysfunction, ie, periosteal pain points (see Chapter 4). Avulsion injuries are the most common pathologic conditions affecting insertion sites. These injuries are caused by rapid loading being applied to the insertional inter-

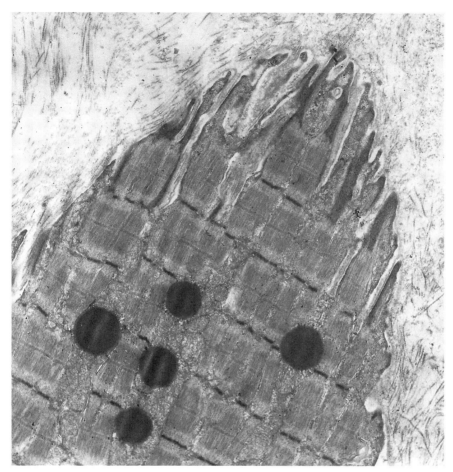

Figure 8–5 Myotendinous Junction. *Source:* Reprinted from Tidball, J.G., Myotendinous Junction: Morphological Changes and Mechanical Failure Associated with Muscle Cell Atrophy, *Experiments in Molecular Pathology*, Vol. 40, pp. 1–12, with permission of Academic Press, © 1984.

face, resulting in its failure. Rarely does separation occur within the junction itself. More commonly it occurs on either side of the junction, in the soft tissue or bone. However, junction or bone avulsion failures have a better outcome than failure in the soft tissues.[29]

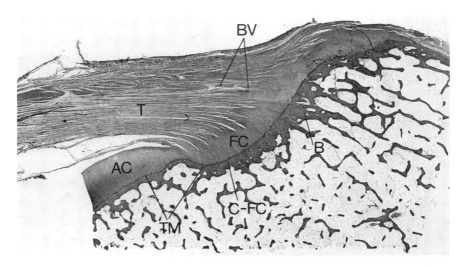

Figure 8–6 Insertional Site. T, tendon; BV, blood vessel; AC, articular cartilage; TM, tidemark; C-FC, cartilage-fibrocartilage; B, bone; FC, fibrocartilage. *Source:* Reprinted from Benjamin, M., Evans, E.J., and Copp, L., The Histology of Tendon Attachments to Bone in Man, *Journal of Anatomy*, Vol. 149, pp. 89–100, with permission of Cambridge University Press, © 1986.

Stress and joint motion are significant factors that support the functional integrity of insertion sites, whereas immobilization has deleterious effects. Woo et al[29] mention that biomechanical studies using animal tissues show that immobilization causes a rapid decrease in soft tissue–bone junctional strength. Conversely, insertion sites become stronger with exercise. The activity must stress the specific insertion site to have a beneficial effect on its strength.

CLINICAL CONSIDERATIONS FOR TREATMENT

In treating soft tissue lesions, it is important not only to localize therapy correctly to the tissue involved but to identify where in the healing process the lesion is. Is it an acute, subacute, or chronic problem? This guides us in administering the appropriate treatment (see Exhibit 8–4).

Acute Phase

The acute phase is marked by the signs and symptoms of inflammation mentioned earlier. Mennell terms this the *healing phase*.[30] Due to inflamma-

Exhibit 8–4 Phases of Healing

Acute	*Subacute*	*Chronic*
• Inflammation	• Inflammation less	• Scar/fibrosis
• Pain before end-feel	• Pain with end-feel	• Pain after stretch, end-feel
• Anti-inflammatory modalities, ice	• Anti-inflammatory modalities	• Ice/heat
• I, II mobilization	• I, II mobilization	• III, IV mobilization
• Gentle transverse friction massage	• Increased transverse friction massage	• Manipulation (V)
• Passive range of motion	• Passive, active range of motion	• Deeper transverse friction massage
• Isometrics	• Increased isometrics	• Active range of motion
		• Isotonics, stretching

tion and pain, movement of the structures is painful early in the range of motion before any tissue resistance is encountered. The patient comments that the area involved stiffens with rest and loosens with movement. However, too much movement exacerbates the condition. This is an important clue to the presence of inflammation, and its disappearance heralds the exit of this phase. The treatment objectives of this phase are to reduce swelling and pain, rest the primary structures involved from function, and maintain the neighboring secondary tissues in as near a physiologic state as possible. For example, if the lesion involves mostly muscle or tendon, active contractions and stretching should be avoided at this time. However, passive joint range of motion (grade I and II mobilizations) can be performed within a painless range of motion to maintain some level of mobility in the related joints. Electrical muscle stimulation or isometric muscle contractions can be used with the muscle in neutral. This causes broadening of the muscle upon contraction and imparts mobility in the forming scar tissue.[31] Gentle transverse friction massage mobilizes the soft tissue scar directly.

Rest from function does not mean complete immobilization but refers to what is termed *active rest*. If a healing joint can be moved 10 degrees in flexion, yet 11 degrees causes pain, then that joint should be passively moved 10 degrees. Immobility creates more morbidity and poor healing of soft tissues and joints. Cryotherapy and cryokinetics play an integral part in the acute and subacute phases and are described below.

Overtreatment results in continued pain after a treatment session for hours, even at rest, and continued signs of inflammation. Easy fatigue and spasm also occur and warn the clinician to slow down and ease up.

Cryotherapy

Cryotherapy is invaluable in this stage and is used to reduce pain and swelling indirectly. For the most part, cryotherapy is beneficial in its ability to limit what is called *secondary hypoxic injury*.[32] When a tissue is injured, the primary site of injury results in cellular destruction, with resultant inflammation and hemodynamic stasis. The tissues adjacent to the injured area suffer from microcirculatory stasis and subsequently become secondarily injured from hypoxia. Cryotherapy, in effect, places these tissues in the secondary hypoxic injury zone in hibernation by slowing their metabolism. This allows them to survive the lower oxygen tension of the inflamed tissue. The net effect is a decrease in further tissue injury and resultant decreased inflammation and swelling.

There are many diverse opinions of ice application protocols, but a survey of the literature suggests that one that works well is 30 minutes of application every 2 hours. Some may be concerned about the Hunting effect or cold-induced vasodilation, which is thought to occur after 15 minutes. However, this response was found to be artifactual and not a factor in therapeutic icing.[32] The real value in cryotherapy is its analgesic effect and induction of hypometabolism of the secondary tissues. Most importantly, the analgesia imposed will allow exercise and movement to be used more comfortably.

Cryokinetics

The combination of cryotherapy and graded active exercise is called cryokinetics and is valuable in hastening recovery.[32] After numbing the injured area with an initial icing of 15 to 20 minutes, light active exercise can be started for 3 to 5 minutes until the numbness wears off. If no pain is experienced, the part is renumbed in 3 to 5 minutes, and a slightly higher level of exercise can be used. Patients motivated to self-treatment will do well with this procedure.

For example, a cryotherapy protocol can be used on sacroiliac joint sprains that is adapted from Knight's work on ankle sprains.[32] First ice is applied to the painful area for 20 minutes or until numbness is experienced. The patient is then asked to perform non–weight-bearing, active hip flexion while supine for only 3 to 5 minutes. The knee is also flexed. If this is tolerable, the patient renumbs the painful area for 3 to 5 minutes and progresses to the next level of difficulty: standing and shifting one's weight from side to side for 3 to 5 minutes. If this is tolerable and painless, the patient renumbs the area again and progresses to the next exercise level, and so on. The idea is to numb the area to allow graduated active exercises to occur painlessly. If the exercise is harmful, pain will be experienced, even through the numbness, and the patient will have gone as far as he or she can progress for that session. Two to 3 hours later, the series of exercise with intermittent icing is tried again to see if the patient can progress further. The exercise difficulty gradually increases after each renumbing. The patient progresses to the next level of difficulty only if the previous level is performed painlessly. A sample list of the graded active exercises for an acute sacroiliac sprain is shown in Exhibit 8–5. The patient is encouraged to perform at least two sessions per day, preferably three. Resting pain, spasm, and continued signs of inflammation signify overtreatment and the need to slow down.

Subacute Phase

The subacute phase is a transitional stage in which inflammation is subsiding and repair is continuing. Painless range of motion is increased, but pain is commensurate with the tissue resistance at or near end range. More motion can be encouraged in the tissues, with transverse friction massage and isometric contractions being used with slightly more intensity. Small-amplitude mobilizations are still used, and possibly manipulation, depending on the clinician's experience. If signs and symptoms of inflammation are minimal, articular dysfunction is very evident, and the patient can tolerate positioning and full slack removal, then a manipulation can be attempted. Keep in mind that manipulation is an impulse movement traversing ⅛ in. Cryotherapy and cryokinetics are to be used. As motion and strength increase, isometric exercises can be upgraded to isotonics.

Chronic Phase

Mennell[30] terms this the *healed phase*. In contrast to the acute phase, patients in this phase will remark that they do not stiffen with rest but hurt more with motion. Pain on range-of-motion testing comes after the end-feel is reached as the tissues are stretched. Remodeling and maturation of scar tissue are occurring. Restoration of function is the hallmark of treatment and includes manipulation, stretching, and progressive resistance exercises. Heat and ice applications can be used to facilitate stretching and ease posttreatment soreness respectively. Pain lasting more than 4

Exhibit 8–5 Cryokinetics Program for Acute Sacroiliac Sprain

Instructions

   Apply initial icing until numb. Exercise for 3 to 5 minutes, with renumbing between levels. Stop at level that causes pain.

Exercise Sequence

   Supine hip flexions
       Renumb for 3 to 5 minutes
   Standing weight transfers
       Renumb for 3 to 5 minutes
   Alternate knee raising when standing
       Renumb for 3 to 5 minutes
   Walking without limping
       Renumb for 3 to 5 minutes
   Sit-downs and stand-ups
       Renumb for 3 to 5 minutes
   Upstairs/downstairs

---

hours after treatment sessions or signs of swelling and decreased strength signal overtreatment.[33] Soft tissue scarring, decreased range of motion, and muscle weakness all need to be addressed in this phase. Transverse friction massage and more vigorous mobilizations (grade IV) are used, and the patient is taught passive and active stretches to increase tissue distensibility. Patients who are treated from the acute phase to the chronic phase are often easier to manage than those who initiate treatment in the chronic phase. But such a situation is ideal at best, for many patients present after months of no formal diagnosis or treatment in a state of pain, stiffness, and weakness. Clinical depression is often a factor in chronic conditions and can unfavorably modulate the clinical picture. It is often necessary to tell patients with chronic conditions that they may not become pain free, despite functional improvements. Setting realistic goals at the beginning of therapy will offset disappointment if 100% success is not achieved.

CONCLUSION

   The soft tissues make up a diverse, complex group of structures that are crucial to the stability and proper function of the locomotor system. Joint dysfunction and soft tissue changes go hand in hand. Immobilization itself is detrimental to the normal health of joints and periarticular soft tissues.

Manual methods, by their very nature, affect these soft tissues directly, speeding their recovery during healing.

Chapter Review Questions

- Describe the acute inflammatory response.
- What is the difference between scarring and fibrosis?
- What effects does immobilization have on the musculoskeletal structure?
- What information from the patient's history characterizes the acute phase of a condition?
- How does cryotherapy affect the tissues?
- What is cryokinetics?
- What information in the patient's history tells us that the acute phase is over and the chronic phase has been entered?

REFERENCES

1. Cantu RI, Grodin AAJ. *Myofascial Manipulation: Theory and Clinical Application.* Gaithersburg, Md: Aspen Publishers, Inc; 1992.
2. Woo SL-Y, Matthews JV, Akeson WH, Amiel D, Convery FR. Connective tissue response to immobility. *Arthritis Rheum.* 1975;18:257–264.
3. Akeson WH, Woo SL-Y, Amiel D, Coutts RD, Daniel D. The connective tissue response to immobilization: biochemical changes in periarticular connective tissue of the rabbit knee. *Clin Orthop.* 1973;93:356–362.
4. Akeson WH, Amiel D, LaViolette D, Secrist D. The connective tissue response to immobility: an accelerated aging response. *Exp Gerontol.* 1968;3:289–301.
5. Binkley J, Peat M. The effect of immobilization on the ultrastructure and mechanical properties of the rat medial collateral ligament. *Clin Orthop.* 1987;203:301–308.
6. Finsterbush A, Friedman B. Reversibility of joint changes produced by immobilization in rabbits. *Clin Orthop.* 1975;111:290–298.
7. Noyes F. Functional properties of knee ligaments and alterations induced by immobilization. *Clin Orthop.* 1977;123:210–242.
8. Herring SA. Rehabilitation of muscle injuries. *Med Sci Sports Exer.* 1990;22:453–456.
9. Katz DR, Kumar VN. Effects of prolonged bed rest on cardio-pulmonary conditioning. *Orthop Rev.* 1982;11:89–93.
10. Nelson DL. Assuring quality in the delivery of passive and active care. *Top Clin Chir.* 1994;1:20–29.
11. Injeyan HS, Fraser IH, Peek WD. *Pathology of Musculoskeletal Soft Tissues: Treatment by Manual Methods.* Gaithersburg, Md: Aspen Publishers, Inc; 1991.

12. Caplan A, Carlson B, Faulkner J, Fischman D, Garret W. Skeletal muscle. In: Woo SL-Y, Buckwalter JA, eds. *Injury and Repair of the Musculoskeletal Soft Tissues*. Park Ridge, Ill: American Academy of Orthopedic Surgeons; 1987:213–291.

13. Jerusalem F. The microcirculation of muscle. In: Engel AG, Banker BQ, eds. *Myology*. New York, NY: McGraw-Hill Book Co; 1986:343–356.

14. Janda V. *Muscle Function Testing*. Boston, Mass: Butterworths; 1983.

15. Faulkner JA. New perspectives in training for maximum performance. *JAMA*. 1986;205:741–746.

16. Saltin B, Gollnick P. Skeletal muscle adaptability: significance for metabolism and performance. In: Peachey LD, Adrian RH, Geiger SR, eds. *Handbook of Physiology*. Bethesda, Md: American Physiology Society; 1983:555–631.

17. Friden J, Sjostrom M, Ekblom B. Myofibrillar damage following intense eccentric exercise in man. *Int J Sports Med*. 1983;4:170–176.

18. Hoppeler H. Exercise-induced ultrastructural changes in skeletal muscle. *Int J Sports Med*. 1986;7:187–204.

19. Garrett W, Tidball J. Myotendinous junction: structure, function, and failure. In: Woo SL-Y, Buckwalter JA, eds. *Injury and Repair of the Musculoskeletal Soft Tissues*. Park Ridge, Ill: American Academy of Orthopedic Surgeons; 1987:171–207.

20. Jarvinen M. Healing of a crush injury in rat striated muscle. *Acta Pathol Microbiol Scand*. 1976;142:47–56.

21. Lundborg G, Myrhage R, Rydevik B.: The vascularization of human flexor tendons within the digital synovial sheath region: structural and functional aspects. *J Hand Surg*. 1977;2:417–427.

22. Gelberman RH, Woo SL-Y, Lothringer K, et al. Effects of early intermittent passive mobilization on healing canine flexor tendons. *J Hand Surg*. 1982;7:170–175.

23. Salter RB. The biologic concept of continuous passive motion of synovial joints: the first 18 years of basic research and its clinical application. *Clin Orthop*. 1989;242:12–24.

24. Kennedy JC, Hawkins RJ, Willis RB, Danylchuk KD. Tension studies of human knee ligaments, yield point, ultimate failure, and disruption of the cruciate and tibial collateral ligaments. *J Bone Joint Surg*. 1976;58A:350–355.

25. Frank C, Amiel D, Woo SL-Y, Akeson WH. Normal ligament properties and ligament healing. *Clin Orthop*. 1985;196:15–25.

26. Frank C, Woo SL-Y, Andriacchi T, et al. Normal ligament: structure, function, and composition. In: Woo SL-Y, Buckwalter JA, eds. *Injury and Repair of the Musculoskeletal Soft Tissues*. Park Ridge, Ill: American Academy of Orthopedic Surgeons; 1987:45–101.

27. Andriacchi T, Sabiston P, DeHaven L, et al. Ligament injury and repair. In: Woo SL-Y, Buckwalter JA, eds. *Injury and Repair of the Musculoskeletal Soft Tissues*. Park Ridge, Ill: American Academy of Orthopedic Surgeons; 1987:103–128.

28. Dahners LE. Ligament contraction: a correlation with cellularity and actin staining. *Trans Orthop Res Soc*. 1987;11:56.

29. Woo S, Maynard J, Butler D, et al. Ligament, tendon, and joint capsule insertions to bone. In: Woo SL-Y, Buckwalter JA, eds. *Injury and Repair of the Musculoskeletal Soft Tissues*. Park Ridge, Ill: American Academy of Orthopedic Surgeons; 1987:133–166.

30. Mennell JM. *The Musculoskeletal System: Differential Diagnosis from Symptoms and Physical Signs*. Gaithersburg, Md: Aspen Publishers, Inc; 1992.

31. Cyriax J. *Textbook of Orthopaedic Medicine.* London: Bailliere-Tindall; 1984.
32. Knight KL. *Cryotherapy: Theory, Technique, and Physiology.* Chattanooga, Tenn: Chattanooga Corp; 1985.
33. Zohn D, Mennell JM. *Musculoskeletal Pain: Principles of Physical Diagnosis and Physical Treatment.* Boston, Mass: Little, Brown & Co; 1976.

Chapter 9

Treatment of Myofascial and Soft Tissue Structures

Chapter Objectives

- to discuss common myofascial pain syndromes and their treatment through such methods as postisometric relaxation, ischemic compression, and stripping massage
- to describe the treatment of tendon and ligament lesions, particularly the use of transverse friction massage
- to describe forms of length-strength treatment, including CRAC and postfacilitation stretching (PFS)

This chapter discusses the more common soft tissue problems of the pelvic and hip regions that are encountered in clinical practice: myofascial trigger points, tendon and ligament lesions, and shortened, tight muscles. The discussion covers both general methods (postisometric relaxation, ischemic compression, stripping massages, transverse friction massage, length-strength treatment) and treatment of specific muscles, tendons, and ligaments.

TREATMENT OF MYOFASCIAL PAIN SYNDROMES

Myofascial pain syndromes share with joint dysfunction the distinction of being one of the more common etiologies of pain afflicting the locomotor system. The pelvic girdle and hip area are very common sites of myofascial trigger points. Most of the material covered in this chapter is derived from the monumental works of Travell and Simons[1,2] and Zohn and Mennell.[3] Their contribution to the understanding of myofascial pain syndromes is immense and must be reviewed in depth for insight into the importance of this problem.

Unlike muscles containing myofascial trigger points, normal muscle tissue does not exhibit tight, painful spots that refer pain on palpation or stretch. Myofascial trigger points (TPs) are defined as hyperirritable spots occurring in bands of skeletal muscle or muscle fascia that refer pain in consistent patterns, often at a distance from the TP. Their location in a given muscle is specific and predictable, and they may occur in any skeletal muscle. They occur in all types of individuals, sparing no occupation, gender, or age group. One 5-year-old girl suffering from "growing pains" was found to have a painful gluteus medius trigger point as the etiology.

TPs can be active or latent. An active TP is symptomatic and painful. The referred pain from the TP is described as deep, achy, and dull. This pain can be elicited by a few seconds of sustained digital pressure on the TP. Patients are usually more aware of the referred pain than of the TP itself. The referred pain from TPs is unique and is not dermatomal, myotomal, or sclerotomal. Active TPs are made worse by ice applications, pressure, strenuous muscular use, passive stretch, cold and damp weather, and a sustained shortened position of the muscle. Patients say that they feel better after a hot shower, especially if they stretch slowly.

A latent TP is like a dormant volcano, waiting to erupt. It is painful on palpation and exhibits all the other characteristics of an active TP, yet it is clinically silent with respect to pain. Although silent, the latent TP can cause stiffness and weakness of the affected muscle. Latent TPs are the more common TPs found. They can very easily be activated to a painful state by acute or chronic muscle overload, chilling (ice applications or cold drafts), sustained postures, trauma, joint dysfunction, and emotional stress.

Satellite TPs are myofascial TPs that become activated because they are located in the pain reference zone of another active TP. A common example is the gluteus minimus TP that arises from an activated quadratus lumborum TP because it lies within its pain referral zone. A secondary TP is one that becomes active because its muscle is overloaded from activities that are synergistic with or antagonistic to those of another muscle with a primary TP. For example, piriformis or gluteus medius muscles can develop secondary TPs as they try to compensate for a gluteus minimus that has active TPs in it. In both these situations, the primary TP must be inactivated along with the satellite or secondary TPs.

On physical examination, palpation will find a band of muscle fibers that harbor a small, discrete area of exquisite pain: the TP. If the palpating finger plucks across the tight muscle fibers, a local twitch will occur and may cause the patient to jump from pain. Stretching and contracting strongly a muscle with an active TP causes pain. The muscle is usually weak on testing. As stated above, sustained pressure on the TP refers pain into a specific area characteristic for that muscle. Referred tenderness is also associated with TPs. Structures within the pain referral district are tender to palpation and may erroneously be incriminated as the etiology. Autonomic phenomena may also be observed in the referral zone. These include skin sweating, piloerection, and vasomotor changes. Skin rolling over the area of a TP is restricted and painful. Joint dysfunction of nearby articulations is common and can be a cause of, or a sequel to, the TP. Strong and near-unequivocal findings leading to the diagnosis of myofascitis are a local twitch response to plucking of the muscle fibers and a reproduction of the patient's symptoms, with radiation of pain into the characteristic referral zone.

Inactivation of Trigger Points

TPs can be inactivated by lengthening the taut bands that harbor the TP through various stretching procedures and enhancing the local circulation with hot moist applications. This is followed by several active muscle contractions by the patient to reestablish neuromuscular "awareness" and signal the muscle that it is all right to function normally again. However, a muscle with a painful active TP in it cannot be just passively stretched. A counterirritant or facilitation technique is often needed to break the pain-spasm cycle. In this regard, Fluori-Methane vapocoolant spray or postisometric relaxation can be used respectively. There is a concern about Fluori-Methane's effects on the atmosphere's ozone layer, as with other fluorocarbons. Ice can be used in its place, or other procedures for inactivating TPs, such as postisometric relaxation, ischemic compression, or stripping massage, can be applied with great success. For an in-depth discussion of Fluori-Methane stretch-and-spray technique, the reader is strongly urged to read Travell and Simons' work.[1,2]

Postisometric Relaxation

Stretching a muscle with a TP to its full, normal length is the most important factor in inactivating TPs. An easy and effective method to accomplish this is described by Lewit[4] and is called postisometric relaxation (PR). It is also used to lengthen shortened, tight muscles found on examination that do not harbor TPs. Postisometric relaxation is gentle, comfortable for the patient, and effective. It can be used on the oldest patients and even on the young. As its name implies, relaxation and stretch are instituted after an isometric contraction of the muscle. The muscle is positioned so that light tension can be induced in the bands of muscle involved. A gentle isometric contraction is performed by the patient, with the clinician resisting. After 10 seconds, the patient is told to relax or "let go," and the clinician stretches the muscle only after relaxation is sensed. The stretch occurs in the direction that stretches the muscle.

Phases of respiration are used to facilitate the contraction and relaxation phases of the stretch. Patients are asked to inhale deeply and slowly while they contract the muscle. They are then told to exhale and relax the muscle while the clinician applies the stretch. Stretching by the clinician is continued slowly and gently until a resistance is met. This could take several seconds. The range of motion gained at the end of the stretch is maintained, and another cycle of contraction-relaxation is performed. The procedure is performed three to five times, with the goal being to lengthen the muscle fully. At no time should the patient experience pain or spasm. This occurs if the stretching is performed too quickly or firmly. The time of contraction can be lengthened to 30 seconds, and a harder contraction can be used to aid in relaxing the muscle. After relaxation is attained, several cycles of active muscle contraction should be performed through the new range.

Whether Fluori-Methane stretch-and-spray technique or postisometric relaxation is used, stretching can cause a painful exacerbation in two common situations. One is when the referred pain is actually radiating radicular pain of neural origin. The stretching will irritate the nerve, and the condition will exacerbate. The other situation is when a muscle is reflexively guarding a joint with damaged ligaments or periarticular structures. When the guarding spasm is temporarily removed, the joint is insulted further, and pain will result. These two situations can be used as diagnostic indicators rather than viewed as therapeutic failures, as long as the clinician realizes the reason for exacerbation.

Ischemic Compression

Ischemic compression can be used to inactivate TPs. It entails the application of direct pressure on the TP until the referred pain is extinguished. It is termed *ischemic compression* because immediately after the compression treatment the skin blanches white before it reddens. After palpating for and finding a band of tight muscle fibers, the clinician searches for the area of maximal pain within the band. Often an area of firmness or a nodule will be found that is exquisitely painful, radiating pain into the TP's characteristic pattern. At first, gentle pressure is applied on the TP with the thumb, the knuckle, the elbow, or a blunt device until the pain starts to refer. At all times the patient must be relaxed and able to tolerate the pressure without wincing, jumping, or contracting the muscle to guard against the pressure. After a few seconds of sustained pressure, the pain will subside, and the patient will be able to tolerate an increase in pressure. This will again create pain, both locally and referred. This new level of pressure is maintained until the intensity diminishes. The process is continued for approximately 1 minute until the TP does not refer any more pain when pressed firmly. Mild, moist heat is applied to increase circulation in the area and help reduce posttreatment soreness.

It must be stressed that at all times the patient is to remain relaxed. The clinician must keep in constant communication with the patient. Such questions as "Am I hurting you? Is this too much? Where do you feel the pain now? Is the pain less now?" should be asked repeatedly until the procedure is done. Instructing patients to focus on their breathing while relaxing on the exhale helps immensely. Working within the patient's tolerance is a must. Months of pain and dysfunction are not going to be cleared up in one painful session. The clinician, too, must be relaxed and not in a hurry. After ischemic compression and heat application, a full, gentle passive stretch should be attempted, with active muscle contractions being performed after this.

Stripping Massage

For this procedure, a lubricating lotion is applied to the skin so that the thumbs, fingers, or elbow can glide over the tight band of muscle and TP. Starting lightly at first, the clinician progressively deepens the strokes as the muscle is stripped along the length of the tight muscle band, toward the TP, and through and over it. The strokes are repeated until the muscle "lets go," the pain reduces, and the TP becomes less palpable. Again, the depth of the strokes and generated discomfort must stay within the patient's tolerance. This procedure is also followed by heat, passive stretching, and active range-of-motion muscle contractions.

Failure to inactivate TPs when using the above techniques commonly occurs if the muscle is not stretched fully or, conversely, if the treatment is too vigorous, causing overstretching and pain. Painful pressures or stretching prevents patient relaxation and affords ineffective stretching. Failure may also occur if the clinician does not use heat or active range-of-motion contractions after the treatment.

Travell and Simons dedicate an entire chapter in their book to factors that perpetuate TPs. They comment: "This is the most important single chapter in this manual; it concerns the most neglected part of the management of myofascial pain syndromes."[1(p103)] Mechanical stresses, nutritional inadequacies, metabolic and endocrine inadequacies, psychological factors, and chronic infection are listed as common perpetuating factors.

Treatment of Individual Muscles

This section concerns the treatment of the more commonly affected muscles and their trigger points. Specific postisometric relaxation, ischemic compression, and stripping massage techniques are described. The reader is referred to the works of Travell and Simons[1,2] for information pertaining to stretch-and-spray technique.

Joint conditions are usually accompanied by myofascial TPs, either for biomechanical or reflexogenic reasons. Sacroiliac joint dysfunction is often associated with TPs in the three glutei muscles, especially the gluteus minimus. Other muscles affected include the piriformis, quadratus lumborum, and erector spinae. One can often observe that if only effective muscle stretching and TP inactivation are performed, sacroiliac joint motion improves. This occurs more often in younger individuals, including children.

Hip joint problems commonly occur with glutei minimus and medius TPs, especially the latter. The tensor fascia lata and hip adductors are also involved. Hip adductor and iliopsoas TPs often masquerade as hip "arthritis," since their referred pain patterns extend into the groin. Pubic symphysis problems are also associated with tension and TPs in the hip adductors.

Gluteus Minimus

This muscle is a very common source of buttock and leg pain, often mimicking a sciatic condition, the so-called pseudoradicular presentation. Travell and Simons[2] state that referred pain into the limb from sacroiliac joint dysfunction is most commonly from activated gluteus minimus TPs. Of the muscles commonly involved about the hip and pelvis, it refers pain the farthest, often to the lateral aspect of the ankle and rarely to the foot.

The anterior and posterior fibers refer different patterns of pain. The anterior fibers are palpated as the patient lies supine with the thigh comfortably extended. The part of the gluteus minimus that lies anterior to the tensor fascia lata is explored for TPs. This is achieved by first finding the anterior superior iliac spine and the tensor fascia lata. By having the patient gently contract the tensor fascia lata with resisted medial rotation of the hip, one can define the borders of the muscle. Palpation is performed just anterior to the edge of the tensor fascia lata. Pain from the anterior fibers is referred to the lateral buttock and down the lateral aspect of the thigh, leg, and even ankle (Figure 9–1).

The posterior part of the muscle is best palpated in the side-lying position, involved side up. The thigh is lightly flexed and allowed to adduct

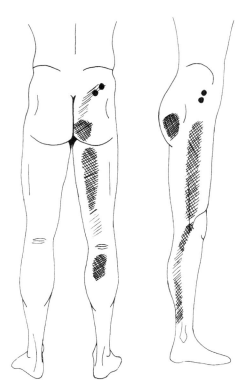

Figure 9–1 Gluteus minimus trigger point pain patterns. Trigger point in the anterior fibers is shown on the right. Trigger point in the posterior fibers is on the left. *Source:* Adapted from *Myofascial Pain and Dysfunction: The Trigger Point Manual,* Vol. 2, by J.G. Travell and D.G. Simons, p. 161, with permission of Williams & Wilkins, © 1992.

toward the table. An imaginary line connecting the most superior aspect of the greater trochanter and the upper free border of the sacrum (near the posterior inferior iliac spine) is used to identify the gluteus minimus and piriformis TPs (Figure 9–2).[2] It is called the "piriformis line" and for the sake of localizing TPs is divided into thirds. The gluteus minimus muscle and its TPs lie above the line; those of the piriformis are below. Pain from the posterior fibers of the gluteus minimus is referred to the posterior and medial buttock, posterior thigh, knee, and proximal calf (Figure 9–1).

To stretch the gluteus minimus muscle using PR, the patient is placed in the side-lying position, involved side up (Figure 9–3). The anterior fibers

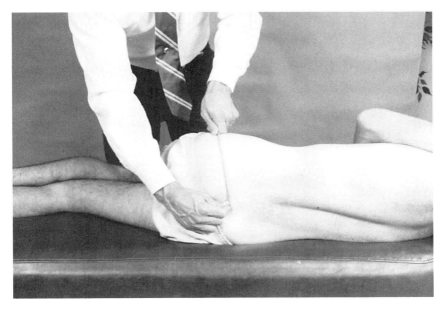

Figure 9–2 The piriformis line runs from the superior aspect of the greater trochanter to the posterior inferior iliac spine. It represents the upper border of the piriformis muscle.

are stretched by placing the upper thigh and leg behind the patient and off the table. The limb is allowed to drop freely until tension is developed in the muscle. The clinician stands behind the patient, places his or her hand just proximal to the lateral aspect of the knee, and gently resists the patient's efforts to abduct the thigh. The patient is instructed to inhale slowly and deeply and to maintain the mild contraction for about 10 seconds. Afterward, the patient is told to exhale and relax or "let go" of the leg so that it descends toward the floor, thus putting the gluteus minimus on stretch. The clinician aids the passive stretching only upon sensing the muscle's relaxing. In this position, gravity greatly assists the process. The procedure is performed three to five times, depending on how tight the muscle is and the response to stretching. The posterior fibers are stretched by dropping the leg off the table in front of the patient and repeating the above procedure.

Ischemic compression of the gluteus minimus is difficult due to its deep location. To be effective, the point of the elbow should be used on larger patients or both thumbs together on average- and smaller-sized patients

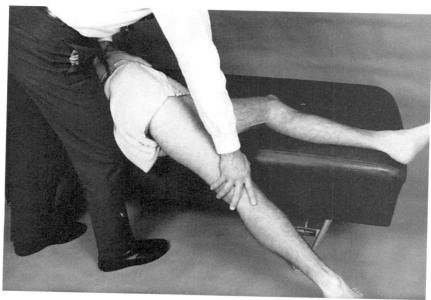

Figure 9–3 Gluteus Minimus PR Stretch

(Figure 9–4). Pressure is increased gradually until pain referral is elicited, and then it is maintained. As the referred pain diminishes, the pressure is increased until the pain reappears. This is repeated over a period of about 1 minute, staying within the patient's tolerance for pain at all times. Heat is applied afterward, and the muscle is actively contracted several times by the patient. On very painful TPs, PR can be used first, followed by ischemic compression.

Patients can be instructed to use a tennis ball or rounded door knob to press into the TP while at home for self-treatment. They can also use gravity-assist PR by dropping the leg behind or in front of them off the bed, inhaling deeply and holding for 10 seconds, and allowing the leg to descend more on exhaling. Ankle weights or a heavy winter boot can be worn to facilitate the stretch.

As stated before, this muscle very commonly harbors TPs in association with sacroiliac joint dysfunction. Other causes of activation and perpetuation are prolonged side lying and standing, intramuscular injections, trauma, lumbar radiculopathy, and overload. Additionally, TPs in the quadratus lumborum muscle commonly activate satellite TPs in the anterior fibers of the gluteus minimus.

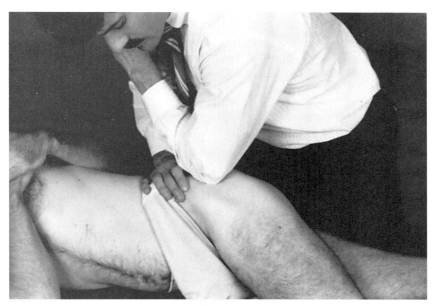

Figure 9–4 Ischemic Compression of Gluteus Minimus

Gluteus Medius

This muscle harbors TPs in three locations that refer pain relatively locally to the lumbosacral region and along the posterior part of the iliac crest (Figure 9-5). One TP is near the posterior superior iliac spine and refers chiefly along the sacroiliac joint, sacrum, posterior iliac crest, and buttock. Another is located just below the midpart of the iliac crest and refers pain into the lateral buttock and sometimes the posterolateral proximal thigh. The third TP is also below the iliac crest but near the anterior superior iliac spine. It refers pain along the crest, lumbosacral, and sacral regions. To palpate for gluteus medius TPs, the patient is placed in the side-lying position with the upper thigh slightly flexed in front of the lower. Gluteus medius TPs are located superior to those of the gluteus minimus, being closer to the iliac crest. Additionally, the gluteus medius TPs do not refer pain as extensively as the gluteus minimus.

Postisometric relaxation of the gluteus medius is performed in the side-lying position and is identical to that of the gluteus minimus. Lewit[4] demonstrates an alternative position with the patient supine. The involved thigh and leg are adducted across the table under the opposite leg. Ischemic compression is also effective in inactivating these TPs.

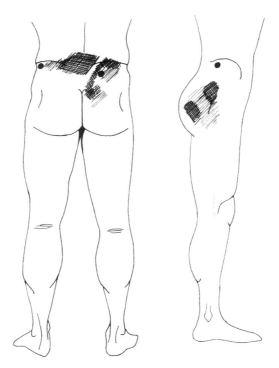

Figure 9–5 Gluteus Medius Trigger Point Pain Patterns. *Source:* Adapted from *Myofascial Pain and Dysfunction: The Trigger Point Manual,* Vol. 2, by J.G. Travell and D.G. Simons, p. 151, with permission of Williams & Wilkins, © 1992.

Factors that activate or perpetuate TPs in the gluteus medius muscle include lower lumbar, sacroiliac, and hip joint problems, leg-length insufficiency, direct trauma, and one-legged stance. Patients frequently complain of trouble sleeping on the affected side. Travell and Simons[2] mention the importance of a short first metatarsal bone (Morton's foot) in the activation and perpetuation of gluteus medius TPs. These TPs are commonly found in martial arts athletes, dancers, and especially deconditioned people starting an aerobics program while doing vigorous and repetitive hip abduction moves.

Gluteus Maximus

Although not as commonly involved as the other two gluteal muscles, TPs in the gluteus maximus muscle do occur often enough, with pain referral patterns that need to be differentiated from sacroiliac joint dysfunction, coccydynia, bursitis, and pain referral from other TPs. The muscle has three distinct areas that harbor TPs (Figure 9–6). One TP is located just lateral to the sacrum and refers pain along the medial part of the gluteal cleft and sacroiliac joint and along the gluteal fold (Figure 9–6A). Another more commonly found TP is just superior to the ischial tuberosity and refers pain throughout the whole buttock and lower sacrum and even to the lateral crest (Figure 9–6B). The third TP lies near the coccyx and is in the most inferomedial fibers of the gluteus maximus (Figure 9–6C). It refers pain to the coccyx, being a source of coccydynia. The first two TPs can be found by palpation across the gluteus maximus muscle fibers, looking for pain referral and a local twitch response. The third TP can be identified by pinching the most inferomedial fibers between the thumb and index fingers and noting for coccygeal pain referral.

PR can be used to stretch the gluteus maximus by placing the patient supine and flexing, slightly adducting, and slightly medially rotating the thigh onto the chest. Another method used to stretch the gluteus maximus is described in Chapter 6 and is beneficial to use in cases of coccydynia. Ischemic compression can be used by grasping the TP between the thumb and index finger and squeezing it.

To differentiate the three gluteal muscles and their TP involvements, the TP location, pain referral, and fiber directions need to be taken into account. Whereas the gluteus minimus commonly refers pain distally and below the knee, and the gluteus medius refers pain near the iliac crest, lumbosacral region, and sometimes the proximal and midthigh, the gluteus maximus pain referral is more localized to the buttock and very infrequently extends into the thigh. The gluteus maximus TPs are more superficial than those of the glutei minimus and medius. Hip flexion is limited in active gluteus maximus TPs, whereas adduction is restricted with gluteus medius and minimus TPs.

Activation and perpetuation of gluteus maximus TPs arise from direct trauma; prolonged sitting; overload, especially when walking uphill or running up stairs; and sitting on a bulky wallet. Sacroiliac joint dysfunction will also perpetuate these TPs.

Tensor Fascia Lata

Myofascial pain from this muscle is often misdiagnosed as trochanteric bursitis and hip joint arthritis. The tensor fascia lata TP is located just below and lateral to the anterior superior iliac spine. To find this muscle, the supine patient is asked to rotate the thigh medially while the clinician gently resists. The muscle and its contour become more prominent, and palpa-

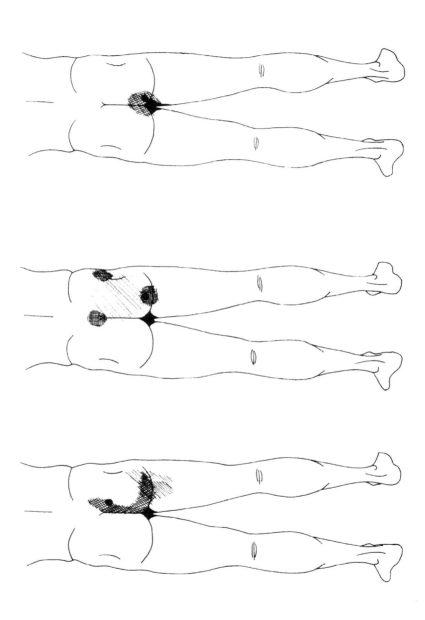

Figure 9–6 Gluteus Maximus Trigger Point Pain Patterns. *Source:* Adapted from *Myofascial Pain and Dysfunction: The Trigger Point Manual*, Vol. 2, by J.G. Travell and D.G. Simons, p. 133, with permission of Williams & Wilkins, © 1992.

tion of its fibers will elicit the TP's pain referral and local twitch response. The pain from the tensor fascia lata TP is referred into the hip joint area and down the anterolateral thigh to the knee (Figure 9–7).

PR is used to stretch the tensor fascia lata. Essentially, the clinician places the patient in the same position as for the Ober's test used for testing a tight iliotibial band (Figure 9–8A). The upper knee is cradled by the clinician while the thigh is extended slightly and allowed to adduct toward the table. Meanwhile the patient stabilizes the pelvis and lumbar spine by holding the downside knee up to the chest, inducing hip flexion. The patient is then asked to raise the thigh against the clinician's light resistance and inhale for 10 seconds. Upon exhaling, the patient is told to relax, and the thigh and leg are lowered to stretch the muscle. This is performed three to five times. The muscle can also be stretched using the same position to stretch the gluteus minimus (Figure 9–8B).

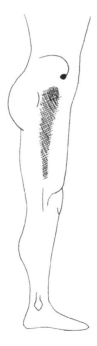

Figure 9–7 Tensor Fascia Lata Trigger Point Pain Pattern. *Source:* Adapted from *Myofascial Pain and Dysfunction: The Trigger Point Manual*, Vol. 2, by J.G. Travell and D.G. Simons, p. 218, with permission of Williams & Wilkins, © 1992.

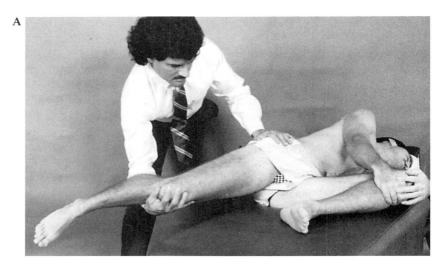

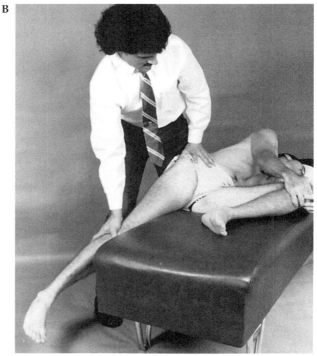

Figure 9–8 (A, B) Tensor Fascia Lata Postisometric Relaxation

For ischemic compression, the patient is in the side-lying position, with the uppermost thigh and leg resting on the table behind the lowermost leg. Pressure is directed into the TP and maintained as explained in the above sections. Heat is applied afterward, and active muscle contractions are performed by abducting and medially rotating the thigh.

Trigger points in the tensor fascia lata are activated and perpetuated by hip joint disturbances, tightness in the iliotibial band, prolonged sitting in a low seat that shortens the muscle, and strenuous running in unconditioned people. The tensor fascia lata TP is commonly activated from TPs in the anterior fibers of the gluteus minimus muscle.

Meralgia Paresthetica (Painful Thigh)

Because of its pain distribution, a tensor fascia lata TP can be confused with meralgia paresthetica, a painful condition due to entrapment of the lateral femoral cutaneous nerve. The entrapment usually occurs as the nerve exits the pelvis either over, through, or under the inguinal ligament near the anterior superior iliac spine. However it can also be entrapped near the spine as it enters the substance of the psoas major muscle or within the pelvis by a tumorous mass. On exiting the pelvis with the iliopsoas muscle, it hooks laterally and proceeds over the sartorius muscle, sometimes penetrating it. This is another potential site for entrapment, although rare.[2] Symptoms include burning pain and paresthesias in the distribution of the lateral femoral cutaneous nerve. Symptoms are increased with standing[5] and hip extension[6] and relieved with sitting or hip flexion.[5] Meralgia paresthetica is often seen in individuals with a pendulous abdomen, ie, from pregnancy or obesity.[5] Tight clothing and belts around the waist are also associated with it.[6] Sensory changes will be noted in the anterolateral thigh, and nerve conduction studies may demonstrate slowed sensory conduction in the nerve where it exits the pelvis.[7]

Because of its close association with the psoas and sartorius muscles, the lateral femoral cutaneous nerve may be affected if they are hypertonic. Lewit[4] mentions that tension in the psoas can be created by dysfunction in the lumbosacral and thoracolumbar segments, hip joint, pelvis, and even coccyx. He also states that by relieving the locomotor disturbance and reducing psoas muscle spasm, the patient with meralgia paresthetica can be helped.

Piriformis

The piriformis syndrome can consist of piriformis myofascial TPs, sacroiliac joint dysfunction, or a neurovascular entrapment of the vessels and nerves exiting the greater sciatic foramen.[2] The signs and symptoms of all three may appear separately or overlap to form a complex clinical presentation.[8] The more common components found are the myofascial pain syndrome and sacroiliac joint dysfunction.

Myofascial Component. Myofascial TPs are located by palpating the muscle in the side-lying position and referring to the imaginary line, the "piriformis line," described earlier with the gluteus minimus muscle. It connects the top of the greater trochanter and posterior inferior iliac spine and corresponds to the upper border of the piriformis muscle. TPs are usually found in the medial and lateral aspects of the muscle and can be palpated externally through the relaxed gluteus maximus. Travell and Simons[2] recommend internal examination via rectal palpation for the medial TP if the clinician is in doubt as to its presence.

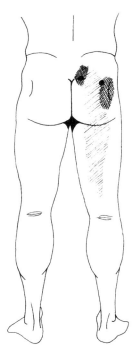

Figure 9–9 Piriformis Trigger Point Pain Patterns. *Source:* Adapted from *Myofascial Pain and Dysfunction: The Trigger Point Manual*, Vol. 2, by J.G. Travell and D.G. Simons, p. 188, with permission of Williams & Wilkins, © 1992.

The medially located TP is found just lateral to the sacrum and refers pain predominantly to the sacroiliac region (Figure 9–9). The TP in the lateral part of the muscle is located just lateral to the joining of the lateral and middle thirds of the piriformis line. Pain referral from this TP extends to the buttock and posterior hip joint region, with some spread into the posterior proximal thigh (Figure 9–9).

Aside from pain and tension in the muscle on palpation, resisted isometric contraction of the piriformis in the sitting position by holding the lateral aspects of the knees with the hips at 90 degrees of flexion exhibits pain and weakness. A positive response and strong indication of piriformis involvement is called the Pace abduction test[9] (Figure 9–10). A tight pirifor-

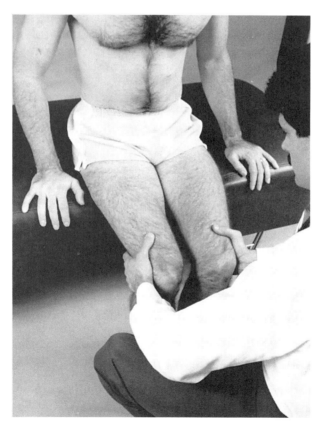

Figure 9–10 The Pace Test for the Piriformis

mis muscle from TPs can display external rotation of the lower extremity by at least 45 degrees while the patient is resting supine.[8] Characteristic pain referral and local twitch response on muscle palpation help distinguish myofascial involvement.

To stretch the muscle, PR in the prone position is easy and effective, especially when combined with ischemic compression.[4] With the patient prone, the knee is flexed to 90 degrees, and the lower leg is pushed laterally, thus rotating the hip joint internally until the piriformis is brought to slight tension (Figure 9–11). The patient is asked to inhale and gently to press against the clinician's laterally directed hold on the lower leg. After 10 seconds, the patient is told to exhale and relax, and the leg is pressed further laterally when the muscle is felt to let go. This is repeated three to five times. Care is taken not to stress the knee or send the muscle into spasm by too vigorous a stretch. Heat is applied afterward, and the patient is asked to contract the muscle actively several times. This is best accomplished with the patient side lying and the upper thigh and knee flexed to 90 degrees. The upper extremity is raised against gravity several times.

An alternative stretch maneuver entails placing the patient supine and flexing the thigh to 90 degrees while adducting it across the body to stretch the piriformis (Figure 9–12). Groin pain signifies hip joint problems and can be most uncomfortable to the patient. PR is conducted by having the patient isometrically resist abduction while the clinician increases the adduction stretch upon relaxation.

A third way to stretch the piriformis is also performed in the supine position (Figure 9–13). The hip joint is held in less than 60 degrees of flexion, the thigh is adducted to tension, and the hip is internally rotated until resistance is met. PR is performed in this position. The patient gently contracts into abduction and external rotation while the clinician supplies counter-resistance. Upon patient relaxation, internal rotation and adduction are gently increased with a careful stretch.

Ischemic compression is effective but must be used carefully so as not to injure the sciatic nerve. Symptoms of shooting pain or tingling down the leg should warn the clinician of this. The clinician must be sure of the TP locations. The point of the elbow can be used, especially on large patients, whereas a double-thumb contact works well on average- and smaller-sized patients.

Factors that activate and perpetuate piriformis TPs are overload, prolonged shortening, blunt trauma, a fat wallet in the rear pocket, and sitting in a slouched position. Positions that shorten the piriformis occur when the hips are flexed and abducted, as in obstetrical examinations and when a woman is supine during sexual intercourse.[2]

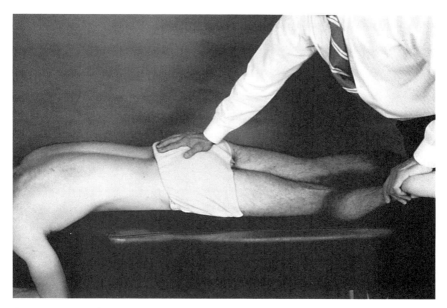

Figure 9–11 Piriformis Stretch Using PR

Sacroiliac Joint Dysfunction Component. Sacroiliac joint dysfunction often occurs with piriformis TPs and can contribute to the clinical picture of the piriformis syndrome.[8] Signs of joint dysfunction are present, ie, articular blockage and positive provocative testing, and must be treated in conjunction with myofascial treatment of the piriformis TP.

Neurovascular Entrapment Component. Approximately 85% of cadavers studied by Beaton and Anson[10] revealed that both the peroneal and tibial portions of the sciatic nerve exit the greater sciatic foramen in front of and below the piriformis muscle. However, in 10% of the cases, the peroneal part passed directly through the substance of the muscle while in 2% to 3% of the cases the peroneal part passed over the superior border before descending down into the leg. In 1% of the cases, the entire sciatic trunk pierced the piriformis muscle. Because of the above anatomic anomalies, the piriformis muscle can entrap the neurovascular structures that accompany it in the greater sciatic foramen. These include the superior and inferior gluteal nerves and vessels, the sciatic nerve, and the pudendal nerve and vessel. Gluteal nerve compression can cause symptoms of pain and paresthesias in the buttock, whereas pudendal nerve compression can create perineal pain, dyspareunia in women, and impotence in men.[8] Entrapment of the sciatic nerve can appear as a lumbar disc syndrome by causing posterior thigh,

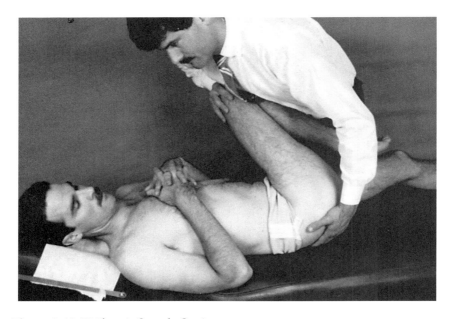

Figure 9–12 Piriformis Stretch, Supine

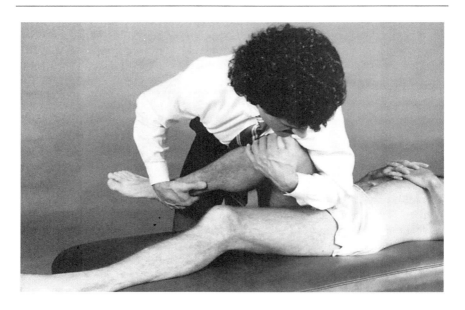

Figure 9–13 Piriformis Stretch, Supine, Using Adduction and Internal Rotation

calf, and foot pain. Electrodiagnostic studies demonstrating slowing of nerve conduction at the greater sciatic foramen coupled with a taut and painful piriformis muscle incriminate nerve entrapment by this muscle.

Differentiating which component is involved can be difficult but the following can serve as a guideline. A myofascial pain syndrome of the piriformis consists of the characteristic pain referral pattern of this muscle, a painful and weak Pace abduction test, and a taut, tender piriformis muscle on palpation. Sacroiliac joint dysfunction is characterized by joint pain, restricted joint motion, and provocative testing that is positive for sacroiliac joint dysfunction. Neurovascular compression is evidenced by paresthesias in the region of the nerve affected and nerve conduction latency localized to the sciatic foramen via electrodiagnostic studies.

Iliopsoas

Because of its "out-of-sight" location, the iliopsoas is an often-overlooked muscle in its role in low back and hip conditions. It is often shortened and tight, especially in people who sit much or have chronic hip joint problems. Iliopsoas myofascial TPs are often found with thoracolumbar and sacroiliac joint dysfunction, especially the former. Lewit[4] is more specific and relates iliacus TPs to lumbosacral joint dysfunction and psoas major muscle TPs to thoracolumbar joint dysfunction.

Travell and Simons[2] describe the palpation of three TP locations in the iliopsoas muscle. The more distal one is in the musculotendinous junction of the psoas muscle just before its insertion into the lesser trochanter and is palpated just lateral to the femoral pulse below the inguinal ligament. Pain from this TP is referred to the low back, groin, and anteromedial thigh (Figure 9–14).

A second TP is found in the iliacus by palpating just inside the rim of the iliac crest near the anterior superior iliac spine (Figure 9–15). If the patient attempts barely to raise the thigh off the table, the iliacus will be felt to bulge on contracting. Pain is usually referred from this TP to the sacroiliac joint and low back.

A third TP is palpated through the abdominal wall just lateral to the rectus abdominis muscle at the level of the umbilicus or below. Pressure is applied downward first and then inward toward the spine. The patient is asked to barely raise the thigh off the table, and the psoas muscle belly can usually be felt to contract. Palpation is more difficult in obese and muscular individuals. The patient must be relaxed, and the palpation must be gentle and slow. Pain is referred typically to the low back.

Interestingly, the psoas appears susceptible to developing hematomas in patients undergoing anticoagulant therapy.[11] This can be visualized with computerized tomography.

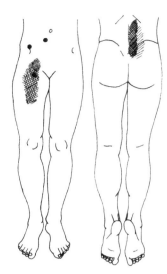

Figure 9–14 Psoas Trigger Point Pain Pattern. *Source:* Adapted from *Myofascial Pain and Dysfunction: The Trigger Point Manual,* Vol. 2, by J.G. Travell and D.G. Simons, p. 90, with permission of Williams & Wilkins, © 1992.

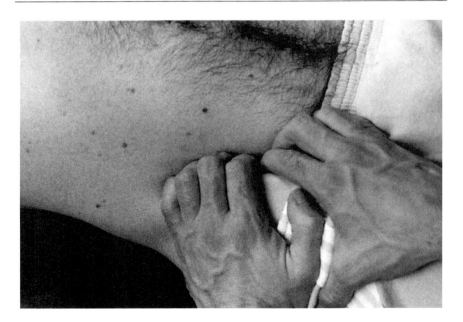

Figure 9–15 Iliacus Palpation

Stretching the iliopsoas with PR is very effective and is accomplished with the patient supine (Figure 9–16). The patient extends the affected thigh and leg off the table while holding the opposite thigh up to the chest. The clinician supports the patient by holding the flexed thigh and gently applies pressure floorward on the extended thigh to stretch the iliopsoas muscle. The clinician can let the foot of the patient's flexed thigh rest against the clinician's thorax to apply a better stretch. The resistance and breathing protocol explained earlier for PR are used. Bilateral involvement is common and should be looked for. TPs in the quadratus lumborum are commonly associated with iliopsoas TPs.[2]

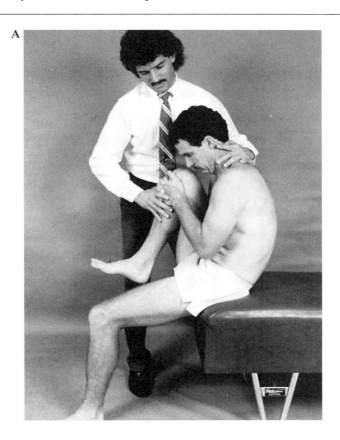

A

continues

Figure 9–16 Psoas PR while supine. **(A)** Pre-positioning before helping patient down. **(B)** Assessing hip flexor length. **(C)** Stretching. Note that patient's foot is against clinician's thorax.

Figure 9–16 continued

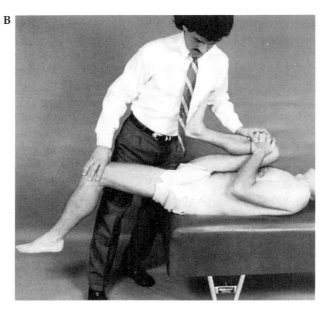

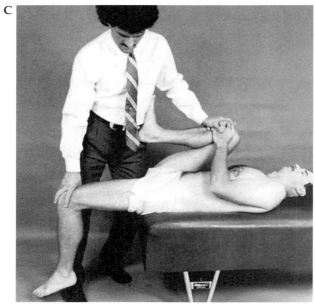

Ischemic compression can be applied at all three TP sites. The transabdominal ischemic compression should be gentle and more akin to firm massage along fibers of the muscle.

Factors that activate and perpetuate iliopsoas TPs include vigorous hip flexion as in sprinting, shortening from prolonged sitting, rapid hip extension, and hip, thoracolumbar, and sacroiliac joint dysfunction.

Quadratus Lumborum

Due to its location and consequent difficult accessibility, this muscle is very commonly overlooked when clinicians are considering myofascial sources of lower back pain. TPs in this muscle are commonly associated with thoracolumbar and sacroiliac joint disturbances.[12] The superficial and deep fibers refer pain to the sacroiliac, hip, and lower buttock regions, simulating other disorders. This is an extremely important muscle to examine routinely.

Palpation of the quadratus lumborum muscle in the side-lying position is discussed in Chapter 5 (Figure 9–17). The upper and lower aspects of the muscle commonly harbor TPs both medially (deep) and laterally (superficial). The upper lateral TP is near the 12th rib attachment and refers pain to

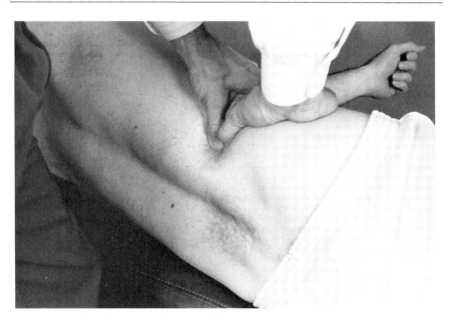

Figure 9–17 Quadratus Lumborum Palpation

the lateral iliac crest and lower abdomen (Figure 9–18A). The abdominal pain referral can be mistaken for visceral disease or inguinal hernia. The upper medial TP refers pain to the sacroiliac joint and is a common cause of misdiagnosed lumbosacral and sacroiliac joint problems.

The lower lateral TP refers pain mostly to the region of the greater trochanter, whereas the lower medial TP refers pain to the sacroiliac and lower buttock regions (Figure 9–18B). These pain referral sites are often tender and cause one to think mistakenly of trochanteric and ischial bursitis respectively.

Factors activating TPs in the quadratus lumborum involve unguarded trunk movements, sustained postures, and activities that demand lumbar spine stabilization. The muscle has attachments to the 12th rib, so vigorous and prolonged coughing can also irritate TPs in it. Combined bending and twisting movements of the trunk are a big offender in stressing the quadratus lumborum. Scrubbing floors, vacuuming, and washing the hood of a car are common mechanisms of TP activation.[12] Side lying while propping the trunk up on an elbow, as in reading or lying on a beach blanket, will stretch the lowermost and shorten the uppermost quadratus lumborum muscle. TPs can activate if this posture is assumed too long. Structural asymmetries, such as leg-length inequality and small hemipelvis, create a situation in which quadratus lumborum TPs will be perpetuated. Joint dysfunction in the thoracolumbar and sacroiliac joints should be manipulated, since these are often associated with quadratus lumborum, especially the former.[12]

The quadratus lumborum commonly initiates satellite TPs in the gluteus minimus, which in turn can create thigh and leg pain.[2] The ipsilateral psoas muscle and contralateral quadratus lumborum often develop secondary TPs in response to a primary quadratus lumborum TP and should be assessed accordingly.

To stretch the quadratus lumborum, Fluori-Methane stretch-and-spray technique in the side-lying posture, as performed by Travell and Simons, works well.[2] DeFranca and Levine[12] use a standing lateral bending stretch-and-spray technique that they find effective with larger and/or very acutely painful patients.

PR can also be effectively used for TP inactivation, with a similar side-lying position used for stretch and spray or the PR stretching of the gluteus minimus muscle (Figure 9–19A). The patient is placed side lying with the involved side uppermost. A bolster or roll cushion is placed under the waist. The upper thigh and leg are allowed to drop behind the patient off the table while being supported by the clinician. The patient holds the head-end of the table with the uppermost arm to afford better stretching.

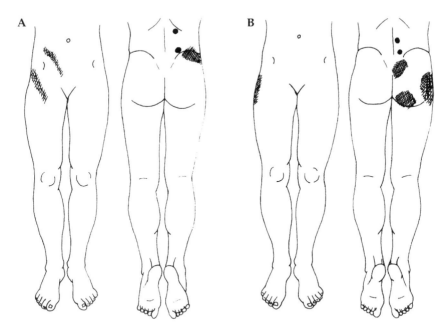

Figure 9–18 Quadratus lumborum trigger point pain patterns. **(A)** Lateral or superficial trigger points. **(B)** Medial or deep trigger points. *Source:* Adapted from *Myofascial Pain and Dysfunction: The Trigger Point Manual*, Vol. 2, by J.G. Travell and D.G. Simons, p. 31, with permission of Williams & Wilkins, © 1992.

The thigh is lowered behind the patient until tension is felt in the quadratus lumborum. The patient then isometrically holds the thigh at that level. The clinician helps to support the thigh to avoid overloading the muscle. After 10 seconds, the patient inhales deeply and, upon exhaling, relaxes and allows the thigh and leg to descend slowly further toward the floor. This new length and stretch is again held isometrically by the patient, and the above procedure is repeated. The clinician can apply an effective stretch by pressing caudally on the patient's iliac crest or greater trochanter and pressing cephalad on the thoracic cage (Figure 9–19B). The thigh and leg are then lowered in front of the body to stretch different fibers of the quadratus lumborum.

Lewit[4] performs a standing PR, which is an excellent home exercise to teach patients (Figure 9–19C). Patients stand with feet apart and laterally flex away from the tight quadratus lumborum. They then inhale deeply to aid isometric contraction of the quadratus lumborum. Looking up with

A

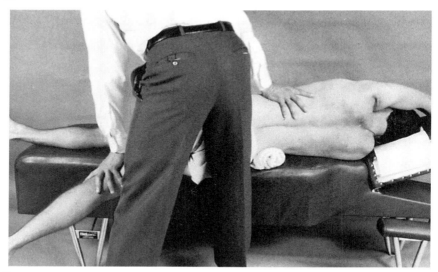

B

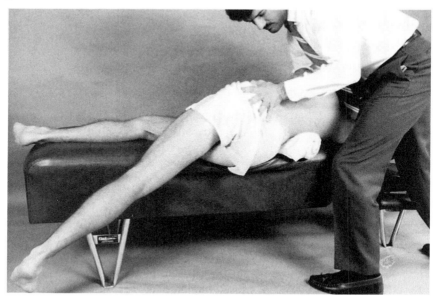

continues

Figure 9–19 (A) Quadratus lumborum PR in the side-lying position. **(B)** Separating the iliac crest and rib cage. **(C)** Standing PR stretch.

Figure 9–19 continued

C

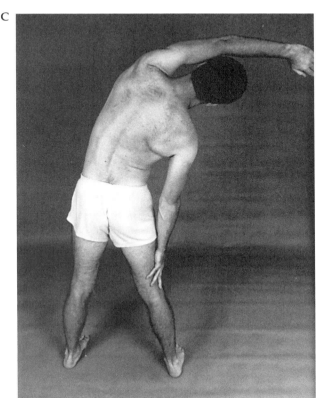

the eyes only and not the head also assists in the muscle's contraction.[2] They then look down with the eyes, exhale, and relax into more lateral bending. This is performed three to five times.

Sitting PR stretching can also be performed by laterally flexing the patient away from the involved quadratus lumborum until it is placed on stretch (Figure 9–20). The patient resists isometrically for 10 seconds, recruits phases of respiration to assist in stretching as above, and relaxes as the lateral bending is increased. This is more effective in medium- and small-sized patients.

Ischemic compression is performed in the same side-lying position that is used in searching for the TPs. The uppermost thigh and leg remain on the table behind the patient, and the uppermost arm holds onto the table

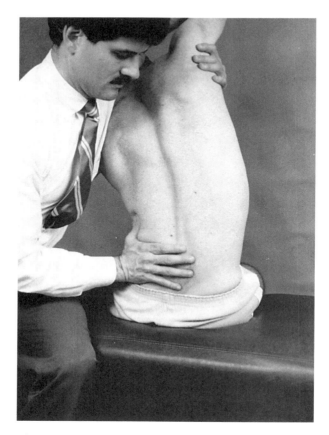

Figure 9–20 Sitting PR Stretch of Quadratus Lumborum

above the patient's head. This allows the iliac crest and 12th rib to separate sufficiently to gain access to the muscle. The entire palpable length of the muscle is explored for TPs that refer pain to their characteristic regions. Ischemic compression is applied until inactivation. The patient must be relaxed, since any muscle guarding response elicited is counterproductive. Ischemic compression can be performed first, followed by PR stretching. Heat is applied, and the patient performs active muscle contraction afterward by hiking the hip upward while standing.

Hip Adductors

The hip adductors often acquire TPs in response to hip joint dysfunction, especially in osteoarthritic joints. The muscles involved include the adductors longus, brevis, magnus, and the "fourth adductor," the perineus. The adductors brevis and longus refer pain to the groin and anteromedial thigh (Figure 9–21). They also refer pain distally to an area just above the knee. The adductor magnus usually harbors a TP at its midpoint that refers pain along the medial thigh from the groin to the knee. Its upper fibers send referred pain deep into the pelvis, mimicking a possible visceral involvement.

TPs in these muscles can become activated after sudden muscle pulls; after prolonged shortening, as in sitting cross-legged; and after activities that demand excessive adductor use, such as skiing and ice skating. Dancers who perform "splits" or people slipping on waxed floors in stocking feet or on ice can easily injure the adductors. Hip joint and pubic symphysis problems can activate these TPs as well.

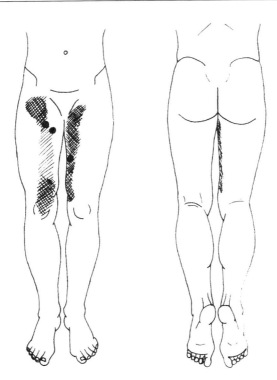

Figure 9–21 Hip Adductor Trigger Point Pain Patterns. *Source:* Adapted from *Myofascial Pain and Dysfunction: The Trigger Point Manual*, Vol. 2, by J.G. Travell and D.G. Simons, p. 291, with permission of Williams & Wilkins, © 1992.

The short adductors can be stretched using PR, with the patient supine and the thigh abducted, flexed, and externally rotated as in the Patrick-Fabere test; however, the foot is placed on the table medial to the other knee (Figure 9–22). Using PR protocol as described before, the clinician presses the knee toward the table to stretch the adductors brevis and longus. To stretch the adductor magnus, the knee is pressed toward the table and then slightly headward.

The straight leg can be abducted to stretch the adductors when using PR. To stretch the adductors brevis and longus, the abducted thigh is pressed floorward (Figure 9–23A). To affect the adductor magnus more, the abducted straight leg is flexed headward, as if performing an abducted straight-leg–raising test (Figure 9–23B). Ischemic compression can also be employed to inactivate these TPs (Figure 9–24).

TREATMENT OF TENDON AND LIGAMENT LESIONS

An effective method for treating soft tissue lesions in tendons and ligaments is *transverse friction massage*, also called *cross-fiber massage*. One cannot do the topic any justice by briefly highlighting its main points; how-

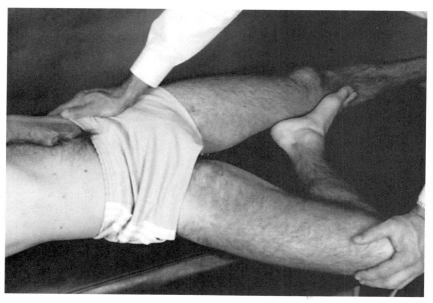

Figure 9–22 PR of Short Hip Adductors

A

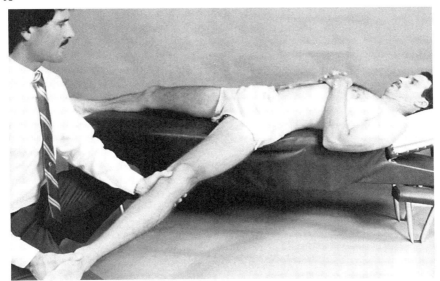

B

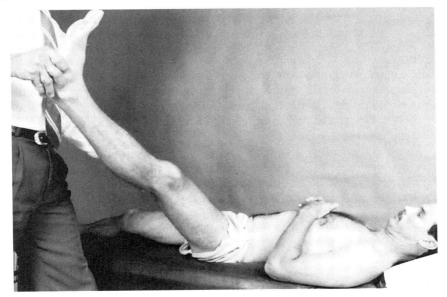

Figure 9–23 (A) PR of adductors brevis and longus. **(B)** PR of adductor magnus.

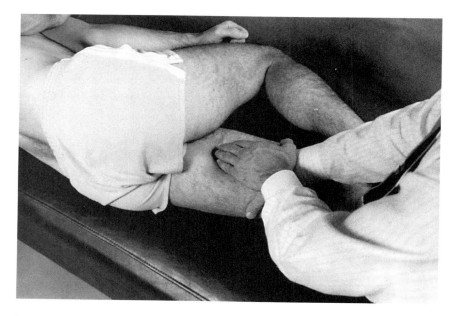

Figure 9–24 Ischemic Compression of Hip Adductors

ever, the reader is referred to an excellent reference written by Hammer.[13] Hammer emphasizes the need for accurate assessment by using selective tissue tension examination. The structure at fault needs to be diagnosed by functional examination rather than by massage based solely on the painful spot's locale. One needs to determine if a tendon, ligament, or muscle is involved. Once the structure is identified, then finding the tender spot becomes more meaningful.

The mechanism of action of transverse friction massage is to break down adhesion formation in healing or healed tissues and to create a reactive hyperemia.[14] The technique is thought to aid in the realigning of collagen fibers in the developing scar tissue (Figure 9–25). Transverse friction massage is to soft tissues what mobilization and manipulation are to joints. In the acute stages of inflammation, when collagen fibers are being laid down, light transverse friction massage imparts the early mobilization so important in reducing scar formation and hastening healing. In chronic conditions, deeper more vigorous transverse friction is needed to break down interfiber adhesions and create mobility between the injured structure and surrounding tissues.

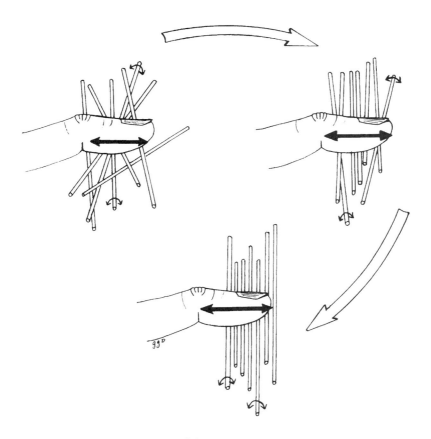

Figure 9–25 Transverse Friction Massage

Four areas where transverse friction massage can be used are the erector spinae insertion site on the sacrum and ilium, the hip abductor tendons at the greater trochanter, the hamstring muscle origin at the ischial tuberosity, and the adductor longus tendon or its origin.

These tendons or insertions are subject to contractile tension and thus are painful on active and resisted ranges of motion on examination. They are also painful when put on stretch. Once the painful tendon or insertion is identified, the most tender spot in that tendon is friction-massaged. The massage occurs across the fibers at right angles and is applied lightly at first. After 2 to 3 minutes of cross-fiber massage, the tissue becomes less painful, allowing deeper massage to take place. This process is continued for up to 10 minutes, followed by ice application and gentle, painless active and passive range-of-motion exercises.

Hammer[13] suggests treating these problems every other day, with most overuse syndromes responding in 2 weeks to 2 months. The addition of manual treatment to any articular dysfunctions or myofascial TPs is also commonly necessary.

TREATMENT OF TIGHT, SHORTENED MUSCLES

Starling's law tells us that muscles need to be at an appropriate length to function optimally. Although it regards cardiac muscle, it can be adapted to include skeletal muscle. In the locomotor system, we find that long muscles are strong muscles and short muscles are weak muscles. "Long" muscles are muscles that are not adaptively or painfully shortened, but are at their appropriate physiological length for optimal strength and function. They are not extra long or overstretched. "Short" muscles, on the other hand, are ones that have adapted to a shorter-than-usual length. This can be caused by myofascitis, which even after painful myofascial TPs are inactivated can leave a "memory" of dysfunction; reflexogenic causes, as when joint dysfunction causes a reflex spasm that lasts for days, weeks, or months; or lack of use or chronic postural overload, as in the case of the hamstring muscles of people who sit far too much. In all these instances, the muscle becomes "immobilized," unable to function optimally and tethering function elsewhere. And in all these instances, the muscle can be reeducated to lengthen painlessly.

Length-strength treatment is treatment of muscle length or distensibility and any related weakness. As discussed in Chapter 4, when one set of muscle groups is short and tight, the antagonist set is often found to be weak and inhibited. It is commonly observed that when the tight, hyperactive muscles are lengthened, the antagonists become released from their reflex inhibition and contract with more strength, sometimes remarkably. This lengthening can be accomplished by postisometric relaxation, contract–relax–antagonist-contract technique (CRAC), or postfacilitation stretching (PFS).

Contract–Relax–Antagonist-Contract Technique

This form of facilitation stretch utilizes both autogenic and reciprocal inhibition phenomena. *Autogenic inhibition* refers to a muscle's becoming inhibited after undergoing a sustained isometric contraction. This is what occurs with PR. *Reciprocal inhibition* refers to a muscle's being inhibited neurologically in response to its antagonist's contracting. This is the added dimension CRAC brings to a stretch. As its name implies, the agonist to be stretched is contracted strongly for about 7 to 10 seconds followed by a relaxation phase. The agonist contraction is about 75% maximal strength. However, a range of anywhere between 50% and 80% of maximal contraction can be used. The patient is then instructed to contract the antagonist to afford active stretching and reciprocal inhibition of the agonist. The muscle is held at this new length and rested for 10 seconds before another cycle of CRAC is initiated. CRAC differs from PR by using a stronger agonist contraction and active stretching supplied by the antagonist (Exhibit 9–1). This form of stretching can be used when trying to lengthen tight hamstrings and adductor muscles, especially in patients who can tolerate stronger agonist contractions. The procedure must be explained beforehand so that the patient knows what to expect.

Hamstring Muscle Group

As a whole, this muscle group can be effectively stretched using CRAC. The patient is placed supine, and the clinician raises the straight leg until the hamstrings come under slight tension (Figure 9–26A). The patient is instructed to push with about half to maximum strength into the clinician's countering resistance. After 10 seconds, the patient is instructed to relax slowly while the clinician stabilizes the part so that no movement occurs. When relaxation is sensed by the clinician, the patient is asked to contract the antagonists and move the part to stretch the agonist (Figure 9–26B). In this case, the patient is told to straighten the knee hard in order to recruit the quadriceps and raise the thigh higher, recruiting the hip flexors. Thus, the patient gets a double "dose" of reciprocal inhibition. The stretched position is maintained for 10 seconds. The procedure is repeated three to five times.

Exhibit 9–1 PR and CRAC Compared

Postisometric Relaxation	*CRAC*
• Minimal agonist contraction	• 50% to 80% agonist contraction
• Isometric hold for 10 seconds	• Isometric hold for 7 to 10 seconds
• Relaxation phase	• Relaxation phase
• Passive stretch by clinician	• Active stretch by patient using antagonist contraction

A

B

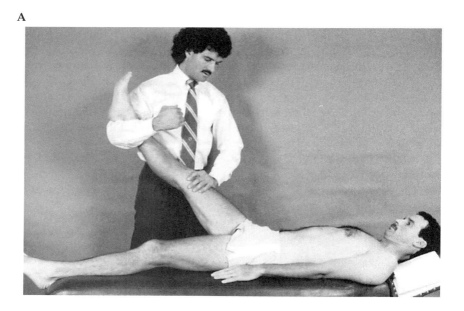

Figure 9–26 CRAC using the hamstrings. **(A)** Muscle is contracted. **(B)** Stretch is applied and held.

Hip Adductors

The adductors are stretched as a group using CRAC. The patient is supine with the clinician supporting and abducting the involved side to tension (Figure 9–27). The opposite leg is dropped off the table, with the foot resting on the floor to help stabilize the pelvis. CRAC is performed as above, but with abduction increased as the hip abductors supply the active stretch. Dysfunctional glutei or tensor fascia lata muscles may cramp if overshortened by their own contractions. On the other hand, if they were being inhibited by tight adductors, reexamination of their contraction strength will show improvement.

Rectus Femoris

Normally when the patient is prone, the heel should be able to touch the ipsilateral buttock if the rectus femoris is of normal length. To lengthen this muscle, PR is used rather than CRAC, since the hamstrings often go into a cramp if actively contracted while in a shortened position. It is common to find patients with pelvic joint dysfunction exhibiting short rectus femoris muscles that create a tethering tension to the anterior pelvis. Trig-

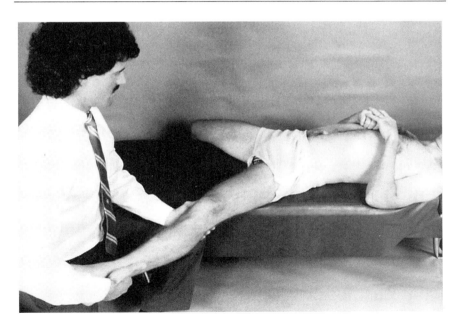

Figure 9–27 CRAC Using the Adductors, Supine

ger points in this muscle refer pain down the anterior distal thigh to the knee (Figure 9–28). To stretch this muscle using PR, the patient is placed prone with a rolled-up towel placed under the distal thigh to impart slight hip extension (Figure 9–29). Grasping the distal leg, the clinician flexes the knee and puts the rectus femoris on a slight stretch. The protocol for PR as described previously is followed. Full lengthening can be attempted by lifting the thigh off the table more when the knee is fully flexed. This technique should only be used with caution in the presence of knee joint problems. Caution should be used with a very tight rectus femoris, for it will cause the pelvis to tilt anteriorly when being stretched, and pain may be experienced in the sacroiliac or lumbar facet joints.

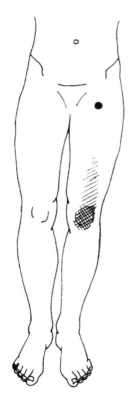

Figure 9–28 Rectus Femoris Trigger Point Pain Pattern. *Source:* Adapted from *Myofascial Pain and Dysfunction: The Trigger Point Manual*, Vol. 2, by J.G. Travell and D.G. Simons, p. 250, with permission of Williams & Wilkins, © 1992.

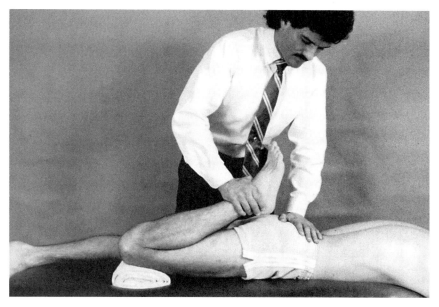

Figure 9–29 Rectus femoris PR stretch. Note roll under distal thigh.

Postfacilitation Stretching

Another type of stretch that can be used to stretch chronically shortened and tight muscles is postfacilitation stretching (PFS). It takes advantage of the inhibition period after an isometric contraction to aid in stretching a muscle. The key aspect to this procedure, as its name implies, is stretching. The muscle is positioned at midrange and contracted strongly for 10 seconds; then it is immediately placed on a quick, strong stretch for 20 seconds. The patient must immediately be able to let go completely after the contraction to afford full relaxation. Since it is a strong stretch, the patient should be told beforehand that he or she will experience pins and needles, numbness, and even discomfort for the duration of the stretch. After the stretch, the muscle is allowed to relax for 30 seconds, and the procedure is repeated 2 to 4 more times. Three sessions of stretching per week for 2 weeks is a suitable trial. The difference between PFS and PR is that the isometric contraction is much more forceful, as is the passive stretching. In using CRAC, the stretching is actively initiated by the patient, whereas in PFS it is totally passive. An example of using PFS on the adductors is shown in Figure 9-30. The patient is in the side-lying position with the

A

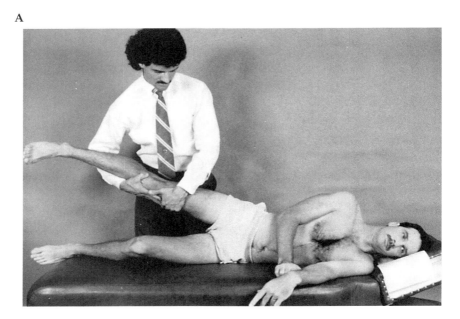

B

Figure 9–30 Postfacilitation stretching using the adductors, side-lying. **(A)** Contraction phase. **(B)** Stretch phase.

involved side up. The upper thigh is passively abducted toward the ceiling until tension is met. The patient tries to adduct the thigh strongly against resistance provided by the clinician. After 10 seconds, the patient relaxes, and the thigh is strongly stretched more into abduction. This is performed three to five times. PR can also be performed in this position.

MISCELLANEOUS CONDITIONS

Iliotibial Band Syndrome

Tight, shortened iliotibial bands are very commonly associated with chronic sacroiliac and hip joint dysfunction (Figure 9–31). They also perpetuate TPs in the hip abductors, tensor fascia lata, adductors, and quadratus lumborum. Ober's test is positive (see Chapter 5), and the groove the band forms on the lateral aspect of the thigh deepens. It is important to treat these structures early, since they are very difficult to release once they have adaptively shortened. Iliotibial band friction syndrome is seen at the lateral aspect of the knee due to a tight iliotibial band rubbing back and forth over the femoral condyle. The snapping-hip syndrome is commonly attributable to a tight iliotibial band, and reduction of

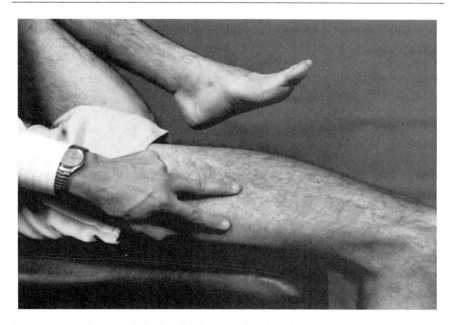

Figure 9–31 Tight iliotibial band. Note the distal end of the band.

symptoms often occurs after sacroiliac joint manipulation and band stretching.[15]

Before stretching tight iliotibial bands, joint dysfunctions and myofascial TPs in the region should be treated. Interestingly, locomotor disturbances in the lower extremity and foot are commonly present, and their treatment often facilitates the progress of the more proximal dysfunction.

The iliotibial band is a thick, tough band of connective tissue that can be hard to stretch. It is often tender to palpation, and the overlying soft tissue often contains small painful nodules. Moist heat applied to the iliotibial bands beforehand facilitates stretching. Next, longitudinal stripping massage strokes can be used until the tenderness subsides (Figure 9–32). The

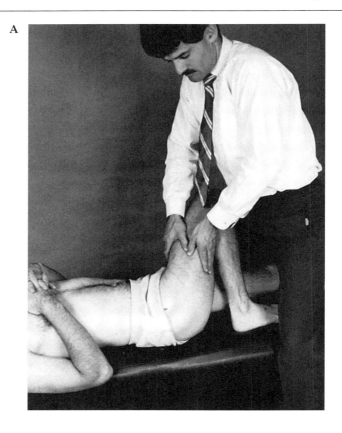

continues

Figure 9–32 (A, B) Iliotibial Band Stripping Massage

Figure 9–32 continued

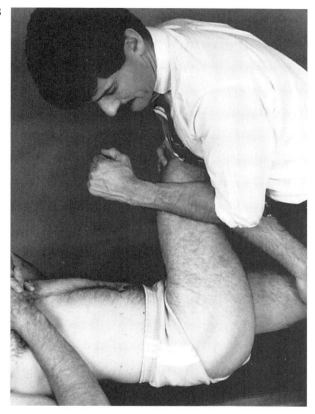

patient is placed supine, with the involved side up and flexed at the knee. The leg is slightly adducted, and the foot rests on the table. The stripping massage strokes start distally at the femoral condyle and proceed toward the greater trochanter. A lubricating lotion can be used but is not necessary. The stripping massage is performed using both thumb pads, with the thumb tips touching, or using the soft part of the proximal forearm. The distal end of the band can be exquisitely painful, and care should be taken to stay within the patient's tolerance.

After longitudinal stripping massage, transverse stretching of the band along its entire length is done, one section at a time. The patient is placed in the above side-lying position. Standing behind the patient, the clinician places the thumbs on the posterior border of the band, thumb tips touching, with the fingers placed on the anterior side. The fascial band is pulled over the thumbs, using the fingers in a motion like that of bending a stick. The thumbs act as a fulcrum over which the band is stretched (Figure 9–33). In this way, the anterior border of the band is put on a localized stretch. After stretching the entire length of the band in this manner, the procedure is repeated, but this time with an attempt to lift the band off the underlying tissues.

Next, the clinician stands in front of the patient and stretches the posterior border of the band in a similar way. The stretching session is finished with skin rolling over the length of the band three to five times. Transverse friction massage is often needed over the femoral condyle and greater tuberosity and should be performed on a separate visit. In conjunction with attending to any articular and muscular dysfunctions in the area, this procedure needs to be performed several times over 2 to 4 weeks. Stretching exercises are also taught to the patient and are discussed in Chapter 11.

Sacrotuberous Ligament Pain

The sacrotuberous ligament is an often-overlooked source of trouble in the case of pelvic joint and muscle dysfunctions. It is not seen with much

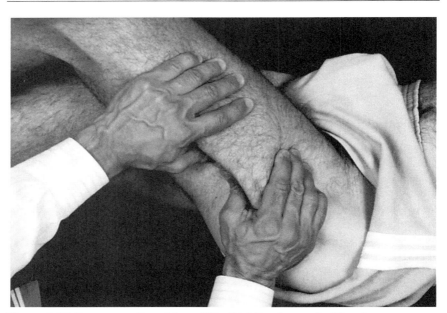

Figure 9–33 Transverse Stretching of Iliotibial Band over the Thumbs

frequency, but when it is present, it can cause much pain and disability for the patient and frustration for the clinician who is unaware of its importance. This is a thick, powerful ligament that can be traumatized from direct falls on the buttock.

Case History

A 44-year-old man attempted to slide down a sliding board with his 4-year-old daughter on his lap. When they reached the end of the slide, the father landed on the ground on his right buttock, falling about 20 in to the ground. His lower back and buttock hurt for 2 weeks and gradually subsided, but he was left with a deep buttock ache that bothered him most with sitting. The pain spread down the back of his thigh almost to his knee. Nothing really bothered it except prolonged sitting. Walking and deep pressure into his buttock seemed to help. Examination revealed right sacroiliac joint dysfunction and gluteus medius/minimus trigger points. However, direct pressure on his sacrotuberous ligament elicited his pain exactly and caused pain referral down his posterior thigh. Sacroiliac joint manipulation and myofascial stretching helped, but most relief was attained after direct pressure techniques were applied to the sacrotuberous ligament.

Another patient, a woman, complained of a painful sacrotuberous ligament after prolonged sitting on a hard gymnasium bleacher during a graduation ceremony. Women commonly experience this, especially after pregnancy and multiparity. Men usually suffer direct trauma, and women, although not immune from traumatic etiology, seem more sensitive to the adverse effects of prolonged sitting in addition to having given birth.

The sacrotuberous ligament refers pain locally in the lower buttock and into the proximal and midposterior thigh (Figure 9–34). It is often described as a deep, achy, sometimes numbing discomfort, especially after long periods of sitting. Getting in and out of a chair is difficult, and the patient prefers to stand.

On examination, postural evidence of pelvic asymmetry is usually apparent, but so is it in many asymptomatic people. Sacroiliac joint motion is restricted, especially in its lower aspect. Straight-leg raising is normal except for restriction due to hamstring tension. The Patrick-Fabere test lateralizes to the side of involvement; however, this is not pathognomonic. In the prone position, palpation of the ligament will reproduce the patient's pain. The ligament is shortened and tight and will feel firm to palpation and almost woodlike.

To treat the ligament directly, strong pressure is applied to stretch it and inactivate any TPs present in the ligament. Contact is taken deep inside the gluteal cleft, and pressure is directly laterally and superolaterally against

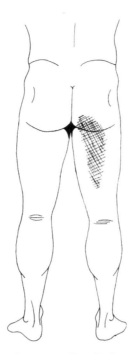

Figure 9–34 Sacrotuberous Ligament Pain Referral Pattern. *Source:* Adapted from *Myofascial Pain and Dysfunction: The Trigger Point Manual,* Vol. 2, by J.G. Travell and D.G. Simons, p. 292, with permission of Williams & Wilkins, © 1992.

several points along the length of the ligament (Figure 9–35). Some authors recommend treating the ligament though the rectum,[16] but externally applied pressure can be just as effective and more comfortable. Strong pressure is maintained for 30 seconds at each point along the ligament or until the referred pain diminishes, whichever is less. Sacroiliac joint manipulations greatly improve the condition, and the patient is counseled in exercises to promote suppleness in the pelvic ligaments (see Chapter 11).

Interestingly, pelvic organ dysfunction is noted to occur regularly in chronic dysfunction of this ligament.[16] Probably because of the stress of childbearing, women experience sacrotuberous ligament problems more often than men. Dysmenorrhea can also be initiated or worsened after a sacrotuberous ligament problem starts and is commonly observed to lessen in most of the cases treated.

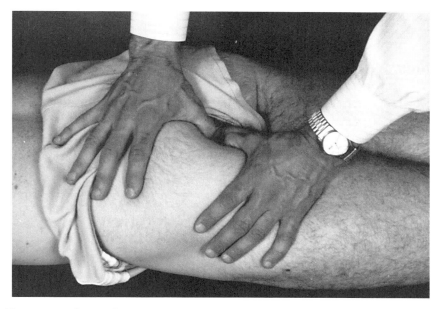

Figure 9–35 Sacrotuberous Ligament Pressure Technique

CONCLUSION

Muscles commonly become dysfunctional in association with pelvic joint problems. This typically manifests as myofascial pain syndromes or adaptive shortening of select muscle groups about the pelvis. Postisometric relaxation, CRAC, and postfacilitation stretch are stretching procedures that can be used to treat these muscles effectively. Ischemic compression and stripping massage aid in inactivating TPs. The sacrotuberous ligament can be an overlooked source of pelvic, buttock, and posterior thigh pain and should be assessed for involvement. The iliotibial bands commonly shorten in the presence of chronic pelvic joint problems and must be addressed therapeutically.

Chapter Review Questions

- What are myofascial trigger points?
- How are trigger points inactivated?
- How is postisometric relaxation performed?

- What is the "piriformis line"?
- Differentiate the clinical presentation of trigger points in the three gluteal muscles.
- Differentiate the myofascial from the neurovascular aspects of the piriformis syndrome.
- How does transverse friction massage work?
- Why is the iliotibial band an important structure clinically?
- How does a patient with a painful sacrotuberous ligament present?
- Contrast postisometric relaxation, CRAC, and postfacilitation stretch.

REFERENCES

1. Travell JG, Simons DG. *Myofascial Pain and Dysfunction: The Trigger Point Manual.* Vol 1. Baltimore, Md: Williams & Wilkins; 1983.
2. Travell JG, Simons DG. *Myofascial Pain and Dysfunction: The Trigger Point Manual.* Vol 2. Baltimore, Md: Williams & Wilkins; 1992.
3. Zohn D, Mennell JM. *Musculoskeletal Pain: Principles of Physical Diagnosis and Physical Treatment.* Boston, Mass: Little, Brown & Co; 1976.
4. Lewit K. *Manipulative Therapy in Rehabilitation of the Locomotor System.* Boston, Mass: Butterworths; 1985.
5. Ghent WR. Meralgia paresthetica. *Can Med Assoc J.* 1972;631–633.
6. Edelson JG, Nathan H. Meralgia paresthetica: an anatomical interpretation. *Clin Orthop.* 1977;122:255–262.
7. Butler ET, Johnson EW, Kaye ZA. Normal conduction velocity in the lateral femoral cutaneous nerve. *Arch Phys Med Rehabil.* 1974;55:31–32.
8. Retzlaff EW, Berry AH, Haight AS, et al. The piriformis syndrome. *J Am Osteopath Assoc.* 1974;73:799–807.
9. Pace JB. Commonly overlooked pain syndromes responsive to simple therapy. *Postgrad Med.* 1975;58:107–113.
10. Beaton LE, Anson BJ. The sciatic nerve and the piriformis muscle: their interrelationship as a possible cause of coccygodynia. *J Bone Joint Surg* (Br). 1938;23:686–688.
11. Nino-Murcia M, Wechsler RJ, Brennan RE. Computed tomography of the iliopsoas muscle. *Skeletal Radiol.* 1983;10:107–112.
12. DeFranca GG, Levine LJ. The quadratus lumborum and low back pain. *J Manipulative Physiol Ther.* 1991;12:142–149.
13. Hammer W. Friction massage. In: Hammer W, ed. *Functional Soft Tissue Examination and Treatment by Manual Methods.* Gaithersburg, Md: Aspen Publishers, Inc; 1991:235–249.
14. Cyriax J. *Textbook of Orthopaedic Medicine.* London: Balliere-Tindall; 1984.
15. DeFranca GG. The snapping hip syndrome: a case study. *Chiro Sports Med.* 1988;2:8–11.
16. Midttun A, Bojsen-Moller F. The sacrotuberous ligament pain syndrome. In: Grieve GP, ed. *Modern Manual Therapy of the Vertebral Column.* New York, NY: Churchill Livingstone; 1986:815–818.

Chapter 10

Clinical Considerations

```
┌────────────────────────────────────────────────────────────┐
│                                                              │
│                     Chapter Objectives                       │
│                                                              │
│   • to discuss treatment categories                          │
│   • to discuss abnormal movement patterns and their treatment│
│   • to describe commonly associated or linked dysfunctions and the │
│     importance of finding and treating primary as well as secondary │
│     dysfunctions                                             │
│   • to discuss the manipulation of transitional segments     │
│   • to discuss hypermobility                                 │
│   • to discuss treatment of children                         │
│   • to discuss the possible effects of treatment of the locomotor system │
│     on somatovisceral disorders                              │
│   • to describe postsurgical or "flat-back" syndrome         │
│   • to list general preventive measures                      │
│                                                              │
└────────────────────────────────────────────────────────────┘
```

In treating pelvic joint and muscle problems, various situations modulate treatment approaches. Is the patient young, with a traumatic first-time occurrence? Is the patient older, with a chronic involvement associated with tissue changes and multiple sites of problems? Are there perpetuating factors that need to be addressed? Is the pelvic dysfunction affecting other parts of the locomotor system and vice versa? Is the patient relatively healthy and in good physical condition or in a deconditioned state, rarely exercising, and leading a stressful lifestyle? The latter situation is not uncommon and presents many therapeutic challenges, most of which involve convincing the patient to take more responsibility for his or her health. In this chapter, observations from clinical practice are discussed that pertain to the above situations and others.

TREATMENT CATEGORIES

The objective in treating joint dysfunction is to restore normal joint play and subsequent motion that is full range and pain free. Similarly, the goal in treating muscular involvement, ie, myofascial pain syndromes, adaptive shortening, injury, etc, is to restore normal length, strength, and conditioning of the affected muscle. Patients are often treated until their pain is gone or much reduced, and then treatment is stopped. This works well in patients suffering from acute conditions. However, their pain can be the tip of the clinical iceberg, heralding deeper, more chronic problems. It is common for patients to seek clinical attention for painful conditions that are actually compensatory reactions of the locomotor system to a more primary, chronic problem. For example, chronic hip joint dysfunction complicated by osteoarthritis is commonly associated with compensatory painful lumbar and/or sacroiliac joint problems. Similarly, sacroiliac joint dysfunction can cause consequent painful muscle reactions or hip joint symptoms, yet itself remain silent to the patient. Although it is important to reduce painful symptoms, they are often only part of the problem. Sole treatment of symptoms often results in failure, especially in the case of chronic locomotor disturbances.

Treatment termed *passive care* pertains to therapy applied by the caregiver (physician or therapist) to a patient, who "passively" receives care.[1] Examples are rest, manual therapy, medications, electrical modalities, heat, and ice. Passive care is appropriate in the acute phase of injury; however, its prolonged use fosters physician dependence and chronicity.

Active care pertains to treatment requiring "active" involvement and responsibility on the part of the patient.[1] Exercise is the foundation of active care and includes stretching, strengthening, and stabilization exercises. A key factor in effective treatment is knowing when and how to shift a patient from passive to active care.

Acute, subacute, and chronic conditions necessitate somewhat different treatment approaches. An acute exacerbation of a chronic condition often occurs and is managed by treating the acute phase first and then focusing on the chronic dysfunctions that were responsible for the flare-up. The Quebec report[2] describes the acute phase as occurring over the first 0 to 7 days, the subacute phase as occurring from the 7th day through the 7th week, and the chronic phase as beginning after the 7th week.

Acute Phase

Acute pain commonly follows trauma from either extrinsic or intrinsic causes, but especially the latter. Inflammation, pain, and spasm predominate in the clinical picture in some cases, but many patients present with just a painful loss of function. The acute symptoms may be new to the patient, or they may be similar to past symptoms but due to a recent injury. However, repeated occurrences, especially with a history devoid of extrinsic trauma as a precipitating etiology, indicate even more an acute exacerbation of a chronic problem. This suspicion is further raised if the condition again presents in the same manner as in the past, or in a manner closely similar.

According to the Mercy guidelines,[1] an initial 2-week trial of manual therapy should be started at a frequency of three to five visits per week. If no documented improvement is seen, a second 2-week trial can then be instituted using a different treatment plan. Failure to respond after a total of 4 weeks of treatment necessitates a referral or discharge.

If improvement is seen and no complications are present that would delay recovery, treatment can progress to 6 to 8 weeks with up to three times per week visit frequency to reach preclinical status. Complicating factors that can increase treatment time by 1.5 to 2 times are listed in Exhibit 10–1 and should be used for prognosticating purposes.

Treatment objectives are to reduce symptoms and disability and to prevent chronicity from developing. Treatment by mobilization and manipulation of joint problems, if indicated, should commence immediately. Joints exist to move and should be encouraged to do so early on in therapy to prevent further morbidity of the joint in question and the surrounding soft tissues. However, movement does not necessarily mean grade V manipulations. An acutely injured joint can be passively moved with gentle grade I and II mobilizations to stimulate mechanoreceptor override of nociception. Nevertheless, nearby dysfunctional joints can be manipulated as long as the manipulation will not disturb the injured joint.

Often, gentle mobilizations are performed on the joint first, and then if the patient can tolerate the positional setup for a manipulation without experiencing pain, one is performed and is usually tolerated well. However, if the patient experiences pain, and especially if it increases when

---

Exhibit 10–1 Factors Complicating Treatment

- Preconsultation duration of symptoms over 8 days
- Severe pain
- Over 4 previous episodes
- Preexisting structural pathology or pathologic conditions

joint slack is taken up, a grade V manipulation is not attempted at that time. Often, the patient presenting with acute sacroiliac joint dysfunction can be instructed in the "three-point" stretch discussed in the next chapter. This is very helpful in cases where weight bearing is painful. Patients in acute pain can often be instructed in this stretching procedure over the phone or on a house call. Usually they can ambulate better and tolerate more of an examination and subsequent treatment after performing the stretch.

Daily applications of ice for 30 minutes every 2 hours are used on the painful area, and if the patient can be motivated to follow a plan for cryokinetics, such a plan can be instituted. This can be nothing more than ice applications until numb, followed by several minutes of walking. See Chapter 8 for a more specific approach.

Manual treatment of joint dysfunction and myofascial trigger points is conducted as explained in earlier chapters on a daily basis for 2 weeks. If dramatic improvement occurs in 24 hours after the first visit, alternate-day visits during the second week suffice. Essentially, aggressive conservative treatment in the short term is effective. The term *aggressive* pertains to the increased frequency of visits and not to the physical nature of the treatment. Children rarely need 2 weeks of daily care and usually resolve on a reduced schedule of visits. Full, painless range of motion, including joint play, negative provocative testing, and normal painless muscle contraction strength and length signal clinical resolution.

Acute cases seem to respond better when the clinician restricts treatment to a few selected problems per visit rather than attempting to treat everything in sight. Attempts to treat compassionately every finding in order to palliate the patient's pain in one visit can backfire with more pain due to overtreatment. Confusion of the clinical picture on subsequent assessments can occur with such an approach.

Take, for instance, a case in which a patient's sacroiliac joints and thoracolumbar joints are manipulated, the quadratus lumborum and gluteus minimus trigger points are treated, and the hip joints are mobilized all in one visit. When the patient returns for assessment and treatment on the following visit, one of three things is observed: the clinical picture is the same, has improved, or takes a turn for the worse. Regardless of the outcome, but especially if the patient worsens, the clinician will be hard pressed to determine what has helped or harmed the case. All of the above areas treated can present similarly when occurring by themselves. This shotgun approach to treatment can often muddle the clinical picture. What is worse, the clinician is unable to tell if the patient improved from the treatment or in spite of it.

The goal in treating the acutely painful lesion, therefore, is to provide pain relief and stabilize the situation. If the case is not clear at first, it will become clear as the intensity of signs and symptoms abates, allowing more assessment to take place.

In general, younger patients who have first-time occurrences without secondary tissue changes respond quickly. However, elderly patients who have truly acute conditions and exhibit only minimal secondary tissue changes can also respond rapidly. Since the major focus in the average acute presentation is pain, treatment success and completion are based on pain relief. Nevertheless, it is also the responsibility of the clinician to restore normal function as quickly as possible to avoid the development of a chronic condition.

Subacute Phase

After the acute phase, the subacute phase comprises the next 7 days to 7 weeks.[2] Treatment frequency should be reduced to two visits per week. A shift from passive care to more active care should be made, and stabilization and rehabilitation exercises should be implemented. The Mercy guidelines describe this period as lasting 6 to 16 weeks, with treatments not to exceed twice weekly. Patients with abnormal illness behavior and tendencies toward chronic pain behavior should be identified at this time (see below).

Chronic Phase

The chronic phase of care can start anywhere from 7 weeks[2] to 12 weeks[3] or 16 weeks.[4] There is widespread agreement that of those patients with pain of more than 3 or 4 months, over 50% will be disabled after 1 year.[4] Hence the importance of preventing chronicity and looking for signs[5] that the patient is at risk of becoming chronic (Exhibit 10-2). Brena and Chapman[6] list the five "D's," a group of symptoms that are commonly seen in chronic pain patients (Exhibit 10–3). Abnormal illness behavior often accompanies and complicates chronic conditions and is defined as a patient's inappropriate or maladaptive response to a physical injury or complaint.[7] Factors that typify abnormal illness behavior are listed in Exhibit 10–4. A multidisciplinary approach is indicated in such cases, and a psychosocial counseling referral should be made.

Chronic joint problems are characterized by stiffness, pain, and soft tissue changes. Often bony changes are observed radiologically, as in osteoarthritis, but radiographic findings correlate poorly with subjective

Exhibit 10–2 Warning Signs for Patients at Risk of Becoming Chronic

- Somatic pain symptoms static for 2 to 3 weeks
- Functional impairment
- Drug abuse (recreational or prescription)
- Emotional distress

complaints. The focus in chronic situations is on stiffness and poor function rather than pain and spasm. However, pain and spasm can occur in an aggravated case. Chronic pelvic joint problems are commonly associated with prior injuries that have healed either poorly or with persistent dysfunctions as sequelae. In addition, sedentary work and lifestyles create, as well as perpetuate, chronic locomotor disturbances.

Involvement of multiple tissues is usually seen, with ligament, capsular, muscular, and/or articular problems. Rapid recovery of function from chronic joint problems is the exception rather than the rule, due to adaptive shortening, fibrosis, and prolonged joint and muscle dysfunction: the hallmarks of a chronic situation.

A prime example of the above is a patient in his 50s who has recurrent lower back and hip pains for 15 years, sits 8 hours a day, and does not exercise or stretch. Examination commonly reveals painfully stiff joints and weak, tight muscles laden with trigger points. Such patients can present with pain or just stiffness. Pain needs to be alleviated, but, more important, function needs to be restored, exercise and stretching need to be implemented, and advice needs to be given to offset the daily postural overload. This patient needs to be taught about dysfunction, perpetuating factors, and prevention.

Treatment objectives involve stretching, manipulating, and exercising function back into the area. Any passive care should be directed at acute exacerbations only,[1] with active care in the form of exercise and advice predominating. A functional demand in the form of treatment and exer-

Exhibit 10–3 The Five "D's" Often Seen in Chronic Pain Patients

- Dramatization: vague, diffuse, nonanatomic pain
- Drug abuse: abuse of pain medications
- Dysfunction
- Dependency: passivity, depression, helplessness
- Disability

Exhibit 10–4 Characteristics of Abnormal Illness Behavior

- Pain avoidance behavior
- Anxiety
- Symptom magnification
- Psychologic distress
- Catastrophizing in order to cope
- Treatment dependency

cise needs to be imposed upon the involved tissues and joints long enough to cause a change in joint mobility, soft tissue extensibility, and muscle strength. Unfortunately, blood supply to many articular structures is minimal, leaving infertile grounds for rapid healing. Modalities and procedures that enhance circulation to the injured part will thus aid healing.

Again, aggressive conservative management is required to establish functional restoration in chronic cases. Even though chronic joint and muscle dysfunctions respond well to manual treatment, some cases respond minimally. Sometimes a 50% improvement is all one can hope for, yet for someone who has had chronic dysfunction and disability for years, even this is a welcome prognosis. The focus should be placed on active versus passive care so that the patient is actively involved in his or her own treatment.

Usually multiple tissues are involved, and compensatory reactions are present. These can confuse the clinical picture, especially if they are treated all at one time. As in acute conditions, 2 to 3 weeks of daily or alternate-day treatments are directed at the major joint and soft tissue components involved. As treatment progresses, observation and assessment allow one to continue with procedures that improve and to ignore those that have no effect or exacerbate the condition. As mobility and pain subside, treatment frequency should diminish, and the patient should be taught stretching and strengthening exercises. However, when acute conditions usually last days, treatment of chronic joint and muscle conditions takes weeks and even months to restore function satisfactorily.

Elderly individuals may be able to tolerate only alternate-day visits or visits twice weekly. If no improvement is seen in 2 weeks followed by another 2-week trial of treatment, then the chances of helping the patient with manual treatments are very minimal. However, suspending treatment for 2 to 3 weeks after an unsuccessful initial clinical trial is sometimes followed by signs of improvement. Treatment can then be reinstituted after reassessment of the situation. This also occurs after weeks of therapy when a patient reaches a plateau and appears to be clinically static. Suspending therapy for 2 to 3 weeks and then reevaluating the situation often facilitates continued improvement.

It is common to find short, tight hamstring muscles and weak glutei muscles in pelvic and hip joint conditions. The ligaments about the sacroiliac and hip joints are usually tight and limit motion. These tissues must be rehabilitated to afford functional return to the area and, more important, to help prevent recurrences and aid the patient in managing the problem. Radiographs of the pelvis should be taken to rule out bony ankylosis of the sacroiliac joints. Manipulating fused sacroiliac joints not only is futile but may impart unwarranted movement to the neighboring lumbosacral spine.

Acute Exacerbation of a Chronic Condition

A common presentation is that of a patient with a chronic pain syndrome that is for the most part tolerable but is punctuated by periods of acute aggravation. The picture is one of an acute presentation, but it is an aggravation of a weakened, dysfunctional condition that has chronically plagued the patient. After the flare-up is treated and the acute signs and symptoms diminish, the patient needs to be assessed for chronic dysfunction. Exercises and rehabilitation are an important part of treatment. Conditions that are improperly managed therapeutically or have healed poorly lead to chronic dysfunction. Recurrent exacerbations of a chronic condition indicate continued poor locomotor function. Perpetuating factors such as postural overload, hypermobility, weakness, and stress need to be addressed. The goals of treatment in this case are to treat the underlying chronic dysfunction, educate the patient about exercises, and limit or try to control any perpetuating factors. Continued frequency of exacerbations indicates lack of patient compliance or therapeutic failure.

ABNORMAL MOVEMENT PATTERNS AND TREATMENT

During the examination, poor joint and muscle function are searched for and then treated with passive and active care methods to restore normal function. Poor movement patterns often coexist with joint dysfunction and muscle trigger points. These should be examined for when the patient is out of the acute stage. In the pelvic region, the three movement patterns examined for are hip extension, hip abduction, and trunk flexion, and the overactive and underactive muscles causing an inappropriate response (see Chapter 5) are identified and treated. Manipulation and mobilization are applied to dysfunctional articulations. Myofascial trigger points are searched for and treated accordingly, and exercises are prescribed to stretch and strengthen the appropriate muscles. Correction of the poor movement pattern facilitates treatment of the regional joint dysfunctions and trigger points, especially in recurrent conditions.

Exercises that enhance peripheral proprioceptive input are very helpful in conditioning the nervous system. Bullock-Saxton et al[8] had subjects walk in balance shoes for 3 minutes five times a day. The shoes were sandals with a hemisphere attached to the bottom of them. They found that in just 1 week, significant increases in gluteal muscle activation were noted as measured on EMG. Peripheral proprioceptive input can also be enhanced by use of wobble or balance boards. A simple home instruction involves using a broomstick handle and a 10×18-in piece of ½- or ¾-in plywood. After placing the broomstick on the floor with its long axis in the sagittal plane under the plywood's center, the patient can stand on the board and try to balance himself or herself using lateral stabilizing strategies. When the stick's axis is placed under the board's center but in the coronal plane, the patient tries to maintain balance using anterior-to-posterior rocking strategies. The balancing movements should come from the ankles and feet and not from bending the trunk. A much more difficult balance board uses a hemisphere attached to the bottom of a board. This forces the patient to maintain balance around an axis of 360 degrees. To enhance proprioceptive input from the peripheral joints, patients should remove visual balancing cues by closing their eyes. Another simple task for patients to perform at home is to see how long a one-legged stance with eyes closed can be held.

If, during the testing of the hip extension movement pattern, poor muscle activation, movement, and contraction sequence are noted, then a search for the cause is performed. Usually one will find tight, overactive iliopsoas, rectus femoris, erector spinae, and hamstring muscles and a weak, inhibited gluteus maximus muscle. Stretching, postisometric relaxation, or postfacilitation stretching techniques should be used first to lengthen short iliopsoas, hamstring, erector spinae, or rectus femoris muscles. Upon relaxation of the overactive muscles, facilitation of the weak gluteus maximus muscle should be performed by appropriate verbal and tactile cues. Scratching or pinching the skin surface over the inhibited muscle heightens cortical awareness. The patient is taught how to become aware of the inhibited muscle and is instructed in contracting it efficiently. Additionally, hip, sacroiliac, and lumbar joint dysfunctions are searched for and treated.

The hip abduction movement pattern usually demonstrates overactive tensor fascia lata, hip adductor, and quadratus lumborum muscles and an underactive, inhibited gluteus medius muscle. Facilitation stretching of the tensor, adductors, and quadratus lumborum should be performed first, followed by activation of the gluteus medius. Joint dysfunction should be searched for and treated in the hip, sacroiliac, and lumbar joints.

The trunk flexion movement pattern usually reveals poor lumbopelvic stabilization, with weak abdominal muscles being substituted for by overactive iliopsoas muscles. Weak and inhibited gluteus maximus muscles are usually present. Overactive erector spinae muscles also inhibit the abdominals and should be assessed for tightness. These tight, overactive muscle groups should be stretched using muscle facilitation stretching techniques. The abdominal muscles should then be facilitated with various pelvic tilting exercises, verbal cues, and tactile stimulation designed to enhance abdominal and gluteus maximus contractions.

ASSOCIATED DYSFUNCTIONS (CHAINS)

As a multilevel system in which all levels are functionally interdependent, the locomotor system exhibits fairly consistent reactions to dysfunction, especially chronic dysfunctions. These seem to occur in chain-reaction fashion, being linked together in function and dysfunction through reflex phenomena. Finding one should lead the clinician to look for the others. Correction of related dysfunctions, if found, is necessary to prevent recurrences of the pelvic joint disturbance. No part of the locomotor system functions without affecting parts elsewhere.

However, confusion arises if one is unaware that pelvic joint and muscle dysfunctions can have far-reaching effects on the locomotor system. How can functional disturbances of the pelvis affect structures as distant as the upper cervical spine? Why is it that if you stomp on someone's foot, the person will scream "ouch" and his or her pupils will dilate—both responses occurring quite distant from the site of physical insult?

The nervous system and its intimate relationship with the locomotor system are what allow these reactions to occur. Often these reactions appear unrelated. For example, as incredible as it may seem, it is quite common to note functional changes in the craniocervical region in response to manipulation of the pelvic joints, especially in children. On the other hand, correction of upper cervical joint dysfunction is often noted to affect pelvic joint function.

Sacroiliac joint disturbances are often associated with joint dysfunctions in the lower two lumbar segments and/or ipsilateral hip joint, especially in adult patients. More common, however, are coexistent craniocervical and thoracolumbar joint dysfunctions, especially the former. Consequently, upon finding pelvic joint dysfunction, the clinician should assess these segments for associated disturbances. In children, more than in adults, craniocervical joint dysfunction is commonly linked with sacroiliac joint problems.

Interdependence of the locomotor system's parts is manifested by treating one end of the spine with manual methods and noticing functional changes at the other end. On the other hand, one can manipulate a sacroiliac joint problem only to have the patient complain of a headache shortly after. In such a case, functional assessment often demonstrates a painfully blocked upper cervical joint that responds rapidly to manipulation, with the headache abating.

Other commonly associated areas of dysfunction are the middle or upper thoracic segments. Often, previously dysfunctional segments here can be observed to move more freely after pelvic joint manipulation. In association with this is often a painful blockage of the right T5-6 costotransverse articulation that self-corrects after correction of the pelvic joint dysfunction. However, it occasionally can worsen and needs direct treatment.

Lower extremity joint dysfunctions are commonly found in association with pelvic joint dysfunctions. Most notably affected are the proximal tibiofibular, subtalar, and midtarsal joints. If dysfunctional, the ankle and foot articulations, being the anchor point of the closed kinematic chain during gait, will force compensatory reactions in more cephalad structures. Strangely enough, stubborn pelvic joint dysfunctions often respond to correction of lower extremity joint disturbances. This is consistently observed in runners and people who stand for most of the day. Subtalar and midtarsal joint function should be routinely assessed. Plantar-to-dorsal joint restrictions in the calcaneocuboid articulation are another important dysfunction to assess. Their correction often has favorable effects on pelvic and hip function. In addition, tight iliotibial bands with myofascial trigger points in the tensor fascia lata frequently coexist with chronic sacroiliac joint dysfunction.

Muscles typically harboring myofascial trigger points that are consistently seen with sacroiliac joint dysfunction include the gluteus minimus and medius, quadratus lumborum, piriformis, and psoas major. As mentioned before in Chapter 4, tight and shortened iliopsoas and erector spinae muscles are often associated with weak and inhibited gluteus maximus and abdominal muscles respectively. Hamstring overactivation is also seen with weak gluteus maximus muscles. Weak gluteus medius muscles are usually associated with overactive and tight hip adductor, tensor fascia lata, and quadratus lumborum muscles. Lewit identified particular levels of joint dysfunction associated with specific muscle dysfunctions (Exhibit 10–5).[9,10] If dysfunction in these joints is not treated, the

Exhibit 10–5 Joint and Muscle Associations

Joint	Muscle
T-10 through L-2	Quadratus lumborum, psoas, abdominals, thoracolumbar erector spinae
L-2, L-3	Gluteus medius
L-3, L-4	Rectus femoris, lumbar erector spinae, adductors
L-4, L-5	Piriformis, hamstrings, lumbar erector spinae, adductors
L-5, S-1	Iliacus, hamstrings, lumbar erector spinae, adductors
SI	Gluteus maximus, piriformis, iliacus, hamstrings, adductors, contralateral gluteus medius
Coccyx	Levator ani, gluteus maximus, piriformis, iliacus
Hip	Adductors

muscle disturbance will continue to occur. Often just treating the joint dysfunction will obviate the need to treat the trigger point or muscle involvement.

Hip joint disturbances are often associated with tight hip adductors and hip flexors. Trigger points in the hip abductors often coexist and need treatment. A weak, hypotonic gluteus maximus muscle is usually present, especially in coxarthrosis.

Lumbar facet and disc syndromes can coexist with pelvic joint disturbances, not necessarily as chain-reaction dysfunctions but as combination lesions. Treatment of pelvic and hip joint dysfunction aids in the healing of these conditions. Bilateral sacroiliac and/or hip joint dysfunctions create more of a demand for motion at the L-4 and L-5 segments than normal. This can result in painful compensatory reactions and possibly premature degenerative changes there. Restoration of pelvic and hip joint function may prevent this decompensation of the lumbar spine and is important in the management of low back pain syndromes.

PRIMARY VERSUS SECONDARY LESIONS

When one finds pelvic joint dysfunction, especially that of long standing, one should assess the abovementioned areas for associated dysfunctions. It is also common to observe adverse reactions in these areas after pelvic joint manipulation, particularly if the pelvic dysfunction is a compensatory reaction and not a primary problem. The following case history serves as an example:

Case History

A 37-year-old woman tennis player presented with thoracolumbar pain of 6 months' duration. Pain was exacerbated by playing tennis, prolonged sitting, standing, and repetitive bending. It was alleviated by stretching the trunk with rotation and extension. The pain was described as a deep "migraine headache" in her back.

The examination revealed a painful dysfunctional thoracolumbar segment associated with extremely stiff sacroiliac joints bilaterally. Quadratus lumborum and psoas trigger points were palpated, eliciting exquisite tenderness that reproduced her symptoms.

The diagnosis was thoracolumbar joint dysfunction with an associated quadratus lumborum and psoas myofascial pain syndrome.

Treatment on the first day entailed manipulation of the thoracolumbar segment. Within an hour posttreatment, the patient experienced extreme pain and spasm. Her back felt weak and vulnerable. The following day she experienced such a feeling of instability she could not get out of bed. Two days later she presented again for treatment. Electrotherapy and myofascial stretching were performed with minimal relief. On the following day, reassessment revealed the same clinical picture as her initial visit. This time, her sacroiliac joints were first mobilized and then manipulated with dramatic relief. On subsequent visits, her sacroiliac joints were treated, and exercises were given to improve joint and muscle function.

The above case history illustrates the consequence of treating a secondary dysfunction (compensation) to a more primary dysfunction: the body's ability to compensate for a more primary lesion is disturbed, and a painful exacerbation often results. It is not uncommon for a compensatory dysfunction or secondary lesion to be painful and therefore receive therapeutic intervention.

This brings up two points. First, the clinician should refrain from treating too many dysfunctions early on in the case. This fosters confusion due to a shotgun approach and makes assessment difficult. Second, there is no substitute for clinical experience. In general, it is helpful to keep in mind that the thoracolumbar and even lower lumbar segments often compensate painfully for sacroiliac joint dysfunctions. If these are treated symptomatically and they exacerbate or remain unchanged, look toward the sacroiliac joints as a possible primary dysfunction. It is always difficult for the clinician to face patients who have just exacerbated from his or her care. However, it is always best to explain to them the dynamics of compensations versus primary dysfunctions and to tell them that clinical trial is often important to determine the nature of their particular biomechanics. This is especially important in chronic musculoskeletal dysfunctions, since compensatory reactions become further ingrained with time and more resistant to change.

Primary dysfunctions are those that are more central in the overall locomotor disturbance. There can be more than one. The pelvis is a very common site for primary dysfunctions, often affecting other parts of the locomotor system. A primary dysfunction, or what Gillet and Liekens[11] and Schafer and Faye[12] call a *major fixation*, is characterized by more chronic signs of dysfunction. A stiff joint limited by shortened capsuloligamentous tissue represents a major or "ligamentous" fixation. The level of major biomechanical dysfunction is usually the most restricted. Motion is blocked in most of the joint's ranges of motion. Complete blockage in all the joint's range of motion is termed an *articular fixation*, with a worst-case scenario being bony ankylosis.[12] Major fixations require the locomotor system to make biomechanical adaptations to them, especially articular fixations. These compensatory changes often become dysfunctional and painful, causing the patient to seek treatment. An example is a sacroiliac joint that becomes painfully hypermobile in reaction to the other sacroiliac joint's hypomobility. Lumbar facet joints often react this way to sacroiliac and hip joint fixations.

Major or primary fixations characteristically respond more slowly to manipulation and often need mobilization initially. Secondary changes are noticed nearby in the form of atrophic skin changes and hypotonic, weak muscles. These fixations are often stiff and palpate with a very firm end-feel. They are not necessarily painful unless injured or stressed during a provocation examination. In the short term, manipulative correction of these fixations yields only partial gains in range of motion, yet changes elsewhere in the locomotor system are often seen to occur. In response to treating major fixations, secondary fixations, which are adaptations to primary fixations, are noted to improve without receiving direct treatment. Only over a period of time, usually weeks and sometimes months, will the chronically stiffened joint adapt to the motion induced by treatment and exercise. As long as a major fixation persists, the patient is at risk for continued exacerbations and maladaptive compensations elsewhere in the locomotor system.

Secondary or *minor fixations* are usually compensatory reactions to major fixations; however, they can occur by themselves, especially in acute conditions or younger patients. They are also called *muscular fixations*, due to the muscular response associated with them. The muscle's hypertonic response creates a joint blockage, but one that is not as restricting as that seen in a ligamentous or articular fixation. Secondary fixations are not as restricted in their range of motion as primary dysfunctions. They are usually symptomatic and respond readily to manual methods, resulting in noticeable short-term relief. Unfortunately, their symptomatic nature often draws attention away from an underlying chronic major dysfunction. However, a clue that one is dealing with a secondary problem is its tendency to recur not only quickly but repeatedly. This situation occurs in the presence of major or primary fixations found elsewhere. Another clue is an exacerbation of the clinical picture within 24 hours of treatment. Sometimes within minutes the patient will complain of pain or spasm, even in areas remote from that treated. The presence of these clues should lead to further assessment and search for more primary dysfunctions. If minor fixations are present in the absence of major fixations, correction is more lasting.

TRANSITIONAL SEGMENTS

The mere presence of congenital anomalies should not lead one to incriminate them as painful etiologies. However, a sacralization with a pseudoarthrosis can become symptomatic just like any other joint. Pelvic and hip joint dysfunction will exacerbate such conditions and need to be addressed. Nevertheless, transitional segments, especially pseudoarthroses, can become irritated with overzealous pelvic manipulations. This is not a fault of the technique as much as its application.

Spondylolisthesis of L-5, although not considered congenital by conventional thinking, can be treated the same way. Instead of trying to reposition L-5 back onto the sacrum, one should try to correct any regional joint and muscle dysfunction. Lower back pain in patients with spondylolisthesis responds well to thoracolumbar, sacroiliac, and hip joint manipulations if these areas are dysfunctional. As with congenital anomalies, seldom does the spondylolisthetic segment itself have to be directly manipulated.

HYPERMOBILITY

Certain situations are associated with joint hypermobility. Hypermobility secondary to lax ligamentous support may be found as a general condition throughout the musculoskeletal system, or it may be due to localized trauma or degeneration. Sometimes it is related to rare, hereditary conditions such as Ehlers-Danlos syndrome and Marfan's syndrome. However, nearly 5% of adults fit criteria that enable them to be called hypermobile.[13] This entails ligamentous laxity affecting the musculoskeletal system in general. Women and children exhibit greater ranges of motion in their joints. Travell and Simons[14] mention that generalized hypermobility is associated with mitral valve prolapse, pelvic floor and abdominal wall weakness, and thin, extensible skin prone to striae.

Muscular weakness, degenerative changes, compensatory reactions, and excessive joint manipulation can contribute to localized hyper-mobility. A dull ache follows activities that place the ligaments under strain. The onset of symptoms is usually delayed, but as the condition worsens, pain occurs soon after the offending posture is assumed. Joint clicking can be heard and is usually referred to in the history as a "catch" occurring during movement. Palpation will reveal excess motion, clicking, crepitus, and pain with sustained overpressure. Muscle spasm may be present to guard any instability. Typically, hypermobile joints tend to cause recurrent problems until they are stabilized, either therapeutically or through natural progression.

In constitutional hypermobility, the patient is able to touch the palms to the floor, hyperextend the knees and elbows, and dorsiflex the fingers to the distal forearm. Pregnancy and the menses can create physiologic hypermobility or exacerbate existing hypermobility.

Regardless, manipulation and strong mobilizations are contraindicated in joints that are hypermobile. A joint that "clicks" on its own is not in need of further external manipulation. Neighboring joints that are hypomobile can be manipulated, affording relief to the hypermobile joint that is com-pensating for the hypomobility. In the pelvis, this can be the opposite sac-roiliac joint, the other pole of the same sacroiliac joint, or one of the hip joints. Lumbar joint dysfunction should also be sought for. Myofascial trigger points in regional muscles are commonly present and require treat-ment. However, strong myofascial stretching across a hypermobile joint is contraindicated, and stripping massage or ischemic compression should be applied instead.

Patients with hypermobile joints are sensitive to sustained postures and prolonged stooping. They need to exercise the regional musculature to in-crease strength and dynamic support. Sustained static postures need to be avoided. Hypermobile sacroiliac joints can be supported with a trochanter belt during acutely painful episodes. The belt is tightened just below the iliac crest and is worn during physical activities over a period of 2 to 3 weeks. To be effective, the belt should be 2 to 3 inches wide, inelastic, and placed about 2 inches below the iliac crest. A chair test can be used to de-termine the need for a trochanter belt and to determine if the person has pelvic ring dysfunction.[15]

The chair test is a simple procedure that tests the functional efficiency of the pelvic ring. Difficulty in performing the chair test is a positive result and indicates pelvic joint and muscle dysfunction, including hypermobility. Wearing a tight-fitting trochanter belt usually makes it much easier to per-form the test, since it affords stability to the pelvic ring. The patient literally feels as if he or she is being catapulted to the standing posture by the strong, stable pelvic ring. This test is positive not only for pelvic joint hypermobility but also for other pelvic joint and muscle problems.

To perform the test, the person should stand just in front of a chair, with the calf muscles touching the chair frame. The arms are held crossed in front of the chest, and the person attempts to sit down slowly and smoothly while keeping the back straight. The feet are kept 6 in apart. After sitting down, the person must return to the standing starting position. The test is normal if the person sits slowly without flopping onto the chair just before sitting down and the back is kept straight. The movement should be performed smoothly without any jerkiness or pain noted. Upon arising, the person should maintain an erect spine and not try to lean or lunge forward to gain momentum. Problems with the joints or muscles about the pelvic ring will make this test difficult to perform. A patient having difficulty with this test will arise jutting the head and chin forward, flexing the trunk in an effort to swing himself or herself out of the chair, or pushing off the thighs with the hands.

If the test is positive, have the patient perform a few simple hip and sacroiliac joint stretches, and then have him or her perform the test again. Almost always an improvement in the test is felt. This serves as a powerful patient awareness and educational procedure and helps demonstrate the importance of exercises. The same response is seen if a trochanter belt is worn.

CHILDREN

Unfortunately, children not only pay the price for the ignorance of adults but, like their parents, are unaware of the hidden costs. This is especially true in the case of functional locomotor disturbances. Parents and clinicians alike must realize that children can suffer from myofascial pain and joint dysfunctions. Pelvic joint dysfunction is a common occurrence in children and is seen more frequently as they enter and progress through their schooling. It is most likely due to excessive sitting in poorly designed seats. Additionally, children are not taught the proper way to sit, stretch, or exercise to prevent locomotor disturbances of the pelvis. It is incredibly important to assess children for pelvic and hip joint dysfunction early on so they do not develop chronic dysfunction and suffer the consequences later. To compound the situation, joint and muscle dysfunction from prior injuries or poor posturing may be clinically latent and therefore asymptomatic. Functional assessment screenings should be performed to identify these dysfunctions, since they are a potential source of future trouble.

Olsen et al,[16] in a study of 1242 children between the ages of 11 and 17, found that 30.4% of them had a history of low back pain and that one third of those experienced limitation of activities due to their pain. The authors also observed that low back pain started early in childhood, increased noticeably after the age of 10, and continued to increase throughout adolescence. They state that by adolescence, low back pain represents a serious public health problem.

In 1988, Balague et al[17] studied 1715 Swiss children ages 7 to 17 and found a history of back pain in 46% of them. Most of this pain was in the lower back. They noted an increase in low back pain as the child aged. Also identified was a correlation between low back pain and smoking, sports, female gender, and time spent watching television.

Mierau et al[18] studied 403 students and found 22.8% of the elementary schoolchildren and 33.3% of the secondary schoolchildren to have histories of low back pain. Interestingly, 88% of those with a history of low back pain demonstrated sacroiliac joint dysfunction on examination, strongly suggesting a correlation between low back pain and sacroiliac joint dysfunction.

These studies contradict the prevalent notion that low back pain is not a problem in children. Yet when one considers the daily events in a child's life that can contribute to dysfunction, it should be no surprise that children suffer lower back pain. Contemplate the numerous falls on the buttocks during the early months of walking, the hours of sitting at school or in front of a television set, the time spent with low-activity computer games, or the physical trauma associated with competitive sports. The potential for injury and dysfunction is just as great as in adults. The following case study illustrates this:

A young ballerina 6 years of age presented with a "pulled groin muscle" as "diagnosed" by her dance instructor. She was told to stretch it out and assured that it would loosen up. After 4 weeks of continued proximal medial thigh pain and tightness, she sought help. On questioning, it was determined that forced stretching to increase her ability to perform "splits" started the problem. However, 1 week prior, she had fallen off her bike and landed on the same hip and leg, causing hip pain that lasted 2 days. She seemed fine until she attempted to stretch her adductors for dance class the next week. On examination, she had sacroiliac and hip joint dysfunction, with a painful trigger point in the adductor longus muscle. Postisometric relaxation with gentle ischemic compression of the trigger point followed by heat was done on the first visit, with only partial relief. The following visit, her sacroiliac and hip joint dysfunctions were manipulated, and the case was completely resolved.

Children who take dance lessons at a young age often present with pelvic and hip joint problems, especially when forced to perform extreme stretches that make them vulnerable to injury. Apparently, this young girl's fall and subsequent joint injuries created undue tension in her adductors that precluded effective stretching. Forced stretching aggravated her adductor muscle, yet she did not complain of hip or sacroiliac pain on clinical presentation. This is a prime example of how underlying joint dysfunctions can remain silent while the patient presents with the more symptomatic secondary reactions. Stretching of the adductor muscles was to no avail, and resolution did not occur for this little girl until primary joint dysfunctions were corrected.

Children who suffer from dysfunction of the pelvic joints and muscles respond quickly with minimal intervention. For the most part, their joints and tissues are more pliable and heal faster. Young patients do not have the chronic tissue changes that we see in adults with long-standing dysfunction. However, a 12-year-old may still suffer from a chronic joint problem of 5 or more years' duration.

The actual treatment of children employs techniques similar to those used with adults except for some modifications. The hand contacts and positioning will differ slightly. For instance, when manipulating sacroiliac joint dysfunctions in small children, one uses finger contacts instead of a pisiform. The small child can lie on top of the parent for security. Children can be incredibly flexible and may present a problem if all joint slack is not removed. However, an audible crack is not often heard with pediatric manipulations, and, as in adults but especially in children, it should not be the goal in treatment. Increased joint mobility is achieved after a successful manipulation, which should be confirmed by a postmanipulative assessment.

A very common complaint in youngsters is a vague pain in the legs with no history of trauma or sickness. If pathology is ruled out, which it almost always is, the infamous diagnosis of "growing pains" is traditionally bestowed. The child is told that he or she will grow out of it, that it is normal, and that there is nothing to worry about. The parents feel relieved and all is well, yet the child still experiences the painful reminder that he or she is growing. Such little patients often exhibit sacroiliac, hip, or lumbar joint dysfunctions that readily correct with good results. Myofascial trigger points in the hip adductors and abductors are surprisingly common and also contribute to the clinical picture.

Pelvic joint dysfunction in children is very commonly associated with craniocervical joint dysfunction, so much so that finding one necessitates looking for the other. The following case report is an example:

A 6-year-old girl complained of lower back pain for 3 months after falling off her swing and landing on her buttocks. Since then, her lower back had bothered her whenever she would run hard while playing. Her family physician had ruled out any serious injury and had prescribed stretching exercises and heat. Upon further

questioning, she did state that after her fall she started to experience mild suboc-
cipital and parietal headaches for 8 weeks. Her parents thought these were due to
her eyes and the need for glasses, but an eye examination failed to show any
problems, and a medical workup was negative for any disease. Physical examination revealed sacroiliac and lumbar joint dysfunction. Manual treatment directed at
these dysfunctions afforded only temporary relief. It was not until a painfully stiff
craniocervical region was mobilized and manipulated that she experienced lasting
relief from both her headaches and her lower back pain.

Often a manipulative correction at the top of the spine results in functional changes in the pelvis and vice versa. Lewit discusses these very
findings.[9] The younger, more supple spine/pelvis adapts readily to functional changes made to the locomotor system. These changes can be observed when comparing pre- and postmanipulative assessments.

Another very common childhood presentation is acute pain attributable
to transient or idiopathic synovitis of the hip. It is the most common cause
of limping and pain in the hip of children in the United States.[19] It is usually a diagnosis of exclusion and self-limits in 7 to 10 days. Septic arthritis,
Legg-Calvé-Perthes disease, and slipped capital femoral epiphysis must
be ruled out first.

Septic arthritis occurs in children usually under 3 years old presenting
acutely ill with fever, malaise, and arrested hip motion. Present are signs
of swelling and inflammation, an elevated white cell count and sedimentation rate, and possibly radiographic findings of joint effusion.

Perthes disease, a form of avascular necrosis, occurs in middle childhood, usually in males. The child presents with persistent pain, a limp,
and restricted hip motion, and radiographic findings vary depending on
the stage of the disease.

Slipped capital femoral epiphysis usually occurs in children older than
10 years of age and is associated with obesity, male sex, and black race. Its
onset can be quick but is usually gradual. A painful or painless limp with
external hip rotation and loss of internal rotation in a child during the vulnerable years strongly suggests a slipped capital femoral epiphysis. Radiographic findings are confirmatory.

In any condition causing hip joint swelling and pain, the hip is held in
an antalgic position of slight flexion, abduction, and external rotation.
Also, it is common in children to experience knee pain with hip joint conditions, therefore necessitating hip examination in all knee complaints.

In transient synovitis of the hip, the child is usually between 3 and 10
years old, male, and presents acutely. Hip pain and limping are predominant. The hip may be held in an antalgic posture, and the range of motion
is limited, although less than that found in septic arthritis. The sedimenta-

tion rate, white count, and X-ray findings are normal. The condition sometimes follows upper respiratory infections. Traditionally, symptomatic care and rest are rendered, and the condition self-remits within 2 weeks. However, often signs of inflammation and swelling are not found, and the clinical picture is one of an atraumatic acute onset of pain without any signs of disease. Functional examination usually demonstrates hip joint dysfunction, particularly in long-axis extension. Sustained long-axis traction interspersed with grade I oscillations of long-axis extension and medial rotation often dramatically relieves symptoms. Accompanying sacroiliac joint dysfunction commonly occurs on the same side and should be manipulated if it persists on follow-up visits.

Infants who present with clicking hips should be assessed for congenital hip dislocation. This misnomer really pertains to the easy ability of the hip joint to dislocate and relocate itself. However, in progressive cases, the dislocations occur more easily, and after 4 to 6 weeks the femoral head can remain outside the acetabulum. After 3 to 5 months, relocation becomes more difficult, if not impossible, without orthopedic intervention. The vast majority of infants with congenital hip dislocation readily self-correct within the first month of life and require no intervention. However, if the tendency to dislocate persists and if the femoral head remains displaced, dysplastic changes will occur. Normal coaptation in the growing hip joint is necessary for proper growth and formation of the femoral head and acetabulum. Dislocation precludes the formation of normal joint architecture and must be corrected.

Clinical suspicion of a continuing dislocatable hip at 6 weeks of age warrants a referral to an orthopedist. With the infant supine and the hip flexed to 90 degrees, the thigh is abducted while pressure is applied medially and upward on the greater trochanter. A click sound signifies reduction of a dislocation and is a positive Ortolani's sign. To test the ease at which the hip can dislocate, the reverse Ortolani or Barlow test is used. The hips are adducted by bringing the knees straight up and applying a posterior shear at 90 degrees of flexion. A clicking sensation signifies dislocation, which can be reduced by performing Ortolani's test. Other associated findings in congenital hip dislocation are decreased normal hip flexion posture, decreased ability to abduct the hips fully while at 90 degrees flexion, short-appearing limb on the affected side, and uneven gluteal and groin creases.

SOMATOVISCERAL REACTIONS

A most interesting and very controversial observation by clinicians experienced with manual treatment of the locomotor system is changes in the viscera. When treating patients for pelvic joint problems, clinicians often notice changes in concurrent organic conditions such as dysmenorrhea, lower-bowel disturbances, and urinary and prostatic problems. Changes seen are those that relate to function rather than pathoanatomy. To date, no clinical trials have been done to substantiate claims of efficacy, but functional changes of the pelvic viscera do occur frequently in treatment of concurrent pelvic joint and muscle dysfunctions. The most well-recognized changes relate to gynecologic problems, with dysmenorrhea being paramount. Although not as consistent as with dysmenorrhea, improvement in the character and frequency of bowel movements and in symptoms related to functional prostatic problems has been known to occur after treating pelvic joint dysfunctions. This is not an appeal to use manipulative therapy as a treatment of choice for organic disorders, but certain conditions seem to respond favorably, and this observation should be investigated further.

Women with dysmenorrhea in the absence of gynecologic disease often respond favorably to pelvic joint manipulation. Manipulation of sacroiliac joint fixations in which sacral contacts are used seem to have more of a favorable effect. In addition, middle and lower lumbar segments are often found to be dysfunctional. Lewit[9] states that menstrual and labor pains felt in the lower back in the absence of disease are usually of locomotor origin and can represent the first clue to the presence of locomotor disturbance. Sometimes pelvic locomotor disturbances cause pain that is mistaken for gynecologic disease. However, visceral disease can manifest as somatic pain and must be ruled out. For example, a woman presenting with lower back pain gained complete relief only after a uterine fibroid was surgically removed.

A statistically significant correlation is found between back pain in pregnancy and subsequent back pain during parturition, also called "back labor."[20] The pain in both of these situations can be significantly reduced when manual methods are applied prenatally to dysfunctional pelvic joints and muscles. This is a most desirable situation, considering the fact that most physicians are reluctant to give medications to pregnant women. Commonly found are sacroiliac and lumbar joint dysfunctions. Myofascial trigger points are regularly observed in the quadratus lumborum, gluteus minimus and medius, and tensor fascia lata. Back labor can often be eased with firm posterior-to-anterior pressure applied to the sacrum during labor. Additionally, squatting and kneeling during labor can ease delivery compared to the dorsal lithotomy position.

Manipulation in third-trimester pregnancies must be judicious, gentle, and performed only in the presence of joint restriction. The vulnerability of this area during this time makes it susceptible to injury from an over-zealous technique. Gentle mobilizations are very beneficial and can be used in place of manipulations when dysfunction is present. A case example is a 34-year-old woman in her 8th month of pregnancy who presented to me with severe sacroiliac joint pain after a vigorous side-posture manipulation was performed by another practitioner. Pain was experienced shortly after a click sound was heard during the manipulation. She found it very difficult to bear weight, getting sharp jabs of pain in the upper aspect of the sacroiliac joint. The upper aspect of her sacroiliac joint was tender and appeared hypermobile. Specific mobilization to the restricted lower aspects of both sacroiliac joints afforded her dramatic relief, manipulation being contraindicated in this case.

Claims abound about the efficacy of manipulative therapy in the treatment of enuresis, yet they remain unsubstantiated. In my experience, results seem to be equivocal at best and sporadic, to say the least. In a study involving 171 enuretic children, LeBoeuf et al[21] achieved minimal results with manipulative therapy. More studies need to be done before opinions on both sides of the issue are confirmed.

POSTSURGICAL OR "FLAT-BACK" SYNDROME

Patients who have undergone surgery with general anesthesia often experience stiffness and lower back pain afterward. The locomotor system is very prone to trauma and dysfunction from static posturing while under general anesthesia due to suppression of muscle tone and protective reflexes. One will commonly find dysfunctional lumbar and sacroiliac joints that need to be manipulated. In cases of lumbar diskectomy, the chances are good that pelvic joint dysfunction was present before the procedure, but postsurgical symptoms are frequently relieved when treatment is directed at restoring functional motion to dysfunctional pelvic or lumbar joints. Abdominal or thoracic surgery involves prolonged supine positioning of the patient and regularly causes lower back complaints postsurgically. Often termed the "flat-back syndrome," this condition presents with an achy, stiff lower back, and patients invariably state that they feel as if they have been run over by a truck. Some patients with postsurgical back pain have had a history of lower back problems before surgery, but many do not. A common presentation is someone who has never had back problems before, undergoes abdominal or thoracic surgery, and starts to experience lower back pain for weeks or months after the procedure.

PREVENTION

The ideal for any practitioner is to prevent the very things that he or she commonly treats. However, reality dictates a totally different situation. First among preventive measures is educating people about the need for maintaining a properly functioning locomotor system. Second, people need to realize that a lack of pain is not a good indicator of function. Unfortunately, people have been indoctrinated into believing that no pain means no problem. This results in silent dysfunctions persisting into symptomatic, chronic dysfunctions. Third, to assume that the locomotor system is not in need of regular exercise and caring is to ignore one of nature's fundamental laws of existence. Indifference to this law will result, sooner or later, in poor function and pain. Last, patients need to be more responsible for their own health and more proactive in their own health care. Otherwise, the practitioner takes on too much responsibility, with the added unenviable task of nagging the patient about noncompliance with exercise or lifestyle changes and being set up for blame when therapeutic failure eventually occurs.

Besides exercises, attention must be given to posture, work and domestic activities, diet, sleep, and stress levels. For instance, repetitive dynamic or static loading of the pelvic ring, especially in the presence of chronic dysfunction, can only serve to perpetuate a locomotor disturbance. It is useless for a patient to engage in treatment of pelvic joint or muscle dysfunction if his or her daily sitting for 8 to 10 hours is not addressed. Walking 30 minutes a day, doing hip extension and pelvic ligament stretching exercises, and limiting prolonged periods of sitting at one time will go far in preventing painful pelvic locomotor disturbances.

A mattress that is too hard or too soft will perpetuate gluteal trigger points and lumbar, hip, and sacroiliac point problems. Typically patients will awaken stiff and sore every morning. The symptoms abate only after being up and about for a short time, and then patients feel fine. The symptom picture repeats itself faithfully the next morning. The pelvis must be allowed to depress into the mattress enough to maintain neutral alignment when recumbent. Sleeping "in" later than usual can precipitate joint and muscle symptoms, and sometimes patients state that they cannot wait to get out of bed because of the impending symptoms they know they will suffer. Any good multicoil mattress that is not too firm should suffice. Foam rubber matting can soften a much too firm mattress, and a sheet of ½-inch or ⅜-inch plywood can firm up a sagging one.

The single most important factor in preventing injury or maintaining adequate functional status is regular exercise. The locomotor system is built for movement, with muscles requiring regular active work, joints needing motion, and ligaments needing stretching to maintain good working order. This is discussed in more detail in the final chapter.

However, even though the onus of prevention falls squarely on patients' shoulders, they are often noncompliant with exercises and other recommendations. They continue to engage in prolonged postures, improper activities, and trauma-inducing sports. There is a high recurrence rate of locomotor disturbances in these situations. In addition, the patient afflicted with a chronic locomotor dysfunction that continually exacerbates regardless of preventative measures requires management.

Manual methods can be applied as a preventative measure to locomotor disturbances, especially for the screening of joint and muscle dysfunctions in the young and for the management of chronic dysfunctions in older patients. Children and young adults need to be assessed less often than older patients. Children, once walking and through their school years, should be assessed every 6 to 12 months, after falls or lower extremity trauma necessitating casting, and more often if they are participating in vigorous sports.

Adults who receive periodic functional checkups and treatment of those dysfunctions found seem to report fewer symptoms and recurrences. This is optimized if the clinician reviews or revises previously recommended exercises and stimulates further commitment to a healthy lifestyle. The goal is for the clinician to treat less as function is maintained more by the patient.

The need for and frequency of continued management are determined by the presence of chronic dysfunctions, permanent structural damage, or congenital anomaly forcing compensatory adaptations in the locomotor system. These categories include physically disabled people in wheelchairs and those walking with a prosthetic limb who are experiencing continued dysfunction from postural, locomotor, or compensatory mechanisms. Repetitive abuse from vigorous sports activities, especially in collegiate, semiprofessional, and professional levels, creates a need for repetitive assessment and possibly treatment.

Chapter Review Questions

- Describe the acute, subacute, and chronic clinical categories as they relate to treatment.
- What is abnormal illness behavior?
- What associated dysfunctions are usually found in each of the abnormal movement patterns about the pelvic-hip region?

- Name three examples of dysfunctions in the pelvic-hip region that are commonly linked or associated.
- What is the difference between primary and secondary lesions?
- What is the significance of hypermobility?
- Discuss pelvic joint and muscle dysfunctions as they relate to children.
- Give an example of a pelvic somatovisceral reaction.

REFERENCES

1. Haldeman S, Chapman-Smith D, Petersen D. *Guidelines for Chiropractic Quality Assurance and Practice Parameters.* Gaithersburg, Md: Aspen Publishers, Inc; 1993.
2. Spitzer WO, LeBlanc FE, Dupuis M, et al. Scientific approach to the assessment and management of activity-related spinal disorders: a monograph for clinicians. Report of the Quebec Task Force on Spinal Disorders. *Spine.* 1987;12(suppl 7):S1–S59.
3. Frymoyer J. Back pain and sciatica. *N Engl J Med.* 1988;318:291–300.
4. Mayer T, Gatchel R. *Functional Restoration for Spinal Disorders: A Sports Medicine Approach.* Philadelphia, Pa: Lea & Febiger; 1988.
5. Vallfor B. Acute, subacute, and chronic low-back pain: clinical symptoms, absenteeism and working environment. *Scand J Rehabil Med.* 1985;11–97.
6. Brena S, Chapman SL. The learned pain syndrome. *Postgrad Med.* 1981;69:53–64.
7. Pilowsky I. A general classification of abnormal illness behavior. *Br J Med Psychiat.* 1979;51:131–137.
8. Bullock-Saxton JE, Janda V, Bulock MI. Reflex activation of gluteal muscles in walking. *Spine.* 1993;18:704–708.
9. Lewit K. *Manipulative Therapy in Rehabilitation of the Locomotor System.* 2nd ed. London: Butterworths; 1991.
10. Lewit K. Chain reactions in disturbed function of the motor system. *Manual Med.* 1987;3:27–29.
11. Gillet H, Liekens M. *Belgian Chiropractic Research Notes.* Huntington Beach, Calif: Motion Palpation Institute; 1984.
12. Schafer RC, Faye LJ. *Motion Palpation and Chiropractic Technic: Principles of Dynamic Chiropractic.* Huntington Beach, Calif: Motion Palpation Institute; 1989.
13. Grahame R. The hypermobility syndrome. *Ann Rheum Dis.* 1990;49:197–198.
14. Travell JG, Simons DG. *Myofascial Pain and Dysfunction: The Trigger Point Manual.* Vol 2. Baltimore, Md: Williams & Wilkins; 1992.
15. Imrie D, Barbuto L. *The Back Power Program.* Toronto: Stoddart; 1988.
16. Olsen TL, Anderson RL, Dearwater SR, et al. The epidemiology of low back pain in an adolescent population. *Am J Public Health.* 1992;82:606–608.
17. Balague T, Dutoit G, Waldburger M. Low back pain in school children: an epidemiological study. *Scand J Rehabil Med.* 1988;20:175–179.

18. Mierau DL, Cassidy JD, Hamin T, Milne RA. Sacroiliac joint dysfunction and low back pain in school aged children. *J Manipulative Physiol Ther.* 1984;7:81–84.

19. Eilert RE. Orthopedics. In: Kempe CH, Silver HK, O'Bren D, eds. *Current Pediatric Diagnosis and Treatment.* 6th ed. Los Altos, Calif: Lange Medical Publishers; 1980:534–556.

20. Ostgaard HC, Andersson GBJ. Previous back pain and risk of developing back pain in pregnancy. *Spine.* 1991;16:4;432–436.

21. LeBoeuf C, Brown P, Herman A, Leembruggen K, Walton D, Crisp TC. Chiropractic care of children with nocturnal enuresis: a prospective outcome study. *J Manipulative Physiol Ther.* 1991;14:110–115.

Chapter 11

Stretching and Exercise

Linda J. Levine

Chapter Objectives

- to discuss general aspects of stretching and exercising
- to describe passive stretching
- to describe dynamic range-of-motion stretching (DROM)
- to describe stabilization exercises

GENERAL ASPECTS OF STRETCHING

This chapter briefly discusses the various aspects of exercises and stretches that assist patients in becoming more effective and therefore more empowered in their own treatment. Joint manipulation serves as a powerful tool in restoring joint function and simultaneously influencing muscle tone. A joint exhibiting joint dysfunction needs to be manipulated first to restore arthrokinematics and offset unwanted arthrokinematic reflexes from occurring. Otherwise recovery can be delayed if exercise is started too early. However, the inexperienced practitioner must be careful not to become overly impressed with the powerful therapeutic effects of joint manipulation lest he or she be lured into thinking that manipulation is all that is needed in the care of joint and muscle dysfunctions. Attention must also be directed to assessing muscles for proper length and strength. From this an appropriate exercise regimen can be formulated. Exercise instruction is a must in the overall care of patients. In a review article on exercise and manipulation and their effects on low back pain, Twomey and Taylor[1] comment that the evidence for exercise in aiding low back pain patients is overwhelming. The relationship between joint and muscle function needs to be acknowledged and addressed when treating patients with locomotor disturbances.

Joint and muscle dysfunctions tend to recur if perpetuating factors are not addressed. Chronically shortened muscles and ligaments are factors that commonly perpetuate articular and muscular dysfunctions. Patients need to be taught stretches and exercises that prevent adaptive shortening, maintain muscle tone, and foster self-reliance. Weak and inhibited muscles also occur in reaction to overactive and tight muscles and need to be treated. To use joint manipulation without teaching patients how to care for themselves with exercise is self-defeating and invites the recurrence of dysfunction. People with joint and muscle dysfunction, especially those who lead a sedentary life or sit too much at work, have no choice but to exercise regularly to avoid continuing bouts of pain. Exercise instruction serves as a tool to enliven those muscles that have been deconditioned via sedentary lifestyles. It also encourages normal joint motion of the associated articulations. Additionally, the nervous system, through exercise, is being bombarded with afferent proprioceptive input while it is receiving a neurophysiologic reeducation. However, this assumes that poor movement patterns have been corrected.

In addition to specific joint and muscle stretches, patients should be encouraged to walk at least 30 minutes a day to include some level of locomotor activity in their lives. This applies especially to middle-aged and older individuals. An aerobic exercise program is a fine adjunct to overall conditioning. Exercising provides a patient with increased energy and vitality. It also elevates a patient's self-esteem and sense of well-being.

To treat muscle dysfunction effectively, patients must be taught stretching exercises for tight, hyperactive muscles and strengthening exercises for the weak, inhibited muscles. The strengthening exercises, in this sense, are actually reeducation or remedial exercises designed to "teach" the muscle to contract properly again. Muscles that have been shortened due to spasm and pain need to be shown that they can painlessly lengthen again and function normally. These muscles are anatomically intact and strong, yet function poorly due to persistent dysfunctional neuromuscular control from injury or maladaptive processes. They need to be reprogrammed on a neurophysiologic basis.

Remedial exercises assist in reprogramming proper movement for the muscle involved.[2] For example, a tight, overactive tensor fascia lata muscle will overpower and inhibit its neighboring glutei minimus and medius muscles, creating poor movement in abduction. The tight tensor fascia lata needs stretching first in order to release its neurologic reign over the glutei muscles. The weak, inhibited glutei muscles need to be selectively trained or reprogrammed to contract optimally again. Remedial exercises help achieve this. The patient is placed in the side-lying position to optimize good contractions and movement from the weak muscle. Gravity alone supplies enough resistance to work against. Sometimes patients with very weak abductors need assistance in just raising the leg. Proprioceptive input from the periphery can be used to facilitate the "learning" process. For example, pinching, scratching, or tapping the muscle involved recruits cortical awareness and facilitates contractions.

The patient needs to be aware of how the muscle is supposed to contract correctly, the wrong movements it performs, and how "cheating" movements come into play. Again in our example above, poor abduction due to weak, inhibited glutei minimus and medius muscles will cause the patient to recruit the tensor fascia lata by rolling the pelvis posterior when in the side-lying position. The patient needs to know that the pelvic rolling is maladaptive to poor hip abductor function. The pelvis should be rolled slightly more anterior than the neutral side-lying posture and stabilized while the patient abducts the leg and thigh. In addition, peripheral proprioceptive input is used to augment contraction. Teaching the patient to recruit and contract the weak muscles properly will aid in reeducating normal movements. Essentially, the patient must be retrained to feel the muscle contract and perform the correct movement. This is performed by the patient over several days or weeks until his or her nervous system "remembers" how to connect with a once-forgotten action.

Four types of exercises and stretches are discussed next: (1) passive stretching, (2) dynamic range-of-motion stretching (DROM), (3) stabilization exercises, and (4) proprioceptive exercises. Their goal is to aid in the effective lengthening of tight muscles and the strengthening of weak ones.

PASSIVE STRETCHING

Passive or static stretching can be used for home exercises to lengthen tight, shortened muscles. The passive static stretches simply place the muscle on stretch for a sustained period of time, usually 15 to 30 seconds or until the patient senses a release in tension. Focusing on breathing is important so that muscle relaxation is maximized on exhalation. No bouncing or ballistic movements should be involved. However, Vujnovich and Dawson[3] found that when ballistic stretching followed static stretching, the neurologic activity related to the muscle in question was decreased more than with static stretching alone. Murphy[4] makes a good argument against static stretching in favor of dynamic range-of-motion stretching, as discussed below. When using static stretching, care must be taken not to take the joint too far beyond its normal range of motion.

Three-Point Stretch

This is the most important versatile passive stretch for the pelvic and hip regions. It stretches the sacroiliac and hip joints and piriformis and gluteus medius muscles. It entails holding the hip joint in three positions (Figure 11–1). While sitting, the patient first pulls the knee up toward the same shoulder and holds it for 30 seconds. Next, a sitting Patrick-Fabere test position is assumed, and the knee is pressed toward the floor for 30 seconds. Finally, the hip is flexed and adducted strongly toward the opposite shoulder while the ankle remains crossed on the other knee. The three stretches are repeated on the other side and are performed once a day. If a

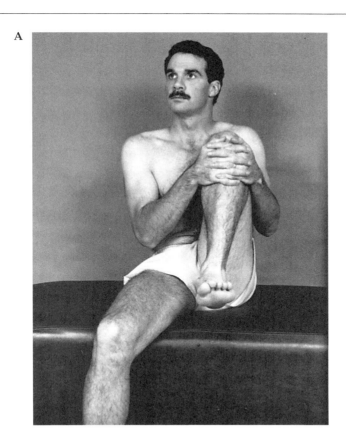

A

continues

Figure 11–1 (A, B, C) Three-Point Stretch

Figure 11–1 continued

B

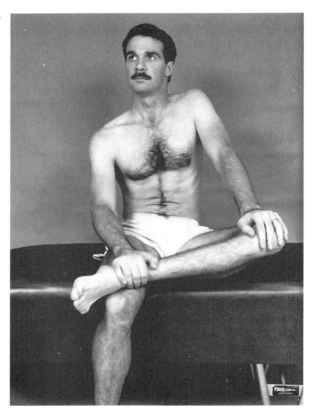

continues

person fails the chair test described in Chapter 10, improvement is usually seen after performing the three-point stretch if sacroiliac and hip joint stiffness are present. This clearly demonstrates to the patient the influence that stretching can have on good function.

Oriental Squat

This stretch is also good for the sacroiliac and hip joints. The person simply squats fully, with the shoulders sinking in between the knees, keeping the feet flat on the floor (Figure 11–2). Patients with stiff pelvic and hip joints will have difficulty performing this maneuver without holding a doorknob or other suitable support to steady themselves. It stretches

Figure 11–1 continued

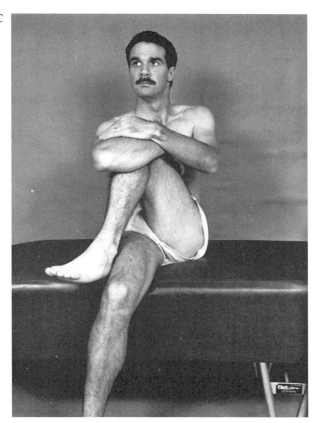

the lower part of the pelvis, lumbosacral spine, hamstrings, and gluteus maximus. It is a good stretch for women to perform during pregnancy and facilitates stretching the bottom of the pelvis for labor. It also aids venous return from the lower extremities back into the systemic circulation. It is a difficult stretch to perform for older patients and those with knee problems. In these instances it should be avoided.

Morning Star

This stretch imparts torque to the low back and pelvis and affects many structures. The limbs are placed so that the patient can stretch into four different quadrants. Too much torsional strain felt by the patient can be

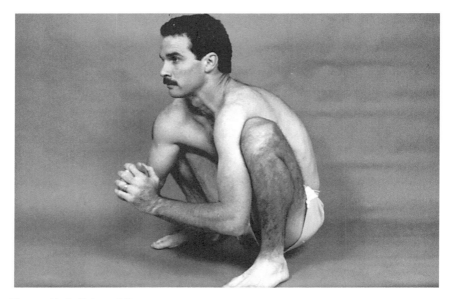

Figure 11–2 Oriental Squat

minimized by bending the crossed-over leg at the knee. The structures stretched on the uppermost side include the sacroiliac and hip joints, hip abductors, piriformis, and quadratus lumborum. Also affected are the lumbosacral and thoracolumbar regions. To facilitate stretching and relaxation, the patient inhales deeply and holds the breath for 10 seconds. While exhaling slowly, the patient relaxes and allows the uppermost leg and arm to stretch floorward (Figure 11–3). Additionally, the patient can try stretching each limb into the direction it points.

William's Flexion Exercises

These classic exercises are a good general stretch for the lumbar spine, pelvis, and hip. While the patient is supine, the knees are flexed onto the chest separately and held for 30 seconds each. Afterward they are flexed upon the chest simultaneously and held again for 30 seconds while a strong pelvic tilt is performed. This imparts a stretch to the lumbosacral joint and erector spinae group.

McKenzie Extension Exercises

These stretches assist in improving lumbar and hip extension. Patients can start off simply lying prone while supporting their upper bodies with

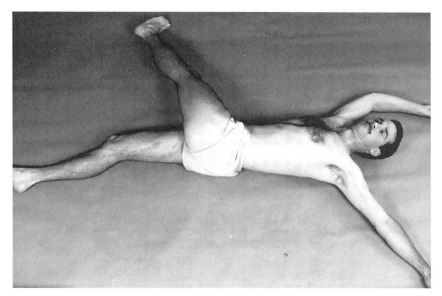

Figure 11–3 Morning Star

their elbows (Figure 11–4A). After 1 to 3 minutes of this, the hands are placed on the floor and a push-up is attempted from the waist up until the arms can lock at the elbows (Figure 11–4B). The buttocks, thighs, and legs remain relaxed. The patient exhales and relaxes the spine and hips, allowing them to sag off the extended arms. Once the spine is felt to sag fully, or near fully, the person returns the upper body to the floor and repeats the stretch. A goal of 10 push-ups at least twice a day is set. This is a good stretch to recommend to patients who sit extensively during the day. If leg pain or pain radiating from the back into the leg is experienced during this exercise, then it is to be stopped. The reader is referred to McKenzie's work for further elaboration.[5]

Adductors

The small adductors are stretched while the patient lies supine, knees bent and abducted outward, with the soles of the feet touching (Figure 11–5A). To stretch the long adductors passively, the patient lies supine with the buttocks and straight legs resting against a wall. Using gravity as an assist, the patient allows the straight legs to spread by sliding along the wall to impart a comfortable stretch. The hip adductors can also be stretched standing. With the feet wide apart, the patient sways to one side,

A

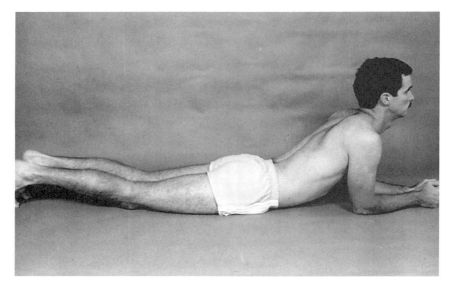

B

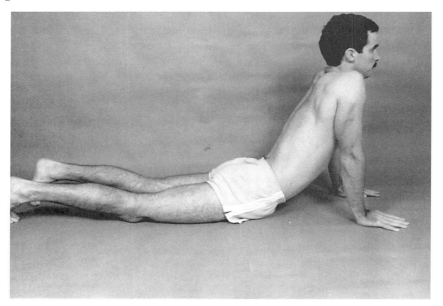

Figure 11–4 (A) Mild extension stretch. **(B)** Full extension stretch.

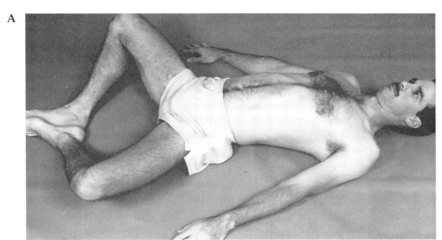

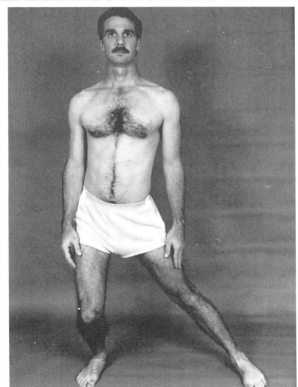

Figure 11–5 (A) Passive stretch for the short hip adductors. **(B)** Passive stretch for long hip adductors.

keeping the pelvis level. A stretch is imparted on the side away from which the pelvic sway occurs (Figure 11–5B).

Iliopsoas

While supine, the patient flexes one thigh against the chest while the other leg is lowered off the foot-end of a bed (Figure 11–6). This essentially is the modified Thomas test reproduced. In the illustration provided, the person is lowering his leg off the side of the couch, which tends to place the person off balance. Lying squarely on the bed while lowering the leg off the foot-end feels more secure. Another way to stretch the iliopsoas muscle passively is to place a foot up on a high stool while the weight-bearing thigh and leg remain extended backward (Figure 11–7). The iliopsoas can also be stretched by assuming a "squat-thrust" or lunge position (Figure 11–8). The side being stretched is extended backward.

Quadratus Lumborum

This muscle can be passively stretched by having the patient prop the torso up on a bent elbow or straight arm while side lying (Figure 11–9).

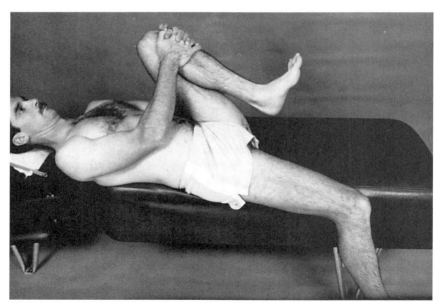

Figure 11–6 Supine Hip Flexor Stretch

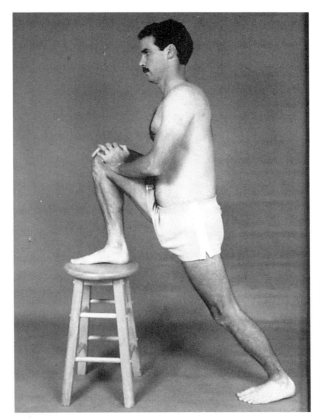

Figure 11–7 Standing Hip Flexor Stretch

The uppermost leg rests on the floor in front of the lowermost leg. The pelvis can be rotated forward or backward to localize the stretch to different parts of the quadratus lumborum. Another stretch can be performed by standing and side-bending away from the tight quadratus lumborum muscle (Figure 11–10). This position can be held statically, or post-isometric relaxation can be used, as discussed in Chapter 9 in the section "Quadratus Lumborum."

Hip Abductors

These muscles are stretched passively in the side-lying posture by having patients lower the uppermost leg and thigh behind them off a couch or

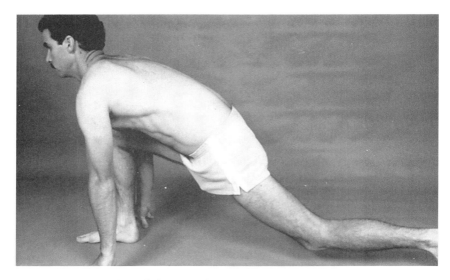

Figure 11–8 Lunge Stretch for Hip Flexors

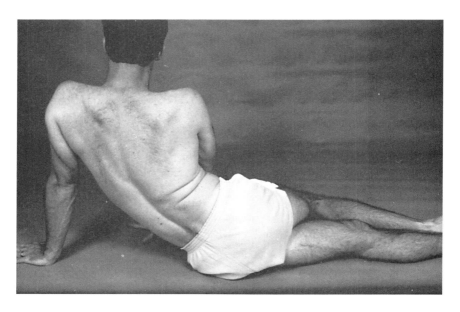

Figure 11–9 Passive Side-Lying Stretch for Quadratus Lumborum

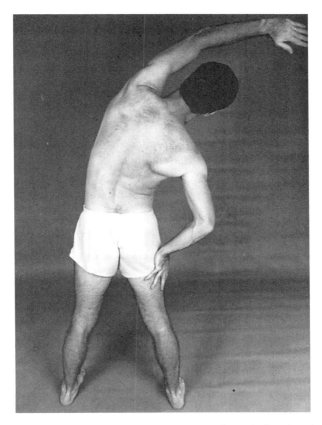

Figure 11–10 Standing Postisometric Relaxation Stretch for Quadratus Lumborum

bed (Figure 11–11). This can be repeated with the leg lowered off the couch in front of the body.

Quadriceps

While standing, the patient brings the heel up to the buttock and extends the thigh straight back, not out to the side (Figure 11–12). Thigh extension should be provided mostly by gluteus maximus contraction. The other hand should hold onto a suitable support for stability. This stretch can also be performed while side lying, with the upper leg being the one stretched as in the standing stretch.

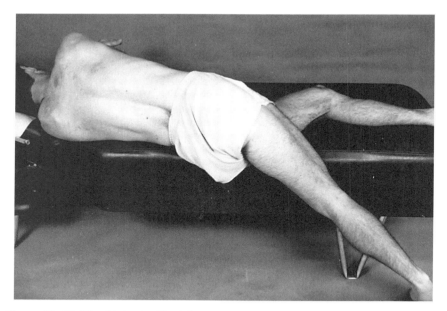

Figure 11–11 Hip Abductor Stretch

Gastrocnemius and Soleus Muscles

The gastrocnemius and soleus muscles are important to consider because of the effect of their shortening on gait and joint dynamics of the lower extremity and pelvis. To stretch the gastrocnemius, the patient leans against a wall and extends the straight leg backward while pressing the heel onto the floor (Figure 11–13A). To stretch the soleus muscle, the same position is assumed but the backward placed knee is bent to relax the gastrocnemius muscle (Figure 11–13B). The bent knee is pressed floorward while the heel remains on the floor.

Iliotibial Band

To stretch the iliotibial band, the patient first stands about 2 ft away from a wall (Figure 11–14). The side to be stretched is nearest the wall. The other leg is crossed over in front of the leg to be stretched, and the patient sways the pelvis toward the wall, keeping it level. The trunk should remain vertical, yet a strong adduction force is applied to the hip region, thus stretching the iliotibial band.

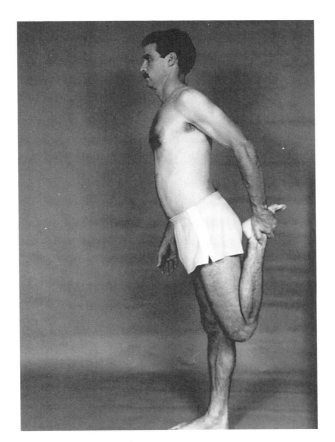

Figure 11–12 Quadriceps Stretch

DYNAMIC RANGE-OF-MOTION STRETCHING

Active facilitative or dynamic range-of-motion (DROM) stretching involves contracting a muscle's antagonist while the associated joint is moved through its full functional range of motion.[4,6] DROM emphasizes slow, controlled movements, allowing the muscle being stretched to be lengthened physiologically. This type of stretching accomplishes two things. First, the antagonist's active contraction supplies a mechanical force that stretches the agonist muscle. Second, the antagonist, via its own contraction, reflexly inhibits and further relaxes the agonist through the process of reciprocal inhibition. The beauty of DROM is that the patient is able to lengthen the muscle while it is simultaneously being reciprocally inhibited. In addition, the joint motion induced is maintained within a physiologic range. In comparison, static or passive stretching has the potential for stretching joints and muscles beyond their physiologic range of motion, thus inviting injury. Also, reciprocal inhibition is not operant during passive stretching.

The following stretch is an example of a DROM exercise. To stretch the hamstrings effectively, the person should lie supine with the hip and knee flexed while both hands support the knee from behind (Figure 11–15A). The quadriceps muscle is contracted and the leg is straightened until the knee locks into extension (Figure 11–15B). If the knee cannot lock into ex-

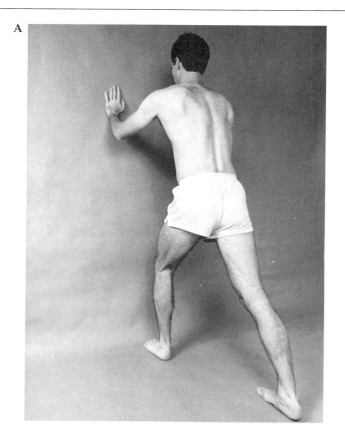

A

continues

Figure 11–13 (A) Gastrocnemius stretch. **(B)** Soleus stretch.

Figure 11–13 continued

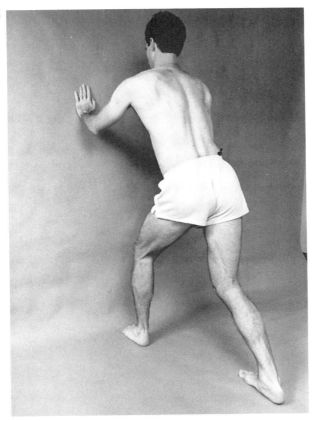

tension because of very tight hamstrings, the thigh should be lowered just until this can occur. The straight-leg position is held for 4 to 5 seconds and then relaxed by flexing the knee. The thigh is then raised slightly more, and active extension of the knee is attempted again to stretch the hamstrings. This is performed three to five times.

Hip Muscle Exercises

Patients with hip and sacroiliac joint dysfunction often exhibit weakness in the muscles about the hip joint, especially the abductors, adductors, and gluteus maximus. The following exercises should be routinely given for

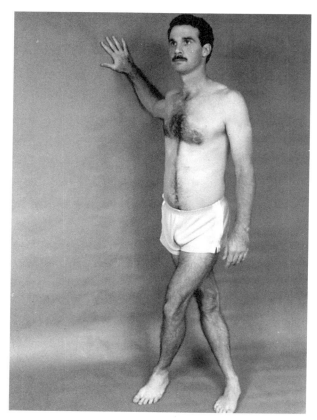

Figure 11–14 Tensor Fascia Lata and Iliotibial Band Stretch

these patients. The hip abductors and gluteus maximus muscles are often inhibited, and their tight, overactive antagonists must be stretched first. Quite often, just the weight of the lower extremity provides enough resistance to exercise with. However, ankle weights can be used for added resistance. Slow, steady contractions should be performed. With a DROM procedure, the contracting muscle is strengthened while its antagonist is stretched. Initially, the patient must be taught proper technique of contraction with close supervision. Afterward, the patient is made aware of his or her responsibility to continue the exercise at home on a regular basis.

Hip Rotation

While supine, the patient raises the straight leg off the floor about 6 inches, strongly internally rotates the entire leg at the hip, and holds it for

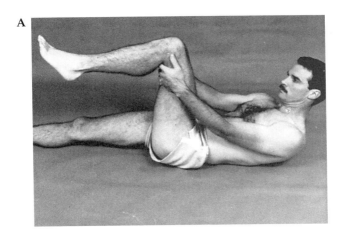

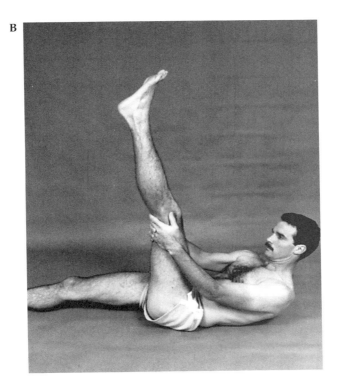

Figure 11–15 (A) Hamstring dynamic range-of-motion stretch, starting position.
(B) Stretched position.

4 to 5 seconds (Figure 11–16). This induces a strong active contraction of the internal hip rotators, thus facilitating them, and it reciprocally inhibits the external rotators, thus lengthening them. Afterward, the entire leg is externally rotated, and the process is reversed (Figure 11–17). This exercise can also be performed supine, with the hip and knee flexed to 90 degrees while the hip is rotated internally and externally. This also serves as a self-mobilization technique for hip rotation.

Hip Abduction

While the patient is side lying, the uppermost leg and thigh are kept straight in line with the trunk and raised about 45 degrees, held for 4 to 5

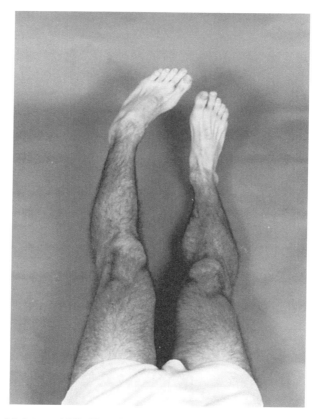

Figure 11–16 Internal Hip Rotation Using DROM, Legs Extended

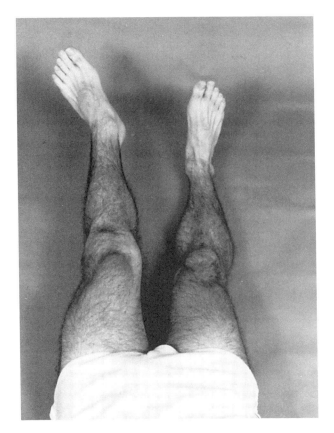

Figure 11–17 External Hip Rotation Using DROM, Legs Extended

seconds, and lowered slowly (Figure 11–18). This exercise places the adductors on active stretch while reciprocally inhibiting them. The bottom leg is flexed at the knee to provide support. The leg should be raised smoothly and in a straight line of abduction. "Cheating" occurs if the leg externally rotates at the hip and the pelvis rolls posteriorly, allowing recruitment of the tensor fascia lata. This also occurs if the leg is raised too high. It is amazing how weak these muscles can be. At times, just the weight of the leg and thigh lifted against gravity entails much effort. Proper movement must be performed. This exercise can also be performed standing by supporting the upright posture when abducting the straight leg.

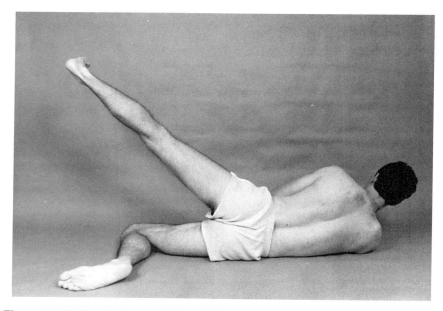

Figure 11–18 Hip Abduction Using DROM

Hip Adduction

While lying on the same side as above, the patient flexes the uppermost leg to place the foot in front of the lowermost knee. The lowermost leg is kept straight and raised as far as it can be (Figure 11–19). This will normally only be several inches. The end position is held for 4 to 5 seconds and slowly lowered. This is performed three to five times. This exercise simultaneously stretches the abductors slightly. A padded surface should be used to lie on to eliminate painful weight bearing at the greater trochanter. The person then lies on the other side and repeats the above two exercises.

Hip Extension

The gluteus maximus is exercised in the prone position, with the knee flexed, foot dorsiflexed, and thigh slightly externally rotated. The thigh is lifted off the floor, not the pelvis, and it is held for 4 to 5 seconds in maximal hip extension (Figure 11–20). This is performed three to five times. The hamstring muscle may cramp due to its being held in a shortened position. Hamstring stretching just prior to this exercise helps alleviate this. If not,

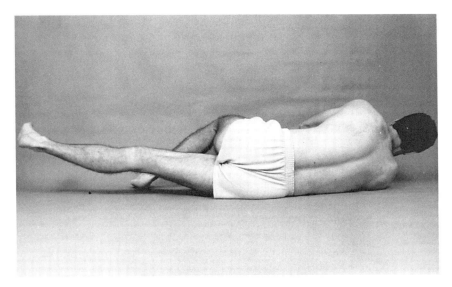

Figure 11–19 Hip Adduction Using DROM

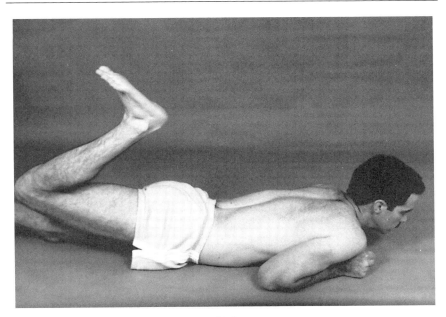

Figure 11–20 Hip Extension Using DROM

the amount of knee flexion held should be reduced. This exercise simultaneously actively stretches the quadriceps and psoas muscles.

Abdominal Crunches

To tone the abdominal muscles, one should place the hip flexors at a disadvantage by flexing the thigh. Any tightness in the psoas and erector spinae muscles must first be addressed. In addition, the feet should not be hooked under any support surface, or the hip flexors will become facilitated. With the patient supine, the legs are bent and spread apart at the knees, with the soles of the feet touching (Figure 11–21). The hands are placed at the sides without touching the floor or being crossed in front of the chest. A chin tuck and pelvic tilt are performed, and the neck and thorax are rolled up until the scapulae come off the floor. The position is held for 4 to 5 seconds and slowly released by unrolling the torso and neck. This maneuver exercises the rectus abdominis and stretches the erector spinae.

To exercise the obliques, the patient is instructed to do as above except that upon raising the torso, one raises the left shoulder toward the right knee and vice versa. At all times, the legs should remain relaxed and

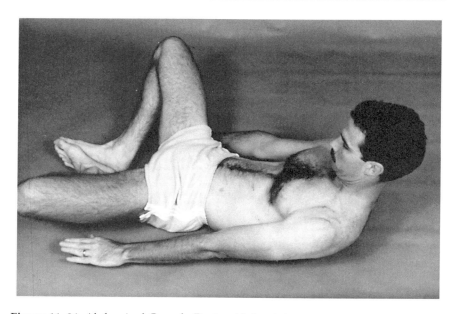

Figure 11–21 Abdominal Crunch, Rectus Abdominis

spread apart. To contract the lower abdominals, one flexes both knees onto the chest and performs a strong pelvic tilt to lift the pelvis off the floor (Figure 11–22). This position is held for 4 to 5 seconds and repeated.

STABILIZATION EXERCISES

Stabilization exercise regimens involve teaching patients the importance of using what is called the "functional range."[7-9] This is the pain-free and biomechanically correct "neutral" position that the lumbopelvic region should assume when performing exercises so as to lessen injury potential. The functional range may be different depending on the task the patient is asked to perform or the position in which it is to be performed. Identifying the functional range is important and depends on ascertaining which movements or positions provoke or relieve symptoms. Evidence for this will usually be found in the history as well as the examination. Static and dynamic loading intolerances as well as weight-bearing and non–weight-bearing difficulties should be assessed.

The functional range concept applies particularly to the lumbopelvic region, allowing the lumbar spine and pelvis to be exercised in a position

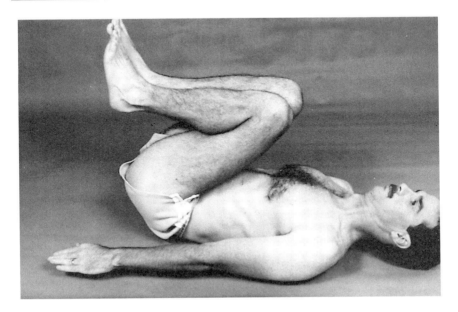

Figure 11–22 Abdominal Crunch, Lower Abdominals

of pain-free stability. Positions that abnormally load the joints and muscles at end range are to be avoided. *End range* pertains to articulations taken to their end range of motion, thus stressing the capsuloligamentous structures. The posterior pelvic tilt offers an excellent strategy for developing the functional range in the lumbopelvic region. Exercises done while a posterior pelvic tilt is maintained will afford a good level of safety for the patient. By maintaining the lumbar spine in the neutral zone or functional range, end-range loading is prevented along with any strain to the associated capsuloligamentous structures. Patients can then be taught to use this functional range when performing activities of daily living, such as vacuuming, gardening, washing dishes, and carrying groceries.

The basis of stabilization exercises is to train patients into seeking and maintaining their neutral zone or functional range while performing exercises or movements or sustaining certain postures. If patients can experience and know when and how to use their functional range, they can prevent injury. This is particularly important for patients who are experiencing pain. As long as they use a pain-free functional range, they will be able to exercise and become active in their own care.

Learning to use a functional range is a psychomotor skill that requires developing a kinesthetic awareness of the position and repetition of its application. The goals of stabilization exercises are for patients to become kinesthetically aware of their functional range and to exercise to muscle fatigue to achieve a training effect. However, emphasis should be placed upon qualitative versus quantitative performance of the exercise. Examples of this type of training are variations of the pelvic tilt and bridges.

Posterior Pelvic Tilt

The posterior pelvic tilt (PPT) is used as a foundation to which trunk and extremity movements can be added for increasing the exercise's difficulty. The PPT aids in training abdominal strength and control. The PPT places the lumbar spine in a safe neutral or stabilization range, and no pain should be experienced. If the PPT is lost during the exercise, low back pain can result either during or after the exercise is performed.

The PPT is performed supine, with the knees bent and feet flat on the floor. This is the original or starting position (Figure 11–23). The arms are placed at the patient's sides. The patient is instructed to tighten the abdominal muscles and flatten the lower back against the floor or against the clinician's monitoring hand placed underneath the lumbar lordosis. Facilitation can be supplied by the clinician in the form of scratching the abdominal muscles, verbally coaching the proper motion ("Flatten your

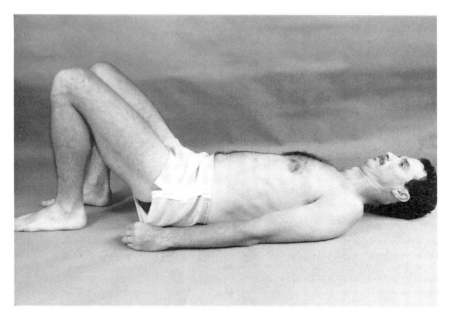

Figure 11–23 Posterior Pelvic Tilt Starting Position

lower back against my hand," or "Roll your tailbone off the floor"), or making the patient aware of the monitoring hand under the lumbar spine by moving the fingers slightly. The clinician may even have to pre-position the pelvis in a PPT position to make the patient more aware of the desired movement.

Once the PPT is attained, the patient is instructed to hold this position for as long as he or she can, with 90 seconds being the target maximum. Lumbar joint mobilization and erector spinae lengthening may have to be done first to allow ease in performing the PPT. Once the patient can hold a strong and sustained PPT, variations of it are added to make it more difficult to hold. All the while, the patient is asked to maintain a strong PPT. For instance, the patient can lie supine with the legs fully extended while trying to hold a PPT for 90 seconds (Figure 11–24). The next level of difficulty would be to ask the patient to raise one arm overhead (Figure 11–25A). Both arms are then tried (Figure 11–25B).

To further increase the level of difficulty, while performing a PPT, the patient is asked to raise one knee to the chest without using the arms to pull it up (Figure 11–26). The foot is then slowly lowered to the table, as in

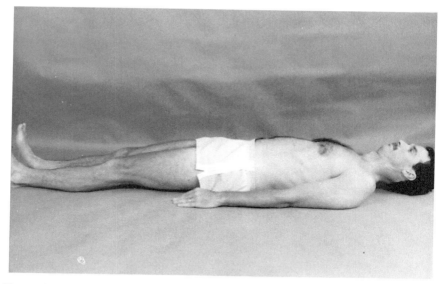

Figure 11–24 Posterior Pelvic Tilt with Legs Fully Extended

the original starting tilt position above. The other knee is raised, and the process is continued for as long as the patient can hold the PPT.

The next level of difficulty involves raising the knee as above while raising the opposite arm overhead (Figure 11–27). More difficult than this would be lowering the leg to a straightened position without resting it on the floor (Figure 11–28). The combination of simultaneously lowering the leg and raising the opposite arm is even more difficult. Arm and ankle weights can be used to enhance difficulty further.

Each level of difficulty is progressed through to see at which one the patient is unable to perform and hold a good PPT. The critical thing to ensure is that the PPT is held throughout the exercise. The patient should then use the next difficulty level that is before this break point. The idea is to bring the patient to the level of difficulty of pelvic tilting at which the muscles are brought to fatigue. The goal is to hold the tilt for up to 90 seconds. Repetitions can be used to aid in training and allow a progression to the next level of difficulty. Each repetition can be held for 5 seconds and repeated 10 to 12 times. Postexercise soreness in the abdominal region should be experienced the following day, but not lower back pain. If low back pain is felt, most likely the PPT is being done incorrectly, or the PPT position is probably being lost during the exercise and the patient is not

A

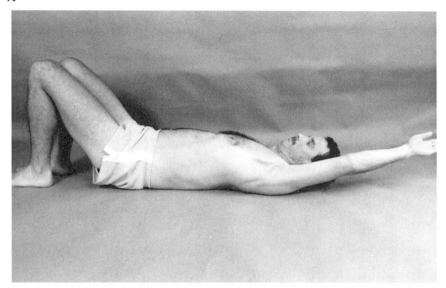

B

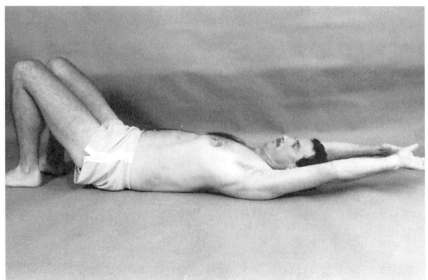

Figure 11–25 (A) Posterior pelvic tilt with one arm overhead. **(B)** Two arms overhead.

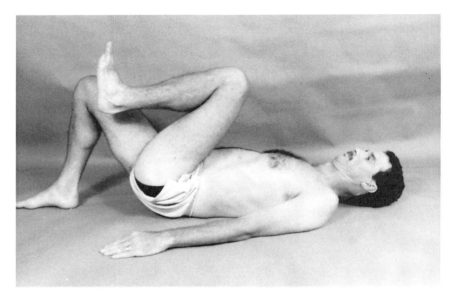

Figure 11–26 Posterior Pelvic Tilt with Hip Flexion

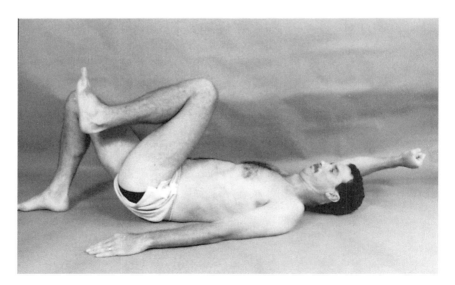

Figure 11–27 Posterior Pelvic Tilt with Hip Flexion and Opposite-Arm Raising

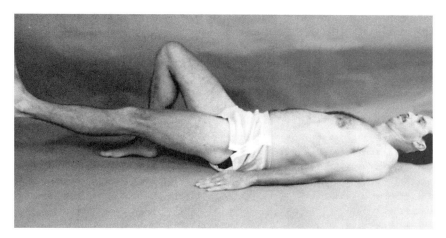

Figure 11–28 Posterior Pelvic Tilt with Straight Leg Held off the Floor

aware of it. Patients should be monitored periodically to ensure proper technique.

Bridge

A bridge exercise is performed while supine by doing a PPT and lifting the buttocks off the floor with gluteal contractions (Figure 11–29). The spine is lifted off the floor one segment at a time from below upward. It is maintained as long as the patient can maintain it, and it can be made progressively more difficult with variations added to it. At no time should pain be experienced. If it is, poor technique is indicated. This exercise is good for training hip extension strength and control.

The first variation involves maintaining a bridged position while raising each heel alternately but leaving the forefoot on the floor (Figure 11–30). This facilitates gluteus maximus contraction. The next level of difficulty entails doing a one-legged bridge, thus making the support-side gluteus medius work more (Figure 11–31A). During one-legged support, the pelvis should remain level. Typically, the pelvis will drop on the unsupported side, indicating weakness in the hip abductors on the weight-bearing side (Figure 11–31B). This should be corrected by bringing it to the patient's awareness and facilitating proper form with positioning or tactile stimulation. One can make the one-legged bridge even more difficult by slowly lowering and raising the legs alternately. Abducting the straight leg while holding a level pelvis will add further difficulty (Figure 11–32).

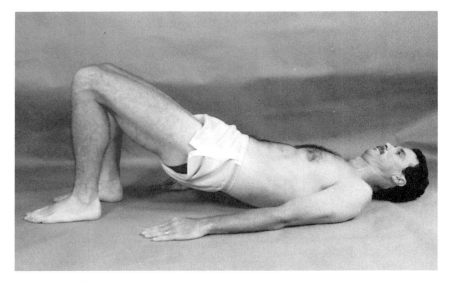

Figure 11–29 Bridge

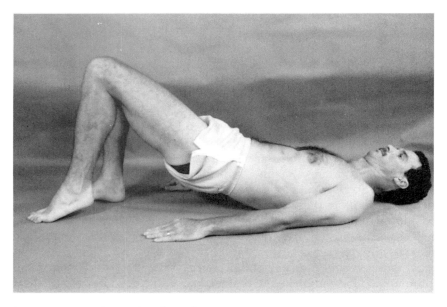

Figure 11–30 Bridge with Left Heel Raised

A

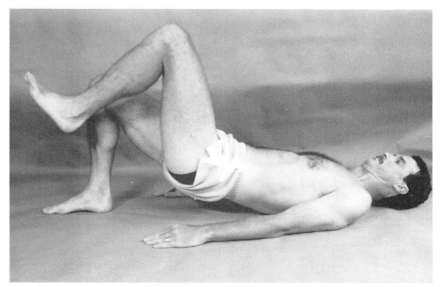

B

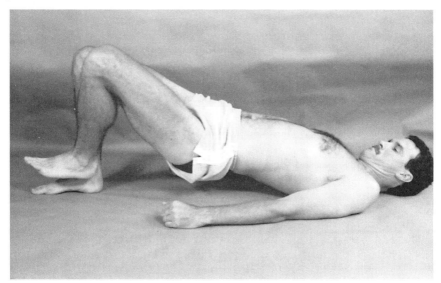

Figure 11–31 **(A)** One-legged bridge. **(B)** Note pelvis dropping on the left.

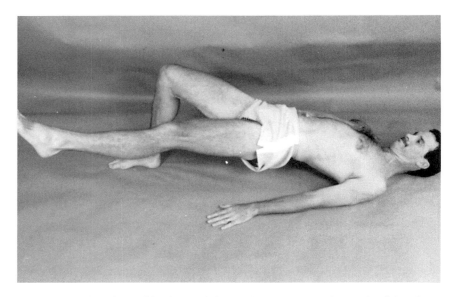

Figure 11–32 One-legged bridge with leg abducted. Due to the angle of the photograph, the left pelvis appears to be inappropriately dropping down.

Again, each level is performed while holding a good bridge position, which includes a PPT. The level at which the patient cannot hold a good position is noted, and the patient is exercised at the next lower level. Contraction times should approach 1½ to 2 minutes. The muscles should become fatigued. Repetitions can be used, with each bridge position held for 5 seconds. Cramping of the hamstrings may occur and indicates the need for their stretching or for positioning the heels further away from the buttocks. Difficulty in performing bridges indicates the need to search for tight tensor fascia lata, quadratus lumborum, piriformis, or hip abductor muscles and dysfunctional hip, lumbar, and sacroiliac joints.

Dead Bug

The dead bug position is held to train abdominal strength and control. A PPT is held as the hips and knees are flexed to 90 degrees and both arms are held upright (Figure 11–33). Difficulty holding this position can be eased by flexing both hips slightly more. To increase the difficulty of this exercise, one can raise the arms alternately overhead (Figure 11–34) or si-

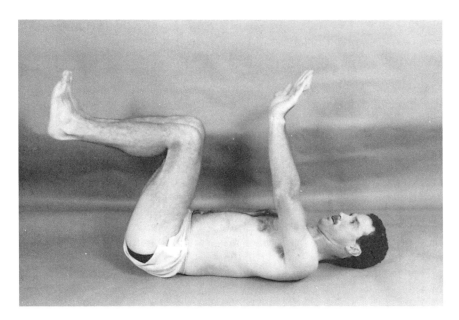

Figure 11–33 Dead Bug Position

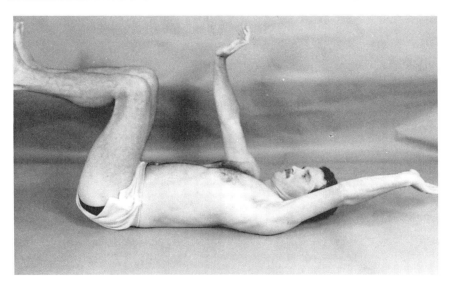

Figure 11–34 Dead Bug Position with Arm Raising Added

multaneously (Figure 11–35) while maintaining the pelvic tilt and leg positions. Further progression would entail lowering the legs alternately (Figure 11–36) by themselves or in combination with raising the arms overhead (Figure 11–37). Again, throughout the exercise, the PPT must be maintained. The leg and arm positions can be held statically or moved rhythmically into and out of their positions.

Gym Balls

A large gym ball can be used to exercise and challenge the neuromuscular system. Exercises such as the pelvic tilt, abdominal crunches, bridges, and spinal stretches can be employed with the ball. The patient is taught to maintain balance on the ball while performing the exercises smoothly. Figures 11-38 through 11-43 demonstrate some exercise positions that can be used effectively. These positions can be statically held or used with repetitions. Again, the goal is to fatigue the muscle to a "burn" without causing pain and all the while maintaining a functional range and proper technique.

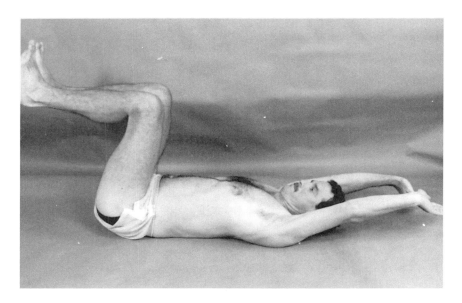

Figure 11–35 Dead Bug Position with Two Arms Overhead

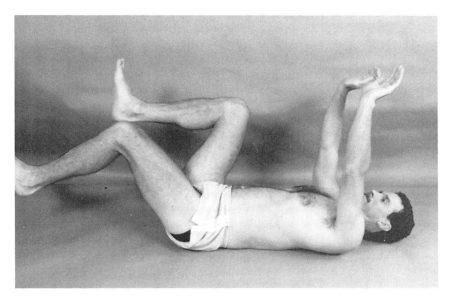

Figure 11–36 Dead Bug Position with Leg Lowering Added

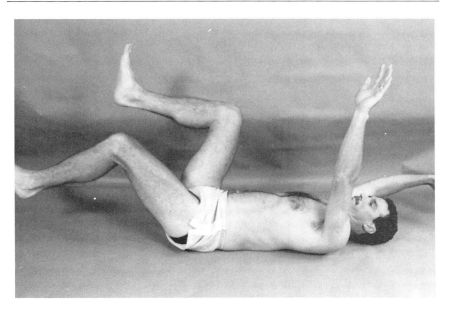

Figure 11–37 Simultaneous Arm Raising and Leg Lowering

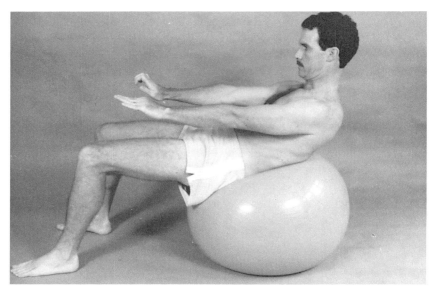

Figure 11–38 Ball Exercises with Pelvic Tilting and Abdominal Crunches

A

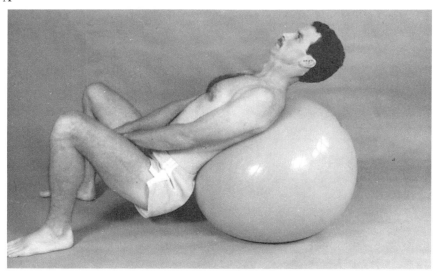

continues

Figure 11–39 **(A)** Squat position, getting ready for transition to **(B)** bridged position. Pelvic tilt is held throughout.

Figure 11–39 continued

B

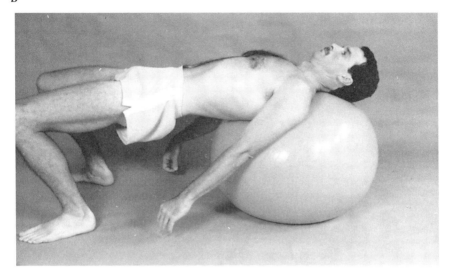

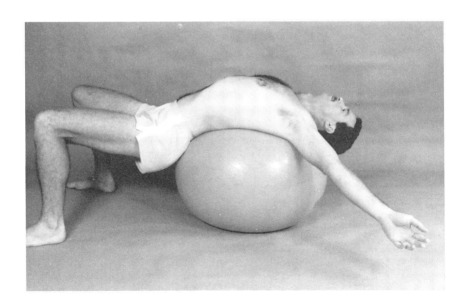

Figure 11–40 Spinal Extension Stretch

A

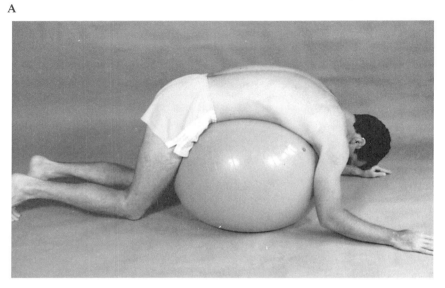

B

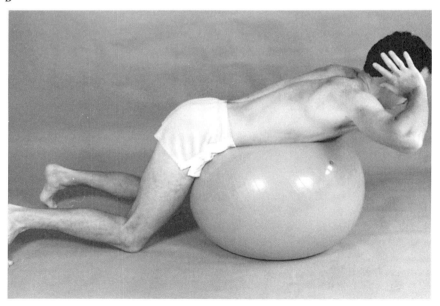

Figure 11–41 (A) Spinal flexion stretch. **(B)** Extension exercises. Feet should be placed against a wall for stability.

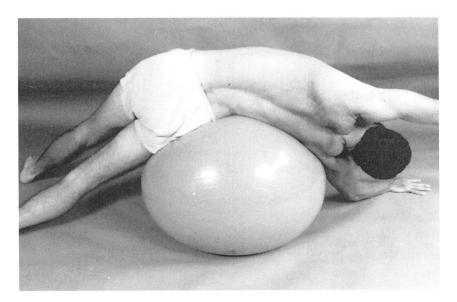

Figure 11–42 Side Stretch

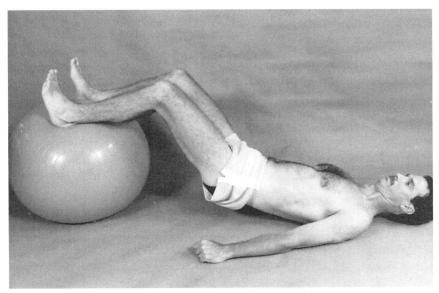

Figure 11–43 Hamstring bridge. Ball can be rolled toward patient.

PROPRIOCEPTIVE EXERCISES

Proprioceptive input from the peripheral joints and muscles can be enhanced to train central pathways and improve activation times and coordination.[10] Bullock-Saxton et al[10] found that reflex activation of the gluteal muscles was achieved by using "balance shoes" that stimulated the proprioceptive mechanisms during walking. Simple balancing strategies can be used by patients to facilitate the cerebellovestibular regulatory pathways to improve muscle activation and coordination. This can lead to improved posture and better neuromuscular control. Freeman[11] used a similar approach in the rehabilitation of sprained ankles. Labile surfaces like balance boards or wobble boards, balance shoes, and one-legged stance exercises can be used to train subconsciously the activity and coordination of postural muscles through sensorimotor stimulation. It is easy and can be fun for the patient to perform balance board or other labile surface exercises for 15 minutes a day. Patients are instructed to use only ankle and leg motions to maintain their balance and not trunk motions occurring at the waist.

Rocker boards or wobble boards can be purchased at various suppliers. Rocker boards allow tilting to occur in one plane and are therefore called uniplanar labile surfaces. With a little time and minimal investment, homemade devices can be made and used as labile surfaces. A broomstick cut to 18 inches or some other similar dowel-like item can be placed under an 18 x 18-inch board. The board should be grooved to hold the dowel in place. This allows tilting to be performed in one plane of motion. Patients can alter their foot position on the board to challenge different axes of balancing motion, ie, anteroposterior tilting, lateral tilting, and diagonal tilting. Tilting exercises can be performed with eyes open or closed. Eye closure removes visual balancing cues and places more of a burden on vestibular and proprioceptive systems. For multiplanar balancing, a hemispherical structure can be attached to a wooden board. A wooden bocci ball can be cut in half and screwed to the bottom of a board. This affords multiple planes of tilting motion in which the proprioceptive system is challenged.

One-legged stance can also be used to train coordination and balance (Figure 11–44). The patient should look straight ahead and not down. The eyes can be open or closed. The patient should attempt to stand as stable as possible for 20 to 30 seconds without wavering too much or losing balance.

MISCELLANEOUS STRETCHES

Coccyx

The postisometric stretch of the gluteus maximus for coccydynia reflexly relaxes the levator ani and subsequently reduces tension in it associ-

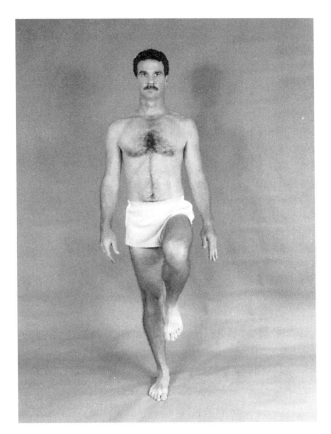

Figure 11–44 One-Legged Stance

ated with a painful coccyx. The stretch can be taught to the patient for use at home and is explained and illustrated in Chapter 6, Figure 6-34B.

Pelvic Floor Muscles

Active isometric contraction of the pelvic floor muscles can be performed to increase tone, especially in women after childbirth. They are called Kegel exercises and entail active contraction of the pelvic floor muscles as if urination or defecation were to be stopped and held back. Women with stress incontinence should perform three sets of 10 to 12 contractions three times a day. Each contraction is held strongly for 3 seconds. Younger women fare much better with these exercises, demonstrating improved urinary control after a period of several weeks. Older patients usually gain only minimal benefit.

Chapter Review Questions

- Why is joint manipulation not enough in the care of musculoskeletal conditions?
- What are remedial exercises?
- What is passive stretching?
- What is dynamic range-of-motion stretching?
- What is the difference between DROM and passive stretching?
- What is a criticism of passive stretching?
- What are stabilization exercises?
- What is the "functional range"?
- How do proprioceptive exercises work?

REFERENCES

1. Twomey L, Taylor J. Exercise and spinal manipulation in the treatment of low back pain. *Spine*. 1995;20:615–619.
2. Lewit K. *Manipulative Therapy in Rehabilitation of the Locomotor System*. 2nd ed. London: Butterworths; 1991.
3. Vujnovich AL, Dawson NJ. The effect of therapeutic muscle stretch on neural processing. *J Orthop Sports Phys Ther*. 1994;20:145–153.
4. Murphy D. Dynamic range of motion training: an alternative to static stretching. *Chiro Sports Med*. 1994;8:59–66.
5. McKenzie RA. *The Lumbar Spine: Mechanical Diagnosis and Therapy*. Waikane, New Zealand: Spinal Publications; 1981.
6. Dominguez RH, Gajda R. *Total Body Training*. New York, NY: Warner Books; 1982.
7. Saal JA, Saal JS. Nonoperative treatment of herniated lumbar intervertebral disc with radiculopathy: an outcome study. *Spine*. 1989;14:431–437.
8. Saal JA. Dynamic muscular stabilization in the nonoperative treatment of lumbar pain syndromes. *Ortho Rev*. 1990;19:691–700.
9. Morgan D. Concepts in functional training and postural stabilization for the low-back-injured. *Top Acute Care Trauma Rehabil*. 1988;2:8–17.
10. Bullock-Saxton JE, Janda V, Bulock MI. Reflex activation of gluteal muscles in walking. *Spine*. 1993;18:704–708.
11. Freeman MAR. Co-ordination exercises in the treatment of functional instability of the foot. *Phys Ther*. 1964;44:393–395.

Appendix A

Case Follow-Ups

CASES

CASE 1: SACROILIAC PAIN

History

A 34-year-old woman, 3 months postpartum, presented with severe "hip" and leg pain of 3 weeks' duration after she attempted to move a refrigerator in order to sweep behind it. She said that in so doing, she twisted her trunk and felt a "catch" (here she pointed to her sacroiliac joint region). The pain was sharp, localized to the left sacroiliac joint and buttock with occasional radiation into the proximal posterior thigh (Figure A–1). Trunk bending and twisting to the left hurt her. Walking and climbing stairs were difficult, since any weight bearing caused jabs of pain to be experienced. The act of arising from a chair was most difficult, although

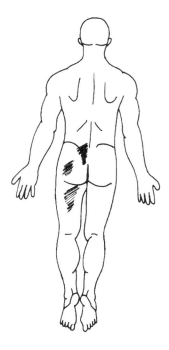

Figure A–1 Case 1: Sacroiliac Pain

---

sitting itself was not. She was able to sleep at night, but at times she would experience her pain upon turning over in bed. Flexing her left knee upon her chest seemed to alleviate the pain for a short period of time. She felt limited in her ability to do normal housework without pain. In the last few days before clinical presentation, she had noticed her entire left leg feeling "heavy" and her calf region feeling sore. She denied any bowel or bladder problems, although she admitted to moderate exacerbation of her pain upon performing a bowel movement.

Examination

- Trunk range of motion was full but painful in flexion and left bending.
- Left PSIS and SI joint line were tender.
- There were left glutei medius and minimus trigger points.
- Left Yeoman's and Gaenslen's tests were painful.
- Sacral apex test was painful and showed lateralizing to the left SIJ.

- Gillet's test showed restricted upper and lower SIJ poles in both flexion and extension.
- Lumbar joint play and range of motion were normal.
- Motor and sensory reflexes were normal.
- X-ray was normal.

Diagnosis

Left SIJ dysfunction with gluteal myofascitis.

Treatment

Visit 1: Ice applications to painful SIJ. Side-lying SIJ manipulation to both upper and lower aspects, using flexion and extension techniques.

Visit 2: Patient felt 70% better. Still achy into leg. Myofascial stretching of gluteals, using postisometric relaxation (PR) and ischemic compression. SIJ manipulation.

Visit 3: Patient felt much improved. SIJ manipulation. Three-point stretching and hip exercises given. Daily walking program.

Case Commentary

This is a straightforward SIJ problem. Provocative testing was positive on examination, and manipulation to the joint greatly improved her condition, thus aiding in the diagnosis. Gluteal trigger points were found; these are very common with SIJ lesions, especially in the gluteus minimus.

CASE 2: "BLADDER INFECTION" AND GROIN PAIN IN A HOCKEY PLAYER

History

A 21-year-old hockey goalie presented with what he called a bladder infection and right groin pain when, after attempting to block a puck with his right leg, he slipped and hyperabducted his thigh. He felt pain in what he described as below his bladder area (Figure A–2) making him think he had a bladder infection. Several hours later, he experienced an achy pain extending into the proximal medial thighs. He found it difficult to walk upstairs and lie on his abdomen. Putting one shoe on at a time by crossing his leg in a sign-of-four position hurt him. Lying on his back and keeping

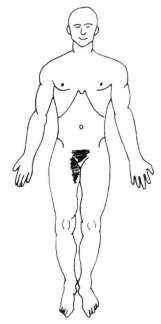

Figure A–2 Case 2: "Bladder Infection" and Groin Pain in a Hockey Player

---

his thighs adducted afforded him relief. Urination was unaffected, and no fever was admitted to.

Examination

- Adductor longus muscles were painful and tight to palpation, passive stretch, and active contraction, especially the right.
- Pubic symphysis was painful to direct pressures.
- Rectus abdominis insertions were tense and tight.
- Gaenslen's test was positive bilaterally.
- There was SIJ dysfunction at the right upper and lower poles.
- X-ray was normal.

Diagnosis

Pubic symphysis joint dysfunction and adductor muscle strain.

Treatment

Visit 1: Ice to pubic symphysis and right adductor tendon until numb, followed by 5 minutes of walking. Repeated every 2 hours.

Visit 2: Patient felt 50% better. PR using general countertorque technique followed by grade IV mobilizations with this technique.

Visit 3: Patient improved by 80%. PR using countertorque technique. Manipulation to dysfunctional SIJs. PR to tense adductor muscles.

Visit 4: Patient felt same. PR using countertorque technique used, since this gave most relief. SIJ manipulation performed, and patient felt much improved.

Case Commentary

This is a good example of a patient's describing one thing, yet it's being something else. "Bladder infection" to this patient was most likely pubic symphysis pain referral to the bladder area. The mechanism of injury is consistent with a pubic symphysis problem. Provocative maneuvers stressing the joint were painful. The muscle strain was evident, since tests stressing the adductor's contractile elements (passive stretching and active contraction) were positive. Interestingly, an SIJ manipulation helped finish the case.

CASE 3: HIP AND GROIN PAIN

History

A 53-year-old housewife presented with right groin pain and stiffness of 5 months' duration after gardening for hours while in a crouched position on her hands and knees (Figure A–3). She found it painful to stand erect and walk the next morning. She could flex her hip to put on socks, but it hurt her and she could not fully straighten it when lying flat. The front of her thigh ached and felt tight. Her groin pain was described as deep and achy. She also noted a diffuse knee ache, yet her knee did not hurt her when she used it. Sitting did not bother her, but bending did. No back pain was present.

Examination

- Hip joint play was painful and restricted in flexion, internal and external rotation, and extension.

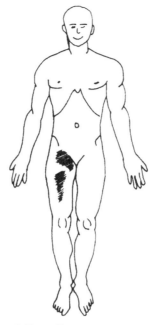

Figure A–3 Case 3: Hip and Groin Pain

- Patrick-Fabere test was painfully restricted.
- Right adductor longus was painful and tense, with trigger points present.
- Right iliopsoas muscles were tense and tender.
- There was joint dysfunction in anterior and posterior glides, flexion, and lateral glide.
- Gluteus medius trigger points were present.
- Lumbar spine examination was normal.
- There was SIJ dysfunction bilaterally, with painful right posterior SIJ ligaments.
- X-ray showed mild degenerative changes in hip joint.
- Knee joint examination was normal.

Diagnosis

Osteoarthritis of right hip with hip joint dysfunction and gluteal and adductor myofascitis.

Treatment

Visit 1: Ice to pubic symphysis and right adductor tendon until numb, followed by 5 minutes of walking. Repeated every 2 hours.

Visit 1: Gentle grade I and II medial rotations, followed by long-axis extension mobilizations. PR of adductor and iliopsoas muscles.

Visit 2: Patient felt good improvement. Grade I and II medial rotation, long-axis extension, and extension; all progressed to grade IV mobilizations. PR of adductor and iliopsoas muscles. Long-axis extension manipulation.

Visit 3: Patient felt 50% better. Long-axis extension manipulation, followed by grade VI mobilizations in long axis. Gluteus medius myofascial stretching with PR and ischemic compression. PR mobilization into full hip extension.

Visit 4: Patient felt the same. SIJ manipulation, hip manipulated in long-axis extension, and extension; anterior-to-posterior (AP) and posterior-to-anterior (PA) glide mobilization grade IV performed.

Visits 5–10: Patient felt 75% better. Repeated hip and SIJ manipulations and mobilizations as per findings. Psoas muscle stretching and hip stretches implemented. Much improved. Daily walking regimen started.

Case Commentary

Hip joint problems, especially in middle-aged and older patients, usually present with groin pain and anterior thigh pain. This woman's knee pain represents pain referral from her hip joint. Mobilizations in the initial phases of care help tremendously in painful hip conditions. SIJ dysfunction is often associated with hip joint problems and needs to be treated. Extension is often limited in hip joint conditions.

CASE 4: PAINFUL TAILBONE

History

Three months previously, a 42-year-old man had slipped on a loose stairway rug and slid down three stairs on his buttocks. He had felt pain in

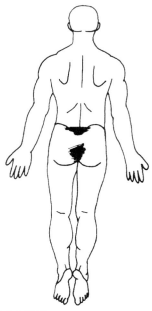

Figure A–4 Case 4: Painful Tailbone

his "tailbone" that was severe and prevented him from arising (Figure A–4). He had been taken to the local hospital where examination findings, including X-rays, had been negative for fracture but he had been told he had a bent coccyx. His pain had subsided slightly since its onset, but he still found it difficult to sit up straight, especially on hard surfaces. He said he was aware of a constant tension around his anus and defecation was painful at times.

Examination

- Trunk range of motion was normal.
- Coccyx was tender, especially on PA pressures and lateral tilts.
- SIJ was painful with Yeoman's and Patrick tests on the left.
- Levator ani was tender and tense.
- Left sacrotuberous ligament was painful and firm.

Diagnosis

Coccygodynia with sacrococcygeal and SIJ dysfunctions.

Treatment

Visit 1: Gluteus maximus PR to relax levator ani. Lateral and PA grade I and II mobilizations to coccyx.

Visit 2: Patient felt sore but slightly improved. Gluteus maximus PR, lateral, and PA mobilizations using grade IVs, SIJ manipulations.

Visit 3: Patient felt 80% improved. Sacrotuberous ligament pressure technique, grade IV coccyx mobilizations.

Visit 4: Patient felt much better. SIJ manipulations, gluteus maximus PR, sacrotuberous ligament pressure technique.

Case Commentary

Typical coccygeal pain involves direct trauma. X-rays are often noncontributory, even if they show a bent coccyx. Many coccygeal X-rays show malaligned segments in normal subjects. Treatment to the sacrococcygeal joint, SIJ, and neighboring soft tissues aids healing greatly. Compassion and understanding for this patient's embarrassment were also much appreciated.

CASE 5: LOW BACK PAIN IN A WEIGHT LIFTER

History

A 39-year-old male weight lifter presented with bilateral sacroiliac pain and lower back stiffness of 2 weeks' duration (Figure A–5). The pain was constant but was worse upon awakening, standing, straightening up and arching his spine, twisting his trunk, and pressing in on his lower abdomen. The pain was alleviated with ice packs, flexing the spine, sleeping on his side in a fetal position, and Advils. It had gradually started after he began lifting extremely heavy weights using a sitting leg sled machine. He noticed his lower back was sore and sensitive to touch where the workout machine's seat met his back. He could reproduce his pain by pressing in on his lower left abdomen, causing it to hurt across his lower back and along each sacroiliac region. Being concerned about this symptom and suspecting visceral disease, his primary care physician ordered blood work and a CT scan of his abdomen/pelvis. Results were normal.

Examination

• Sacroiliac and thoracolumbar joints were stiff and painful.

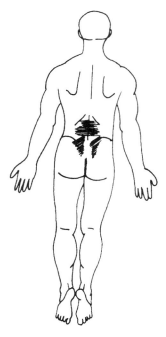

Figure A–5 Case 5: Low Back Pain in a Weight Lifter

- Sacrospinalis trigger points were present bilaterally.
- Iliopsoas muscle belly was very tender and reproduced much of his pain in the back even upon light palpation.
- Upper lumbar spinous processes were very sensitive, and thickened skin was found over the spinous processes.

Diagnosis

Iliopsoas myofascial pain syndrome, thoracolumbar joint dysfunction.

Treatment

Visit 1: Trigger point massage of sacrospinalis and sacroiliac joint manipulation. Gave moderate but only temporary relief.

Visit 2: Iliopsoas trigger point work and myofascial stretching. Much relief gained.

Visit 3: Condition still painful but better. Thoracolumbar manipulation performed with more myofascial stretching of iliopsoas muscles bilaterally.

Visit 4: Patient felt much better and continued to feel better. Further iliopsoas stretching was performed, along with thoracolumbar manipulation. Patient was shown iliopsoas stretches and told to decrease weights to a more reasonable amount.

Case Commentary

It is interesting to note that very light palpation of this man's psoas muscle was enough to elicit his pain pattern. Obviously, visceral disease needed to be ruled out in such a case, as it was by his medical doctor. Thoracolumbar joint dysfunction often accompanies psoas muscle problems, and treatment needs to be directed at both.

CASE 6: RIGHT HIP AND BUTTOCK PAIN IN AN 11-YEAR-OLD BOY

History

An 11-year-old boy presented with right buttock pain of 2 days' duration after he had turned a sharp corner while running. He said that in doing so, he had twisted his trunk and heard a loud snap that resulted in buttock pain. The pain was sharp, localized to the left lateral hip and sacroiliac joint regions (Figure A–6). Bending, extending, and twisting his trunk to the left were painful. He walked with a limp, lunging his left leg forward, since weight bearing was painful. Rolling over in bed and getting up from a sitting position were the most painful. The pain felt better while he was supine with both knees flexed to the chest. He felt an achy pain in his left groin and was worried he had a hernia. He was unable to play any sports due to his pain. He denied any bowel or bladder dysfunction.

Examination

- Trunk flexion was limited to 90 degrees, and left rotation was limited.
- Left PSIS and SI joint line were exquisitely tender to palpation.
- Left gluteus medius trigger point was found that referred pain to his hip region.
- Left Yeoman's test was painful, and left straight-leg raise was positive at 60 degrees.

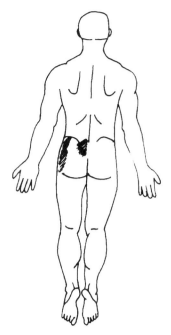

Figure A–6 Case 6: Right Hip and Buttock Pain in an 11-Year-Old Boy

- Gillet's SIJ palpation demonstrated restricted motion in left SIJ.
- Motor and sensory reflexes were normal; no nerve tension signs were present.
- X-rays of the hips were normal.

Diagnosis

Left sacroiliac joint dysfunction and gluteal myofascitis.

Treatment

Visit 1: Prone, supine, and side-lying SIJ mobilization grades I through III; cryokinetics at home recommended, consisting of ice applications until numb, followed by 15 minutes of walking every 2 hours.

Visit 2: Patient felt 50% better. Myofascial stretching of gluteus medius and SIJ manipulation were performed.

Visit 3: Patient felt much better. Wanted to participate in sports again. SIJ manipulation repeated. Patient was given stretching exercises for hip, SIJ, and tensor fascia lata.

Visit 4: Patient felt no pain. Myofascial stretching of tensor fascia lata and hamstrings performed. Patient was instructed in proprioceptive exercises and balance board use.

Case Commentary

It is important to rule out a slipped femoral epiphysis with this history of a limp, hip, and groin pain in a young person. However, his examination directed attention to his SIJ, and he responded well to treatment.

CASE 7: LOW BACK PAIN AFTER A TENNIS SERVE

History

A 47-year-old tennis player presented with low back pain after serving tennis balls for an hour 1 week previously. The pain had come on over the course of that evening. The pain was located over the right flank region and SIJ area and was worse with bending and left bending (Figure A–7). Sitting erect or lying supine lessened his pain. Sneezing and sudden trunk movements created sharp, stabbing pain in the back. His right buttock also ached. No bowel or bladder dysfunction was present.

Examination

- Trunk flexion and left lateral flexion were limited and painful.
- Quadratus lumborum trigger points were found that reproduced his back and hip pains.
- Additional trigger points were found in the gluteus minimus and tensor fascia lata.
- Hip abduction showed an abnormal movement pattern, with hip hiking initiating the movement.
- Thoracolumbar joint dysfunction was palpated.

Diagnosis

Quadratus lumborum myofascitis with thoracolumbar joint dysfunction.

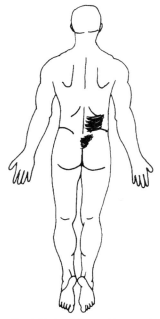

Figure A–7 Case 7: Low Back Pain After a Tennis Serve

Treatment

Visit 1: Stretch and spray of quadratus lumborum with heat applications.

Visit 2: Patient felt less achy, with no radiation into hip, but stiff in lower back. Thoracolumbar region manipulated, and stretch and spray of quadratus lumborum repeated.

Visit 3: Patient was much improved and was given home stretches for quadratus lumborum.

Case Commentary

The quadratus lumborum (QL) muscle is often overlooked in lower back pain patients. Flank pain and coughing pain are not unusual symptoms with QL trigger points but also signal other problems. The abnormal movement pattern of hip hiking during hip abduction gives us a clue that the QL is overactive and vulnerable to developing trigger points. Thoracolumbar joint dysfunctions are also linked with QL trigger points.

CASE 8: A GOLFER WITH THIGH PAIN

History

A 25-year-old golf player presented with right anterolateral thigh pain of 2 weeks' duration. The pain came on insidiously after he had played nine holes of golf. It was described as a "migraine" headache in the thigh that spread from the upper anterolateral thigh to the distal lateral thigh (Figure A–8). The pain was worse with walking, sitting, and sleeping on that side. The pain was temporarily eased with warm baths and by lying on his side and letting his painful leg and thigh hang off the bed behind him. He also mentioned that he had had lower back pain in the past that was alleviated by yoga stretches.

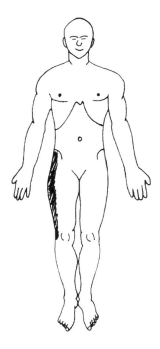

Figure A–8 Case 8: A Golfer with Thigh Pain

Examination

- Side-lying hip abduction was painful and exhibited a poor movement pattern, with the tensor fascia lata contracting well before the gluteus medius while the patient attempted to roll the pelvis backward.
- Modified Thomas test demonstrated positive testing for a tight tensor fascia lata, with slight flexion and abduction noted in the dependent thigh. A notable groove was observed along the iliotibial band.
- Tensor fascia lata was tight and painful with very painful trigger point in it that reproduced the patient's pain pattern upon palpation.
- Hip adductor shortness was noted.
- Yeoman's, Patrick-Fabere tests were positive for right side, with pain localized to right SIJ.
- SIJ palpation was positive for joint dysfunction.

Diagnosis

Tensor fascia lata myofascitis with sacroiliac joint dysfunction.

Treatment

Visit 1:   Postisometric relaxation of the right tensor fascia lata was done. Postfacilitation stretching of the right hip adductors was performed.

Visit 2:   Patient felt 50% better, with no leg pain radiation down thigh. Hip pain developed about 2 hours after last treatment. SIJ dysfunction present on assessment, and manipulation was performed. Tensor fascia lata and adductor stretching also done.

Visit 3:   Patient felt 75% improved. Right lower back pain same. Right quadratus lumborum trigger point found on assessment. Stretch and spray to quadratus lumborum and SIJ manipulation performed.

Visit 4:   Patient felt much improved. He was given stretches for SIJ, tensor fascia lata, quadratus lumborum, and hip adductors.

Case Commentary

The tensor fascia lata often causes anterolateral or lateral thigh pain. It commonly participates in a chain reaction of dysfunction involving the quadratus lumborum, gluteus minimus, hip joint, and SIJ, as we see also in the next case.

CASE 9: A ROLLERBLADING EXECUTIVE WITH HIP PAIN

History

A 43-year-old male executive presented with hip pain of 2 days' duration after 2 hours of Rollerblading. The pain came on gradually and worsened as the day went on. The pain was deep and achy. It was localized in the left lateral hip region with no radiations (Figure A–9). Any movements hurt him, and he said he noticed a swelling in the area. Ice helped, and lying on the area hurt, as did any hip movements, climbing stairs, and getting in and out of his car.

Examination

- Active and passive hip movements were painful in any range.
- A slight swelling was detected over the left greater trochanter that was both painful and slightly reddened.

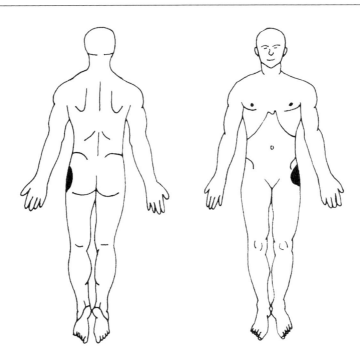

Figure A–9 Case 9: A Rollerblading Executive with Hip Pain

Diagnosis

Left trochanteric bursitis secondary to overuse.

Treatment

Visit 1: Ice and interferential current therapy were applied to the bursa. The patient was instructed to continue icing every 2 hours until numbness was experienced.

Visit 2: Patient was 70% improved. Further examination was possible and showed hip joint dysfunction, TFL and gluteus minimus trigger points, and SIJ dysfunction. The hip was mobilized and the SIJ was manipulated.

Visit 3: Patient felt much improved. Swelling reduced and bursa palpated as painless. Postisometric relaxation to TFL and gluteus minimus performed. Hip mobilized.

Visit 4: Patient was pain free. Exercises were given to stretch hip and SI joints, TFL, and gluteus minimus.

Case Commentary

The diagnosis of bursitis is often handed out too freely. A prerequisite is that the pain must be in a known anatomical site of a bursa. This case affords us that, as well as painful movements in all ranges, whether active or passive. This patient was too uncomfortable to continue with an in-depth examination on the first visit. After his pain subsided, further examination revealed other dysfunctions that were successfully treated. This case seems to represent a bursitis secondary to overuse in the presence of related joint and muscle dysfunction. However, it should be remembered that bursitis may be a harbinger of a collagen-vascular disease.

CASE 10: "GROWING PAINS" IN A 7-YEAR-OLD DANCER

History

A 7-year-old girl experienced vague leg pains after 3 weeks of dance classes. The pains were described as achy and located in the lateral thighs and lower legs, predominantly on the right side (Figure A–10). Vigorous running bothered her, and rubbing her legs helped. Sleeping was uncomfortable. No trauma was recounted, and her medical doctor diagnosed her as having "growing pains." Treatment was restricted to children's Tylenol and watchful waiting.

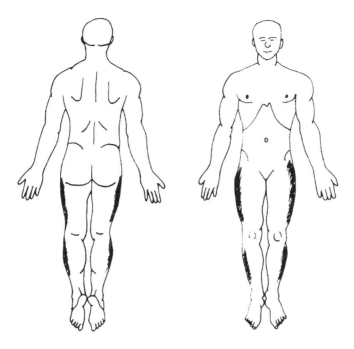

Figure A–10 Case 10: "Growing Pains" in a 7-Year-Old Dancer

Examination

- Trunk range of motion was normal.
- There was right SIJ dysfunction and restricted hip extension joint play.
- Right SI joint line and PSIS were tender.
- Gluteal and hip adductor trigger points reproduced her leg pains.
- Hip abduction movement patterns were poor, with weakness of motion and tensor fascia lata and quadratus lumborum substitutions.

Diagnosis

Sacroiliac joint dysfunction with gluteal and adductor myofascial trigger points.

Treatment

Visit 1: SIJ manipulation and postisometric relaxation of the adductors and gluteal muscles.

Visit 2: Patient slept better, but her legs still ached. SIJ manipulation, hip mobilization, and tensor fascia lata stretching.

Visit 3: Patient felt much better. She had no night pains, ran much better, felt minimal discomfort. Hip mobilization. Stretching advice given to her dance teacher. Patient discharged.

Case Commentary

Children very often do suffer from leg pains that are commonly diagnosed as growing pains. The clinician who is versed in functional assessment of the locomotor system will find relevant dysfunctions in a large majority of the cases. Children too can benefit greatly from this type of treatment, often dramatically so. Pelvic joint and muscle dysfunctions are commonly at fault in a "growing pains" diagnosis, specifically the sacroiliac and hip joints and gluteal and hip adductor muscles. Young dancers, as well as older ones, often do not have the coordination and strength for certain dance routines. This is especially so with hip abduction movements. Compensation and poor movement patterns can result if a child is forced to perform beyond his or her developmental capabilities.

CASE 11: A "TURNED-OUT FOOT" IN A 12-YEAR-OLD BOY

History

A 12-year-old boy presented with the concern that for the past 3 years his right foot had flared out as he walked. His mother commented that he seemed clumsy but thought it was normal for his age. She also expressed concern about his right foot turning outward when he walked. He admitted to experiencing occasional hip and lower back achiness after playing soccer or running. He also experienced headaches at a frequency of one per week. No history of significant trauma was present. An orthopedic physician advised them to do nothing, as it would straighten out with time.

Examination

- Postural examination revealed an anterior tilt to the pelvis. Patient sat with a pronounced slouch. He appeared moderately uncoordinated in his movements.

- Gait examination revealed an externally rotated and pronated right foot.
- Trunk flexion was limited due to hamstring tightness and discomfort.
- Modified Thomas test showed substantially short psoas muscles bilaterally, especially on the right.
- Sacroiliac and hip joint dysfunction was found on the right, especially in extension. The right SIJ line was tender to palpation, and Yeoman's and Patrick-Fabere tests were positive on the right.
- Hip flexion with adduction was very limited and painful bilaterally, especially on the right.
- Straight-leg raising was tight and limited due to hamstring shortness.
- Hip adductors were shortened and tight.
- Craniocervical joint dysfunction and poor cervical movement patterns were exhibited.

Diagnosis

SIJ and hip dysfunction with psoas and hamstring myofascial shortening.

Treatment

Visit 1: Psoas stretching using proprioceptive neuromuscular facilitation (PNF) techniques, SIJ manipulation.

Visit 2: Patient felt looser. Still "stiff" in hips. Psoas stretching using PNF. Hip mobilization, adductor stretching. Hip and SIJ stretches were given.

Visit 3: Patient felt difference in hips while running; not as achy. Felt as if foot did not flare out as much. On observation of gait, foot still externally rotated. Psoas, adductor, hamstring PNF performed. Hip and SIJ manipulated.

Visit 4: Felt a big difference. However, headaches seemed worse. On gait observation, foot displayed noticeably less of an external rotation. Craniocervical manipulation performed. Psoas, adductor, hamstring PNF.

Visit 5: Patient felt much better with headaches, and major difference with walking. No achiness in lower back with running. Felt much looser overall. Foot only slightly externally rotated with gait, almost not noticeable. SIJ manipulation performed. Patient taught psoas, hamstring, adductor stretches. Pelvic tilting exercises were given. Wobble board exercise for proprioceptive input was given.

Visit 6: 1 month follow-up: No headaches since last time, and walking with no external rotation of right foot. Psoas and hamstring PNF and hip and SIJ manipulation performed. Exercises reviewed. Discharged.

Case Commentary

It is not uncommon to find young people who seem to be neuromuscular "illiterates." They seem incoordinated and display jerky movements. They have a difficult time relaxing and fully letting go when they are examined and treated. Movements patterns are poorly performed, and joint/muscle dysfunctions are prevalent. The above case is a good example of this. Although the patient presented with no real painful complaint, his concern of an unsightly gait led to the uncovering of key joint and muscle dysfunctions that related to his major concern. As with most cases, multiple factors were operant. His major problems seemed to be extremely tight hip flexor, hamstring, and adductor muscles. This is a common pattern seen in young patients who are "challenged" proprioceptively. Their coordination is faulty, and they exhibit jerky motions, finding it hard to relax in response to examination commands. The hip and SIJ dysfunctions were also key. Interestingly, his craniocervical region seemed to be linked to his pelvic problem, since his headaches worsened as work on his pelvis was undertaken. He experienced a noticeable overall difference after the upper cervical manipulation. Pelvic and craniocervical dysfunctions are often linked, and the discovery of one should alert clinicians to look for the other. It would have been interesting to see what would have happened if just the craniocervical region was manipulated first.

Index

Page numbers in *italics* denote figures and exhibits;
those followed by "t" denote tables.